Epidemiology

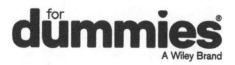

for
dummies®
A Wiley Brand

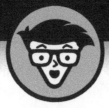

Epidemiology

by Amal K. Mitra, MD, DrPH
Professor of Epidemiology and
Biostatistics

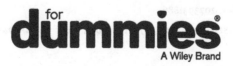
for dummies®
A Wiley Brand

Epidemiology For Dummies®

Published by: **John Wiley & Sons, Inc.**, 111 River Street, Hoboken, NJ 07030-5774, www.wiley.com

Copyright © 2023 by John Wiley & Sons, Inc., Hoboken, New Jersey

Media and software compilation copyright © 2023 by John Wiley & Sons, Inc. All rights reserved.

Published simultaneously in Canada

For general information on our other products and services, please contact our Customer Care Department within the U.S. at 877-762-2974, outside the U.S. at 317-572-3993, or fax 317-572-4002. For technical support, please visit https://hub.wiley.com/community/support/dummies.

Wiley publishes in a variety of print and electronic formats and by print-on-demand. Some material included with standard print versions of this book may not be included in e-books or in print-on-demand. If this book refers to media such as a CD or DVD that is not included in the version you purchased, you may download this material at http://booksupport.wiley.com. For more information about Wiley products, visit www.wiley.com.

Library of Congress Control Number: 2023931886

ISBN: 978-1-394-17070-8 (pbk); ISBN: 978-1-394-17071-5 (ebk); ISBN: 978-1-394-17072-2 (ebk)

SKY10043638_022823

Contents at a Glance

Table of Contents

Introduction

As a beginner in public health, you may be on a quest to know about diseases that are affecting your community, other countries, and the world. If you desire to build a career in a field of epidemiology, you want to know more about what causes certain diseases and how they're transmitted, or as a public health professional, you want to advise people about disease prevention.

You've come to the right place. Epidemiology has been a hot topic in the past few years with the Covid-19 pandemic, but there's so much more to it. Getting a degree in epidemiology is a good choice because the concepts and skills of epidemiology will prepare you for plenty of jobs in public health. Even if you aren't a researcher or a data analyst, epidemiology can help you get a sense about numbers when you hear that the Covid-19 rates are rising or coming down, or when you hear that Forest County of Hattiesburg, Mississippi is the hot spot of lead poisoning.

About This Book

Epidemiology For Dummies emerged from the needs of undergraduate and graduate students in public health, especially in the field of epidemiology. During the Covid-19 pandemic, almost all face-to-face classes were closed and classes were only offered online. Some students faced challenges in fully understanding some difficult topics during this online format.

This handy guide isn't a textbook or workbook in epidemiology. Rather, I wrote this book based on my decades of experience in practicing medicine, conducting health research, and teaching public health for undergraduate as well as graduate students to help explain the concepts of epidemiology in plain English with plenty of real-life examples, calculations, and illustrations.

Here you can read about an array of concepts, starting from Epidemiology 101 to more advanced research methods to ethics in conducting human research. I focus on the following areas:

>> The history of the development of public health and epidemiology

>> The epidemiologic triangle

- Person-place-time distribution of diseases
- Causal association and Hill's criteria
- The three levels of prevention
- Vaccine-preventable diseases
- Disease surveillance
- Steps of outbreak investigations
- Screening methods
- Epidemiologic study designs
- Bias and confounding
- Population projection
- Ethics in human research

I also provide step-by-step explanations and answers to practical issues like the following:

- Investigating outbreaks and analyzing data
- Solving problems of sensitivity, specificity, and predictive value
- Calculating commonly used rates, ratios, and proportions
- Calculating incidence, prevalence, and standardized mortality ratio (SMR)
- Calculating country-level data for population projection

Foolish Assumptions

When writing this book, I've made a few assumptions about you, my dear reader. I made the following assumptions:

- You're bored or somewhat disappointed by reading textbooks with small fonts, full of concepts after concepts, with few examples of topics that don't provide real-life examples of epidemiologic applications.
- You've struggled understanding some of the technical terms and concepts in epidemiology, but you see your future working in public health.
- You're excited about applying what you've studied in your epidemiology courses, but you need a little extra help with the calculations.

>> You've been working a few years in a health department and you've faced many issues, such as choosing the right study design based on your resources, preparing a questionnaire, or investigating and controlling an epidemic.

>> You're a silent learner, and you don't ask questions in a class.

Icons Used in This Book

Throughout this book, you can find icons — small pictures next to the text that point out extra-important information. Here's what they all mean:

TIP

For gems of accumulated wisdom — quite often the kind learned by painful experience! — follow this icon.

WARNING

Consider this icon like a stop sign. When you see it, stop and pay extra attention because you might make a mistake — perhaps in a math calculation or something extra important — if you're not careful enough.

REMEMBER

You're trying to do things correctly and efficiently. Problem is, you may not always know what's right and what isn't. When you see this icon, pay attention to the text.

TECHNICAL STUFF

This icon is used for more advanced material that you don't need to read to understand the concept at hand. It's information that's interesting but not absolutely essential.

REAL LIFE EXAMPLE

This icon points out concepts with practical examples, some from my own research.

Beyond This Book

This book is chock-full of tips and other pieces of helpful advice you can use as you study epidemiology. I provide links where you can go online for more information. In addition, check out the book's Cheat Sheet at www.dummies.com and search for "Epidemiology For Dummies Cheat Sheet" for information to reference on a regular basis.

Where to Go from Here

This book represents a starting point for concepts and uses of epidemiology. Your new learning curve in public health is just beginning. So, now what? You can flip through the Index or Table of Contents to find a subject that interests you.

Or you can turn to whatever section looks to have the answers and information you're wanting most. No matter where you start, you can read a section or two, stop, and then come back when you need more guidance. I tell my students, "Epidemiology is easier than you think and more fun than you can imagine."

1

Getting Started with Epidemiology

Gain a basic knowledge about infection and infecting agents such as bacteria, viruses, parasites, yeasts, molds, and others; how diseases occur, and why you are *not* sick all the time despite living in a world with so many infecting agents.

Get background information about how the science of modern-day epidemiology came into play through different stages of legendary works in the field.

Understand the scope of epidemiology, two major functions of epidemiology, and the importance of epidemiology in measuring health status, searching for disease causation, and controlling and preventing diseases and events in humans.

Identify sources of epidemiologic data such as the Centers for Disease Control and Prevention (CDC), the World Health Organization (WHO), census data, vital statistics, and others.

Explore older and modern theories of diseases causation and important contributions of people in laying foundation and the development of different branches of public health.

Uncover milestones in public health, such as James Lind's study of finding the treatment for scurvy, the cholera investigation of John Snow, Joseph Goldberger's study of the cause of pellagra, the famous influenza pandemic, the eradication of smallpox, the connection between smoking and cancer, the development of theories of causal association, and more.

Recognize the means and ways of controlling several common infections, such as waterborne diseases, airborne diseases, vector-borne diseases, parasitic diseases, and sexually transmitted infections.

Chapter **1**

Entering the World of Epidemiology

You're about to enter the wonderful world of epidemiology — an adventure of hunting for five million trillion trillion (that's a five with 30 zeroes after it) bacteria, about six million parasites, and nearly 7,000 virus species that are prevailing in the world. Thank goodness not all of them are harmful to you. The vast majority of them either live on the planet or inside you harmlessly or keep at bay like microscopic superheroes. Fewer than 100 species of bacteria, 300 species of parasitic worms, about 70 species of protozoa, and more than 200 viruses are known to cause disease in humans.

Most of the disease agents, which are infectious in nature, are controllable, either by antibiotics, vaccines, or by other public health preventive measures, such as personal hygiene, safe water supply, proper sanitation, healthy food habits, and by improving your resistance to infecting agents.

This chapter gives you an overview of this world of epidemiology and serves as a jumping-off point into this book. This chapter previews the concepts of epidemiology, mentions the importance of crunching numbers, addresses disease prevention, and discusses disease prevention, and more.

Introducing Epidemiology

Epidemiology is the study of human diseases and events. Epidemiologists are disease detectives whose jobs include the following:

>> **Searching for the cause of diseases in humans:** All associations aren't causal. Chapter 16 provides concepts on knowing if an association between an exposure and a disease is causal or not.

>> **Identifying people who are at risk:** Certain host factors are associated with diseases. Descriptive epidemiology (see Chapter 7) deals with person, place, and time factors that are associated with diseases. Chapter 5 addresses the risk of people in getting different types of diseases.

>> **Determining how to control or stop the spread:** Knowing the chain of disease transmission helps you prevent or control the spread of a disease. Refer to Chapter 5 for more information about chain of disease transmission.

>> **Preventing the disease from happening again:** Chapter 11 explains the different levels of disease prevention with practical examples.

Recognizing How Numbers Can Help Study Disease

Epidemiology and biostatistics are like cousin sisters. However, epidemiology isn't learning about math. I often ask my students whether they like math, and most of the time, they respond no and sometimes emphatically that they hate math. That's okay. Epidemiology doesn't deal with hard-core math problems. These sections explain that epidemiologists use a basic knowledge of algebra to calculate numbers.

Grappling with the epidemiologic triangle

The concept of the *epidemiologic triangle* includes these three factors of a disease:

>> **Agent:** The causative factor (such as a bacteria, virus, or parasite). In other words, the what that causes the disease.

>> **Host:** Humans and non-human animals can harbor a disease. They're called *disease hosts*.

» **Environment:** Factors in the environment such as temperature (hot or cold), noise, moisture, dusts, and others cause diseases. Also, agents and hosts both live in the environment, which makes a balance between disease and health.

When germs enter and grow in the human body, it's called an *infection*. The germs may be bacteria, viruses, parasites, yeasts, fungi, or other microorganisms. They're agents for an infectious disease. These agents live and multiply in the environment that humans live. But an infection doesn't necessarily lead to a disease. The favorable conditions in the environment help agents grow.

On the other hand, when a person's immune system is strong enough, it can fight the germs and cure an infection without causing a disease. If immunity is low, the germ gets the upper hand, and the person fails to resist the infection, which in turn leads to a disease. In a chronic disease model, as I describe in Chapter 6, you can find that the causes are multifactorial — they are called *risk factors*, instead of agents. Chapter 16 explains the concept of multiple risk factors for a noncommunicable disease.

Classifying epidemiology

Two broad classifications of epidemiology that you need to know are as follows:

» **Descriptive:** *Descriptive epidemiology* provides you answers for what, when, where, and who questions. Most health surveys, censuses, and case reports are descriptive in nature. In descriptive studies, you can identify risk groups or *hot spots* (or areas where diseases and agents cluster). Descriptive information can be highly valuable in generating a hypothesis and conducting a future study to evaluate the hypothesis through experimental studies, interventional studies, or a randomized controlled clinical trial (RCT) (you can find details in Chapter 17).

» **Analytical:** *Analytical epidemiology* deals with the why and how questions. Some statistical tests (called inferential statistics) are used for answering these questions. Analytical epidemiology is used to prove the hypothesis.

Understanding epidemiologic transition

The changing nature of diseases is a continuous process, and it depends on several factors including the ecology, public health measures, vaccine development, antibiotic use, genetics, and other host factors. The transition of disease occurrence from acute and infectious diseases to chronic and noncommunicable diseases (NCDs) is called the *epidemiologic transition*. Chapter 8 describes in greater detail this changing pattern of diseases.

Consider the following: The worldwide pandemic of Covid-19 has evolved as one of the most fatal diseases in human history. Similarly, a few other pandemics including plague, influenza (flu), smallpox, and HIV/AIDS have caused devastations and killed a large number of people. Some other infectious diseases such as pneumonia, diarrhea, malaria, and tuberculosis are still common causes of morbidity and mortality in many developing countries.

On the other hand, noncommunicable diseases such as heart disease, cancer, stroke, unintentional injuries, chronic obstructive pulmonary disease (COPD), Alzheimer's disease, and diabetes are the leading causes of death in the United States. Developed countries have curtailed mortality rates from infectious diseases. Some of the infectious disease has been eliminated (such as smallpox) in the world or reduced to a minimum level (such as polio, tetanus, measles) in developed countries. Polio is expected to be eliminated soon.

Connecting demography and disease

Changes in demography are certainly affecting the disease pattern and the healthcare costs. Health consequences of aging are many, including pain and arthritis, osteoporosis, falls and accidents, hearing defects, eye problems, heart disease, diabetes, depression, Alzheimer's, and senile dementia.

The burden of healthcare costs is also escalating. For example, in recent years, one-fifth of older Americans spent more than $2,000 out of pocket on healthcare. Chapter 9 looks at different demographics, including a comparative picture of the population structure of several countries, a list of the ten most populous states in the United States, and the top ten countries with the largest proportion of senior citizens. In addition, you can discover how to project step by step the future population of several countries.

Figuring out rates and risks

One of the focuses of descriptive epidemiology is to calculate rates and risks. Epidemiologists summarize health reports and describe the risks based on numbers. Chapter 10 explains how to calculate important rates such as crude birth rate, crude death rate, age-specific rates such as infant mortality rate, neonatal mortality rate, post-neonatal mortality rate, and perinatal mortality rate, cause-specific rates such as cancer- and heart-diseases mortality rate, and gender-specific rates such as breast cancer rates and prostate cancer rates.

Some of the rates, such as mortality rates, often need to be standardized to compare with similar rates of an entire country or another nation — this process is called *standardization*. This same chapter shows you how to standardize mortality rates by using direct and indirect methods.

Focusing on Prevention Rather Than a Cure

The three levels of disease prevention include

>> Averting a disease before it attacks you

>> Detecting a disease early enough so that you can reduce the disease severity

>> Preventing disabilities and promoting quality of life

The following sections discuss the specifics.

Identifying prevention levels

Three levels of prevention include primary, secondary, and tertiary prevention. By a simple method of hand washing you can prevent a number of diseases, such as waterborne diseases and Covid-19. Chapter 11 discusses what diseases can be prevented and what the levels of prevention are.

Using vaccines

Vaccines give you a type of immunity which lasts long, sometimes life-long (such as measles) — this is called *artificially acquired immunity* — in contrast to *natural active immunity* acquired from exposure to a disease. Chapter 12 explains the importance of vaccines and provides a vaccination schedule by age-group. I also explain what vaccines you shouldn't get if you're pregnant.

Surveilling disease

The National Notifiable Disease Surveillance System (NNDSS) is currently surveilling about 120 diseases. The primary purpose of disease surveillance is to predict, detect, and minimize harm caused by an outbreak, epidemic, or pandemic of diseases, and to inform people about possible preventive measures from a future epidemic. Chapter 13 is about methods of conducting disease surveillance.

Studying an outbreak

Some diseases occur in low numbers in a community at any given time. These diseases are called *endemic*, such as sore throat, ear infection, skin disease, urinary infection, and others. Some diseases can appear suddenly in a large number beyond the normal limit. The diseases are called *epidemics*; when epidemics occur in small scale or in a confined area, it's called an *outbreak*.

Chapter 14 gives you step-by-step methods about conducting an outbreak investigation. I describe my real-life example of investigating an epidemic of blood dysentery (also called shigellosis) in rural Bangladesh. I explain how to prepare your team, how to establish the existence of an outbreak, how to find the sources and the cause of the epidemic, and how to properly collect and analyze data to develop a hypothesis and suggest further studies to prove the hypothesis.

Relying on screening

A number of valid and reliable screening tests are available to detect diseases from apparently healthy individuals. Here are some characteristics of a good screening test:

>> **Safety:** Almost all screening tests are safe and don't have any side effects. Screening tests also don't increase risks to individual's health.

>> **Convenience:** Some screening tests are comparatively more convenient than others. For example, a urine test for glucose is more convenient than a blood glucose test.

>> **Acceptability:** The screening test must be acceptable to the general people.

>> **Sensitivity:** Sensitivity is measured by the proportion of true disease-positive individuals who test positive by the screening test.

>> **Specificity:** This is measured by the proportion of true disease-negative individuals who are tested negative by the screening test.

>> **Predictive values:** The two kinds of predictive values are positive predictive value and negative predictive value. They measure the quality of a screening test.

Through screening tests, you can detect a disease before clinical symptoms appear. Chapter 15 discusses some commonly used screening programs, including mammogram, breast self-exam, Pap test, colonoscopy, PSA for prostate, occult blood test for stool, and more.

Delving into Study Finding

Here I provide snapshots of topics related to studies in this book:

>> **Finding criteria of causal association:** Bradford Hill developed several criteria by which you can determine if an association is causal or not (see Chapter 16).

>> **Using different types of epidemiologic studies:** Epidemiologic studies are two types: descriptive and analytical or experimental. Several epidemiological studies fall under these two groups (refer to Chapter 17).

>> **Tackling bias and confounding:** Factors like bias and confounding affect study results. These factors must be controlled at different stages of a study (see Chapter 18).

>> **Examining ethical procedures in research:** People rely on the findings of a scientific research. You need to follow proper ethical procedures when conducting a study so that the research findings are valid and reliable. (Chapter 19 discusses ethics in greater detail.)

Figuring Out What You Know about Epidemiology: Some Q&As

How much do you really know about epidemiology? Are you taking an epidemiology course with plans to work in public health, or are you just interested in what causes diseases? No matter, work through these questions to see how much you know about epidemiology.

Before you read a certain chapter, read the corresponding question (I include ten questions for ten different chapters) and try to answer the question. After you read that chapter, you can flip back here and check your answers.

1. What does epidemiology help you do? (Chapter 2)

   (A) Epidemiology helps in measuring health status.

   (B) Epidemiology deals with disease prevention.

   (C) Epidemiology looks for the cause of a disease.

   (D) All of the above

2. Who is considered the Father of Medicine? (Chapter 3)

(A) Hippocrates

(B) Joseph Goldberger

(C) John Snow

(D) James Lind

(E) Noah Webster

3. Who investigated the famous cholera epidemic in London's Golden Square? (Chapter 4)

(A) Hippocrates

(B) Joseph Goldberger

(C) John Snow

(D) James Lind

(E) Noah Webster

4. In case of infectious diseases, the capacity of an agent in causing a disease is called what? (Chapter 5)

(A) Infectivity

(B) Pathogenicity

(C) Virulence

5. Climate change and global warming can increase the risk of what? (Chapter 6)

(A) Waterborne disease

(B) Airborne disease

(C) Parasitic disease

(D) Vector-borne disease

(E) All of the above

6. Rotavirus is most common among children of what age? (Chapter 7)

(A) Younger than 2 years old

(B) Between 2 and 12 years old

(C) Adolescents

7. What is the top cause of deaths in the United States? (Chapter 8)

(A) Heart disease

(B) Stroke

(C) Cancer

(D) Pneumonia

(E) Covid-19

8. Which country has the largest proportion of senior citizens? (Chapter 9)

(A) United States

(B) United Kingdom

(C) France

(D) Sweden

(E) Japan

9. True or false: Infant mortality rate (death rate in children younger than 1) is one of the best indicators of health of a nation. (Chapter 10)

10. By using a screening test (such as colonoscopy) you can early detect colon cancer. What kind of disease prevention can a screening test offer? (Chapter 11)

(A) Primary prevention

(B) Secondary prevention

(C) Tertiary prevention

Answers: 1.) D, 2.) A, 3.) C, 4.) B, 5.) E, 6.) A, 7.) A, 8.) E, 9.) True, 10.) B

VIRUSES CAUSING OBESITY: IS IT REAL?

Obesity in the United States has reached epidemic proportions with a steady rise in prevalence rates over the last 20 years. This epidemic however isn't limited to the United States — worldwide obesity has nearly tripled since 1975. In 2022, more than 1 billion people worldwide are obese — of them, 650 million are adults, 340 million adolescent, and 39 million children.

(continued)

(continued)

The causes of obesity are multifactorial. Although obesity is primarily thought of as a condition brought on by lifestyle choices, recent evidence has made researchers start to look at whether a link between obesity and viral infections in humans exists.

Numerous animal models have documented an increased body weight and a number of physiological changes, including increased insulin sensitivity, increased glucose uptake, and decreased *leptin* (a hormone that inhibits food intake and increases energy expenditure) secretion that contribute to an increased body fat. Of several viruses, *adenovirus-36* (Ad-36) infection is more commonly found an obesity-causing agent in animals. Other viral agents associated with increasing obesity in animals include *canine distemper virus (CDV), rous-associated virus 7 (RAV-7), scrapie, Borna disease virus (BDV), SMAM-1,* and other *adenoviruses.*

Some of these mechanistic theories were proven by experimental studies in animals, which are outlined here:

- CDV infection causes damage to the hypothalamus, which regulates a person's energy intake. Damage to the hypothalamus disrupts the carefully coordinated balance between energy intake and expenditure, often leading to increased calorie intake and/or decreased calorie burning, and thereby to rapid weight gain.

- The thyroid hormones are important for regulating weight. RAV-7 infection causes lymphoblastic infiltration in the thyroid, leading to an underactive thyroid. *Hypothyroidism* (an underactive thyroid) is a known cause of slower metabolism and weight gain.

- Scrapie infection causes damage to the adrenal gland, hypothalamus, and pituitary gland. All these factors combined cause weight gain.

- BDV infection also causes damage to the hypothalamus.

- In an experimental study, chickens infected with SMAM-1 had 50 percent more abdominal fat than control chickens.

- Although Ad-36 is a virus that largely infects humans, it's the first human virus that has been found to cause obesity in animal models. Ad-36 infection was found to increase the amount of adipose tissue. Leptin expression and secretion in adipocytes was observed to be lower and glucose uptake was increased. Both of these effects can be attributed to the development of obesity. Two epidemiologic studies found such an association between Ad-36 and obesity in humans.

Further epidemiologic studies and possibly experimental studies are needed to establish whether a causal link exists between obesity and virus infection. However, a virus infection could be one of the many factors that cause obesity. Each of the many factors that cause a disease is called a *component cause.*

Chapter **2**

Epidemiology 101 — Understanding the Basics

From your classwork, you probably know epidemiology is a core component of public health. Here I want to make sure you have a strong foundation about your coursework in epidemiology.

Chapter 1 gives you an overview to this book whereas this chapter addresses what to expect from your studies in Epidemiology 101 and beyond, focusing on how the field of epidemiology is applied in epidemic control and in disease prevention. This chapter also provides you what you need to know if you plan to work in this field, including what's necessary for conducting research.

Defining Epidemiology — What to Expect from Your Coursework and Beyond

Epidemiology is what epidemiologists do. And what's that specifically? They're scientists who study diseases and events in humans. As an epidemiologist, you're considered a disease detective in the world of public health. In other words, an epidemiologist searches to identify and measure a disease, its risk factors, and what caused it.

If you dissect the term, *epi* means *upon*, *demos* means *people*, and *logy* is the *knowledge or education*. Therefore, epidemiology is the science of diseases or events that happen in humans.

Like any other investigators at the scene of a crime, epidemiologists begin by looking for clues. As an epidemiologist, you'll work as a fact-finder. Epidemiology helps you to design studies, conduct systematic methods of investigations, gather data, interview people, create spot maps, and use several other procedures. By studying epidemiology, you not only understand concepts but also get the know-how and their applications in real-life situations.

The following sections deal with *descriptive epidemiology*, which describes data distribution in terms of time, place, and person and *analytical epidemiology*, also called *experimental epidemiology*, to find out the determining factors of diseases.

Describing distribution

When you're trying to get information about a disease, a few questions come to mind:

>> What happens?

>> When does it happen?

>> Where does it happen?

You get these what, when, and where answers by analyzing information or data about a disease. This type of analysis is called *descriptive epidemiology*. Suppose you're hearing about a new disease called mpox (formerly called monkeypox) that occurred in humans in 2022. Descriptive epidemiology answers the following questions:

>> What is mpox?

>> What are the symptoms of mpox?

>> Who is affected by mpox?

>> When did mpox appear in humans?

>> Where was mpox found first?

>> Which U.S. states have the most cases of mpox?

>> How many people are affected by mpox?

>> How many people have died from mpox?

>> What lab methods are used to diagnose mpox?

>> What is the treatment for mpox?

Descriptive epidemiology refers to describing the characteristics of the disease, the people at risk, morbidity and mortality from the disease, the locations, and the time-trend of the disease. In descriptive studies, you use some statistical tools that are called *descriptive statistics*. Chapter 7 discusses descriptive epidemiology in greater detail.

Determining determinants

After you know answers to the questions in the preceding section, you can further compare the transmissibility or infectiousness, *pathogenicity* (whether the agent can cause a disease), and *virulence* (disease severity and mortality) of mpox with other similar diseases and conduct experimental studies (such as using a vaccine) in controlling the disease. The type of epidemiologic analysis that deals with this kind of in-depth study is called finding *determinants* of a disease. Refer to Chapter 17 where I discuss different epidemiological studies such as case-control study and cohort study. These types of analytical studies and clinical trials or experimental studies are appropriate for knowing why a disease occurs and how to control it.

Avoiding errors when conducting an epidemiological study

To be successful in conducting an epidemiologic study, even if it's a small-scale survey for your classwork, be aware of some common mistakes that you can avoid:

>> **Know the population.** All sciences make mistakes, and epidemiology is no exception. The most common mistake is to start a study without knowing the population well. Hippocrates, the Father of Medicine, mentioned in his treatise on *Airs, Waters, and Places* that whenever you enter a new place, know the population characteristics and their mode of life.

>> **Describe when, where, and what.** Don't forget to provide the context and definitions of your study population. Define when, where, and what — the time frame of your study, the geographical area, and the type of study design. Also, describe how you get your samples.

>> **Make comparisons.** Some types of studies (such as interventions or experimental studies) need a comparison group. Even a historical control is useful when you evaluate the effect of some interventions. However, for descriptive studies, such as a cross-sectional study, you may not bother about having a comparison group. Chapter 17 discusses the different types of epidemiologic studies.

>> **Estimate causality.** As an epidemiologist, you should be very cautious in calling an associated factor causal. Chapter 16 discusses Bradford Hill's criteria of causality.

>> **Calculate sample size.** Inadequate sample size fails to produce valid results.

>> **Recognize generalizability.** Recognize the limitations in your study. For example, if you only study Mississippians, you may not always be able to generalize your findings to the entire United States.

Realizing Why Epidemiology Is Important

Epidemiology is one of the basic sciences of public health that affects almost everyone's life. This section helps you understand how epidemiology contributes to important issues affecting people's health.

Here I give you highlights of some important contributions of epidemiology that have impacted human health and survival, such as measuring health status, discovering vaccines and preventing diseases, using epidemiologic methods for identifying a causal association, and suggesting methods for controlling epidemics.

Identifying and measuring health status

John Graunt, an English statistician, was the first person who birthed the concept of vital statistics in London in 1603. He systematically recorded all deaths in London and published his data in the *Bill of Mortality* — the first book on counting numbers and measuring health status. His initial work has developed the field of vital statistics that is a backbone of measuring health status.

Focusing on disease prevention

The primary objective of public health is to control and prevent diseases that are prevailing in the world. Refer to the section, "Preventing diseases before they hit," later in this chapter for specifics about what an epidemiologist does.

With present-day scientific knowledge, scientists are still struggling to prevent cancers, heart disease, diabetes, and many disability-causing chronic illnesses. The discovery and uses of vaccines for common infectious diseases have decreased childhood mortality and increased life expectancy of people. These vaccine-preventable diseases include chickenpox, diphtheria, flu, hepatitis A, hepatitis B, Hib, HPV infection, measles, meningitis, mumps, polio, pneumococcal pneumonia, rotavirus, rubella, tetanus, and whooping cough. Epidemiology is continuously looking for vaccines for controlling many more diseases (for example, dengue, Ebola, and malaria).

Searching for causes

As an epidemiology student, you'll find it fascinating how scientists discovered the causes of diseases. In older days when the actual cause of a disease was unknown, people believed in supernatural forces such as witchcraft, sorcery, and evil spirits causing diseases. Then came the *miasma theory* — the belief where a noxious form of bad air entering the body caused diseases. That was 20 years before the development of the microscope and a few years before the birth of the germ theory!

You need to be familiar with the germ theory that revolutionized the causal theory of infections. In fact, the germ theory of disease is the currently accepted scientific theory for many diseases. Chapters 3 and 4 discuss the different scientists and discoveries.

In addition to causes of infectious diseases, you should also know the development of the concept of "risk factors" for noninfectious diseases. In 1950, Richard Doll and Austin Bradford Hill suggested that the risk of lung cancer was related to the number of cigarettes a person smoked per day. The famous longitudinal study known as the Framingham Heart Study is another milestone that you need to be aware of because of its far-reaching impacts in public health.

Controlling epidemics

Some people tend to link epidemiology with epidemic control. *Epidemic control* is just one of many important tasks that epidemiologists do. The Centers for Disease Control and Prevention (CDC) play a pivotal role in controlling the introduction and spread of infectious diseases, providing consultation and assistance to other nations and agencies in improving their disease prevention and the control and health promotion activities, and advocating for vaccination and other disease control activities.

In 1958, the CDC sent a team of Epidemic Intelligence Service (EIS) officers to Southeast Asia for the control of smallpox and cholera epidemics. In 1980, smallpox was eradicated from the world. In 1988, the World Health Organization (WHO), together with Rotary International, UNICEF, and the CDC passed the Global Polio Eradication Initiative (GPEI), with a revised target to end polio by 2026.

Epidemiologists help in controlling disease. As an epidemiology student, you'll know what diseases have been controlled because of the introduction of vaccines (refer to Chapter 12).

Currently, the WHO recommends the limited use of a malaria vaccine for children living in Sub-Saharan Africa and other regions where *Plasmodium falciparum* (a severe type of malaria parasite) is highly prevalent. Chapter 12 describes vaccine-preventable diseases and vaccines that are needed for travelers.

Understanding How Epidemiology Tools Are Applied

You should expand your skills by applying epidemiologic tools in community-based research in the following ways:

>> Apply epidemiologic research designs based on the outcome measurements (see Chapter 17).

>> Measure rates such as incidence, prevalence, odds ratio, relative risk, and others depending on the types of the data (see Chapters 10 and 17).

>> Apply screening methods, depending on the disease conditions (refer to Chapter 11).

>> Investigate an epidemic (check out Chapter 14).

>> Project future populations and control future health problems (see Chapter 9).

These sections focus on the role of epidemiology in identifying risks, measuring disease morbidity and mortality, identifying the impact of experimental studies, and in preventing diseases.

Using epidemiologic methods to identify risks

One of the major tasks of epidemiologists is to identify any risk factors for disease, injury, and death. An epidemiologist describes a disease in terms of person, place, and time to identify specific populations (age, sex, race, and occupation) who are at risk and the places (rural or urban, type of housing, environmental conditions, and others) where the public health problems are greater and the time when the disease reaches a peak. Furthermore, epidemiologists measure potential biological, chemical, physical, and behavioral exposures for diseases to identify risk factors. Refer to Chapter 7 for more details.

Measuring morbidity and mortality

Epidemiologists monitor diseases and other health-related events over time. If you monitor a disease in a locality over time, you can describe the level of the cases (*morbidity*) and deaths (*mortality*) from the disease. A proper monitoring system can identify when an epidemic is impending before it hits. Based on the rates of morbidity and mortality of the prevailing diseases in your community, you can prioritize the top diseases of public health importance and allocate resources accordingly. Chapter 8 deals with the assessment of disease patterns.

Describing the impact of an intervention

Experimental studies and community-based interventions are part of epidemiologic studies. Here are a few examples of what epidemiological studies have shown:

>> A low dose of aspirin can reduce the risk for a second heart attack and certain types of strokes, mainly by preventing blood clots from forming within blood vessels.

>> Supplementation of low-dose iron in low-income postpartum women is effective in reducing anemia.

>> Different Covid-19 vaccines are effective in reducing hospitalization, ICU admission, and death in fully vaccinated populations.

The scope of epidemiological research is wide — from descriptive studies, analytical studies, and experimental studies. Chapter 17 deals with different types of epidemiologic studies such as an ecological study, a cross-sectional study, a case-control study, and a cohort study.

Preventing diseases before they hit

Epidemiology plays a vital role in all levels of disease prevention. When studying prevention, you need to be familiar with these three pillars of disease prevention (refer to Chapter 11):

>> **Primary prevention:** It refers to preventing a disease from happening. Examples include

- Giving vaccines for diseases such as measles, polio, tetanus, diphtheria, whooping cough, and others

- Hand washing, social distancing, and using face masks to prevent Covid-19 and many other communicable diseases such as Ebola, influenza, and tuberculosis

- Providing safe water and sanitation for the control of diarrheal diseases

>> **Secondary prevention:** This refers to reducing the duration of a disease and preventing complications and deaths. Screening is such a tool used in epidemiology for early detection of diseases. Examples include

- Regular self-exams and mammograms to detect breast cancer

- A Pap smear test to detect cervical cancer

>> **Tertiary prevention:** This refers to preventing disabilities of people who have suffered from major diseases and injuries. Tertiary prevention also aims to provide people with a quality of life, through new job placement or rehabilitation, depending on the disabilities the person might have suffered. Examples of tertiary prevention include

- Rehab program after cardiac bypass surgery

- Chronic disease management program (such as for diabetes complications)

- Support group sessions for improving coping skills from a major episode of depression

Furthermore, several types of epidemiological studies are effective in predicting risk factors and controlling diseases. Ecological studies, case-control studies, and population-based longitudinal studies are examples of epidemiological studies that have established the role of identifying risk factors and taking measures in the prevention of diseases. For example, epidemiological studies have been used in identifying and determining the risk factors for mental health outcomes such as suicide and suicidal behaviors.

Investigating epidemics of unknown cause

By conducting a continuous scrutiny or vigilance of diseases, you can identify when a new disease has appeared in your locality. A recent outbreak of mpox is a perfect example. Scientists have started learning about the risk factors and mode of transmission of the disease. After a disease appears in the form of an epidemic, the epidemiologists are who's called to investigate the epidemic.

Here's what an epidemic investigation team does in a thorough investigation (Chapter 14 describes them in greater detail):

>> **Establishes the existence of an epidemic.** Epidemic investigation starts when a large number of cases are reported. Based on the clinical observations and laboratory results, epidemiologists come up with a case definition of the probable cause of the epidemic. They conduct further investigations to establish the existence, route of transmission, and the disease agent for the epidemic.

>> **Describes the type of the epidemic.** The two types are

- **Common source:** A disease like watery diarrhea is spread from a contaminated water source such as a river or a pond.

- **Propagated source:** In this case, the disease (such as blood dysentery) is spread from one infected person to another.

>> **Describes the risk factors in terms of person, place, and time.** Your initial descriptive data analysis helps in developing a hypothesis. You'll conduct further studies to prove the hypothesis — the latter studies are analytical epidemiologic studies.

>> **Finds out sources.** In this difficult step, you'll collect environmental samples that you had suspected as possible sources of the agent. Sometimes isolating the disease pathogen from the environmental samples, such as water, is difficult.

>> **Looks for the cause.** This step of an epidemic investigation is important. You gather all the clues such as symptoms of patients, onset of the disease, the nature of the epidemic curve, and the pathogen (bacteria or virus) to establish the cause of the epidemic.

>> **Identifies the modes of transmission.** From the case history, the nature of the epidemic curve, and the source, you can find the mode of transmission: person-to-person spread or a common source spread of the disease.

>> **Intensifies the surveillance system to find new cases.** New case-finding and contact tracing are a few techniques of the surveillance system. By door-to-door search, you can find out new and ongoing cases.

>> **Takes measures for controlling the disease.** Control measures include the treatment of cases, the prevention of the further spread of the disease from the primary cases (the first few cases), and health education such as proper hand washing, sanitation, and others.

Evaluating public health programs

Quality assurance and quality control activities are key components of epidemiologic research. While evaluating public health programs, you'll measure quality assurance and quality control in every step of the program. In essence, this evaluation ensures validity (or accuracy) and reliability (or precision and reproducibility) of the public health program.

Quality assurance

The purpose of quality assurance activities before data collection is to standardize the procedures and thus prevent or at least minimize systematic or random errors in collecting and analyzing data. The activities involved in this process include the following:

>> A detailed protocol preparation

>> The development of data collection instruments

>> The development of operation manuals

>> The training and certification of staff

The design of quality assurance activities should follow pretesting and pilot studies.

REMEMBER

One of the tools of data collection is a well-designed questionnaire. As a program evaluator, you'll ensure the program uses a data collection instrument that's valid and reliable. Choose data collection instruments and procedures that have been used effectively in previous studies to measure both suspected risk factors and disease outcomes. On occasion, even though the questionnaire is a well-established data collection instrument, you may need to pre-test it and validate it in another country population because the characteristics of the two populations may be different. For further information, read Chapter 17.

Quality control

Activities of quality control generally begin after data collection and data processing starts. However, monitoring the data collection process may also ensure quality data. As an epidemiologist, you should follow certain standard quality control strategies:

>> Observe the procedures performed by staff members.

>> Identify obvious protocol deviations.

>> Carry out special studies of validity and reliability in samples of subjects at specified intervals throughout data collection. These procedures include

- Periodic checking of the equipment

- Field monitoring the use of the instrument

- Checking for missing data

>> Coordinate quality control in data analyses. In this process, make sure your team members know how to use the statistical software and that they're using correct statistical methods and avoiding bias.

>> Ensure avoiding bias in all steps of the study including data analysis and the report writing to minimize any reporting or publication bias.

REMEMBER

If you're assigned to evaluate a public health program, your job isn't to find out errors but rather to recommend a coordinated, properly conducted, public health program with clear objectives, a proper study design, standardized procedures, and unbiased methods of data collection, data analysis, and reporting. A properly conducted public health program is intended to promote people's health. You, as a program evaluator, are assisting in the process.

Contrasting the Roles of a Physician and Epidemiologist

Public health is a multidisciplinary field whose goal is to promote the health of a population through organized community efforts. As a field of public health, epidemiology focuses mainly on preventing illnesses in the community, whereas medicine focuses on treating illnesses in individuals. A physician, who reduces a patient's ailments and sufferings and cures a disease by using medicine, gets immediate rewards compared to the achievements of epidemiologists (and other public health workers), which are difficult to recognize because identifying people who have been spared illnesses isn't easy. This section describes the major functions of a physician and an epidemiologist.

Eyeing the differences

When you're studying epidemiology, you may need to know the differences between a physician and an epidemiologist; Table 2-1 helps.

TABLE 2-1 Differences between a Physician and an Epidemiologist

Physician	Epidemiologist
Primary job is to provide treatment and cure of a disease.	Primary job is to prevent a disease.
Deals with the individual patient.	Deals with a group of people or an entire population.
The mode of approach is a passive process in the sense that patients take the initiative to visit a doctor's clinic or a hospital.	The mode of approach is an active process because an epidemiologist initiates programs to prevent a disease.
A physician initiates the process in finding the cause of a disease in an individual.	An epidemiologist initiates the process in finding the risk factors and the causes of a disease affecting a population.
A physician directly helps an individual.	An epidemiologist indirectly helps a community.
A physician is involved in basic science such as drug development, efficacy trials, and the underlying disease pathology.	An epidemiologist is involved in research, mostly in applied science, such as collecting and analyzing data to investigate health issues, determining whether populations at high risk for a disease, and identifying the effectiveness of a drug among a population.

Helping people

Physicians save lives and make a difference in helping patients minimize pain and suffering. They get patients early relief by diagnosing and treating the disease as soon as possible and preventing complications with proper patient management. For example, a patient is having fever, chills, cough, sore throat, muscle or body aches, headaches, and fatigue. A physician can quickly distinguish between a cold and the flu and can provide appropriate medicines, which can help the patient get better in a few days.

The flu virus is highly contagious with the potential of affecting anybody, especially children younger than 2 and the elderly people older than 65. Epidemiologists conduct research in developing an effective vaccine depending on the prevailing flu strains; each season's flu vaccine can be different. Epidemiologists provide preventive services such as conducting epidemic investigation and disease management, initiating disease surveillance, screening a disease for early diagnosis, conducting research to identify the cause, mode of transmission, disease occurrence, and mortality, and predicting disease outcomes. People get long-term benefits from the work that epidemiologists do.

Describing diseases differently

A physician makes a provisional diagnosis based on the patient's medical history, symptoms or complaints, and signs identified during an examination. A physician then can confirm the diagnosis by doing several blood tests or diagnostic tests. A physician, being an expert and a specialist in identifying and treating a wide range of health conditions, describes a disease in a clinical perspective and the prognosis of the disease in terms of recovery, complications, or death.

On the other hand, an epidemiologist studies how often diseases occur in different populations and why. Using statistical approaches, they seek to find answers to questions how a particular health problem has been introduced in the population. They identify new diseases that have never been seen before and what causes them, such as Legionnaire's disease, Ebola, and MERS. Epidemiologists also help health planners act in preventing a disease.

Grasping the difference between acute and chronic disease

Physicians determine treatment based on how long the patient has been sick. Some diseases start acutely and last for a few days whereas other diseases with similar symptoms are chronic, meaning they last for months with remissions and relapses. Suppose a patient has diarrhea; if the symptoms last for three to four days, the most common cause of watery diarrhea in an adult is *E. coli* diarrhea, unless the patient lives in a country where cholera is common. On the other hand, if the patient has been suffering from diarrhea for a few months, physicians will look for causes of chronic diarrhea, such as irritable bowel syndrome (IBS), food allergy, or some serious illnesses like Crohn's disease or ulcerative colitis. A physician can give treatment according to the diagnosis of the cause of the symptoms.

An epidemiologist most commonly defines a disease based on the length of the incubation period (or induction period) of the disease. The *Incubation period* is the time from the point a germ is introduced in the body until the time when the person developed symptoms. An epidemiologist identifies whether they can use a screening test early enough before the onset of symptoms to easily control the disease.

Another example is the case of an outbreak investigation. The nature of the outbreak and the cause depend on the disease's incubation period. For example, consider an outbreak due to food poisoning, which has a very short incubation period.

An epidemiologist investigates this time difference between the intake of food and the start of symptoms to discover the possible cause of the outbreak.

Table 2-2 gives you an idea about how a physician and an epidemiologist identify a few acute and chronic diseases. Both identify cholera as an acute disease and alcoholism as a chronic disease. However, based on their nature of work, epidemiologists and physicians identify a few diseases such as AIDS and spinal injury differently. This happens because the action plans to control or cure the disease could be different between the two. Bottom line: For almost all cases, an epidemiologist and a physician work as a team — for example, investigation of Covid-19 or the management of a cholera epidemic.

TABLE 2-2   Identifying Diseases by a Physician and an Epidemiologist

	Epidemiologist	
Physician	Acute	Chronic
Acute	Cholera	AIDS
	Staph infection	
Chronic	Spinal injury	Alcoholism

Seeking Medications

Based on the nature of medicines, some are available only with a prescription, such as an antibiotic or a steroid. Some medicines are available without a prescription — over-the-counter. As a public health professional, you should also know that several countries in the developing world are yet to control the use of several medicines and get them available to the public only with a prescription. These sections examine medications and what you may encounter in your epidemiology courses.

Eyeing over-the-counter (OTC) and prescription medication

Over-the-counter (OTC) drugs are medications that are available with or without a prescription, whereas certain medications, known as prescription drugs, are available only when a doctor recommends them. Some medications are available both as a prescription and over-the-counter drug. OTC drugs are available in pharmacies, grocery stores, discount stores, gas stations, and airports.

In the United States, FDA regulations ensure that OTC drugs are safe and that the labels are easy to understand. Before using any OTC medicine, a patient should consider the benefits and the risks.

Here are some examples of commonly used OTC medications that patients can purchase without a prescription:

>> **Pain relievers:** acetaminophen (Tylenol) and ibuprofen (Advil, Motrin)

>> **Cough and cold medicines:** Robitussin, Nyquil

>> **Allergy medicine:** Claritin, Benadryl

>> **Heartburn medicines:** Prilosec, Tagamet HB, Maalox, Tums, Zantac 75

>> **Laxatives:** Dulcolax, glycerin suppositories

>> **Diarrhea remedies:** Immodium A-D

>> **Diet pills:** Alli

>> **Acne remedies:** retinoid (vitamin A derivatives), benzoyl peroxide (BP), glycolic acid, lactic acid, beta-hydroxy acid (BHA)

>> **Hair regrowth solutions:** Minoxidil

If a patient's insurance doesn't cover OTC medicines, sometimes they may cost higher than prescription medicines. Table 2-3 lists the top ten prescription drugs in the United States. This list has remained fairly consistent.

TABLE 2-3 **Top Ten Commonly Used Prescribed Drugs in the U.S.**

Drug Name	Brand Name	Primary Use
Atorvastatin	Lipitor	Cholesterol
Amoxicillin	Amoxil, Trimox	Antibiotic
Levothyroxine	Synthroid, Levoxyl	Thyroid
Metformin	Glucophage, Fortamet	Diabetes
Lisinopril	Prinivil, Zestril	Blood pressure
Amlodipine	Norvasc	Blood pressure
Metoprolol	Lopressor, Toprol XL	Blood pressure
Albuterol	Ventolin, Proventil	Asthma
Omeprazole	Losec	Stomach ulcer
Losartan	Cozaar	Blood pressure

Examining the role of traditional healers

Many societies have an acute shortage of qualified doctors. For example, in 2019 Bangladesh had only 0.6 qualified doctors per 1,000 people. For the economically marginalized village people in a developing country, such as Bangladesh and some parts of India, people first go to unqualified traditional healers called a *palli chikit-shaks* or a homeopathic practitioner because the treatment is cheaper. In remote villages where no qualified doctors are available to help, these traditional healers are the only people to diagnose, treat, and refer patients to the nearest health centers.

Some other forms of treatments offered by traditional healers are traditional Chinese medicine, Ayurvedic medicine, Kabiraji medicine, Unani medicine, spiritual therapies, amulet therapy, and others. Traditional birth attendants (TBAs) provide home-delivery services. TBAs (usually old mothers) are individuals within the community who assist mothers in maternal care and conduct deliveries at home.

In South Africa, traditional healers fulfill different social and political roles in the community, including healing physical, emotional, and spiritual illnesses, directing birth or death rituals, protecting warriors, counteracting witchcraft, narrating the history, and continuing aspects of their tradition. They also work as educators, counselors, social workers, and psychologists.

REAL LIFE EXAMPLE

In 2003, the government of Bangladesh initiated the community-based skilled birth attendant (CSBA) program to increase accessibility of skilled delivery at home. They targeted to train 13,500 government field staff as CSBAs who are trained TBAs to take care of pregnant women, conduct deliveries, and provide postnatal services because of a shortage of qualified obstetrics/gynecologist doctors in Bangladesh.

THE ROLE OF COMPLEMENTARY AND ALTERNATIVE MEDICINE (CAM)

Complementary and alternative medicine (CAM) is the term for medical products and practices that aren't part of standard medical care. Complementary medicine, sometimes referred to as *natural, holistic, home remedy,* or *Eastern Medicine,* is used along with standard medical treatment whereas alternative medicine describes medical treatments that are used instead of traditional (mainstream) therapies. As an epidemiology student, you should know people's choice of different treatments, including CAM.

More than half of adults in the United States say they use some form of CAM, and total visits to CAM providers exceed total visits to all primary care physicians. In fact, out-of-pocket costs for CAM are estimated to exceed $27 billion.

In the United States, some of the most frequently used and well-known CAM therapies are relaxation techniques, herbs, chiropractic care, and massage therapy. Many states do require licenses in chiropractic care, acupuncture, and massage therapies; fewer states require licenses in naturopathy and homeopathy. Numerous other therapies and modalities are considered unlicensed practices and at present few or no formal regulations apply to these therapies and modalities. The New York State Office of Regulatory Reform and CAM have identified more than 100 therapies, practices, and systems that could be considered CAM. One of the most widely used classification structures, developed by The National Center for Complementary and Alternative Medicine (NCCAM) of NIH (2000), divides CAM modalities into five categories:

- **Alternative medical systems:** Examples include traditional Chinese medicine, Ayurvedic medicine, homeopathy, and naturopathy.

- **Mind-body intervention:** Examples include meditation, prayer, and mental healing.

- **Biologically based treatments:** They include specialized diets, herbal products, and other natural products such as minerals, hormones, and biologicals. An example of a nonherbal natural product is fish oil for the treatment of cardiovascular conditions.

- **Manipulative and body-based methods:** Examples include therapies that involve movement or manipulation of the body. Chiropractic care is the best known in this category, and chiropractors are licensed to practice in every U.S. state. Massage therapy is another example of a body-based therapy.

- **Energy therapies:** Examples include the manipulation and application of energy fields to the body. In addition to electromagnetic fields outside the body, it's hypothesized that energy fields exist within the body. The field of energy that surrounds and extends out from the body (about 8 feet) is called a *biofield*. The existence of these biofields hasn't been experimentally proven; however, a number of therapies include qi gong, Reiki, and therapeutic touch.

Medical schools, nursing schools, and schools of pharmacy are teaching their students about CAM. The National Institute of Health (NIH) provides research support for CAM through the National Center for Complementary and Integrative Health. The first large, multicenter trial of a CAM therapy was conducted in 1997 by the Office of Alternative Medicine (OAM), the National Institute on Mental Health, and the NIH Office of Dietary Supplements. The trial tested the effect of *Hypericum* (St. John's wort) for depression. More research is needed to demonstrate the efficacy of CAM in human health.

Considering How a Disease Is Transmitted

When you study epidemiology, you need to know how people get sick. The following sections examine some of the different ways that a disease can be transmitted.

Defining key infection terms

Some of the terms are somewhat confusing when you mention infectious diseases, communicable disease, and contagious disease. Here I help you keep track of these words:

>> An *infectious disease* is caused by a minute germ called bacteria or virus. Some of the infectious diseases can spread from one person to another but some don't.

>> Those infectious diseases that spread directly from person to person are called *contagious diseases.* Therefore, an infectious disease may or may not be contagious, but all contagious diseases are infectious.

>> You may hear the terms *communicable* and *noncommunicable* diseases. Don't worry though because the terms *communicable* and *contagious* are interchangeable, meaning they're the same.

Noncommunicable diseases are chronic diseases, and they can't spread infection from one person to another (except hereditary or genetically transferred diseases). Noncommunicable diseases (NCDs) are non-infectious, meaning that they aren't transmissible directly from one person to another. NCDs include heart diseases, stroke, most cancers, diabetes, chronic kidney disease, osteoarthritis, osteoporosis, Alzheimer's disease, asthma, autoimmune diseases, and several others.

Here are a couple examples of infectious communicable diseases:

>> **Measles:** This highly infectious viral disease occurs mostly in children. If one child is infected with measles, it's likely that other siblings in the family will get infected.

>> **Influenza:** This is another viral infection, and it is highly communicable from one person to another. The transmission is through air droplets by sneezing and coughing.

Here are a couple examples of infectious noncommunicable diseases:

>> **Urinary tract infection (UTI):** This is usually a bacterial infection although it's not transmitted from person to person. If a person gets a UTI after sex, more than likely they didn't adequately clean their genitalia.

>> *E. coli* **infection:** *E. coli* is a bacteria that's transmitted through the fecal-oral route. You can get it by drinking contaminated water or by eating infected food, especially raw vegetables or uncooked ground beef.

Spreading infection of an outbreak from person to person

Several infectious diseases can cause a threat as an epidemic. At the time of writing this book, the world is facing such an epidemic of Covid-19. When an epidemic crosses the boundary of one country and affects several countries simultaneously, it's called a *pandemic*.

Covid-19 is a large pandemic that has caused about 637 million cases and more than 6.6 million deaths as of early 2023. The virus that causes Covid, SARS-CoV-2, spreads from person to person via respiratory droplets. (An epidemic spread from person-to-person is also called a *propagated source epidemic*.) Because of the nature of person-to-person transmission, the disease is lasting longer. Another significant reason for the number of cases and deaths is a result of the changing nature of the virulence and transmissibility of the virus because of newer strains.

Human factors play a big role in the control of a disease that's transmitted from person-to-person like Covid-19. The containment of this pandemic will only be successful when people follow proper preventive measures and until a large majority of the people get immunity from the disease by vaccination and through natural infections.

Here are a couple other examples of diseases that are transmitted from person to person and have also caused epidemics from time to time:

>> Shigellosis is a bacterial disease caused by several strains of *Shigella*. When people's immunity decreases, the bacteria can flare up and infect many people, especially young children. Because of person-to-person spread, the disease affects many people in a family and many families in an area, causing an outbreak. Hand washing is the best method of preventing shigellosis, and antibiotics are the first line of treatment. However, multiresistant strains of the bacteria make it difficult to treat the patients.

» Ebola hemorrhagic fever, a viral disease, caused an epidemic that killed thousands of people, mainly in western Africa in 2014. The virus spread through human contact with contaminated body fluids.

Getting infection of an outbreak from a common source

A common-source outbreak occurs when a group of people get sick simultaneously after being exposed to an infection from the same source. This type of outbreak can be caused by a bacteria, virus, toxin, or other infectious agents. One of the diseases of a common source origin is cholera, caused by a bacteria called *Vibro cholera*. The transmission of the bacteria is through the fecal-oral route. The disease usually originates from a contaminated source of water.

REAL LIFE EXAMPLE

When I was working as a medical officer in a diarrheal disease treatment center at a remote village of Matlab, Bangladesh in 1985–1986, a huge number of people were admitted to the hospital with symptoms of diarrhea, vomiting, abdominal cramps, and fever. All of them developed similar symptoms after eating a common food prepared with raw milk, banana, and *sabu* grains (a kind of cereal). The infection was a severe form of food poisoning due to *Salmonella* enterocolitis.

Relating infections with cancers

Cancer is a chronic disease. A few bacterial or viral infections can cause cancer, including the following (refer to Chapter 12 for further information):

» **Human papillomavirus (HPV):** This virus is associated with cervical carcinoma and carcinoma of nasopharynx.

» **Hepatitis B and Hepatitis C:** These viruses can cause hepatocellular carcinoma (liver cancer).

» *H. pylori* **infection:** This bacteria harbors in the stomach and commonly causes gastritis. Only a few (about 1 to 3 persons out of 100) go to develop stomach cancer and gastric mucosa-associated lymphoid tissue (MALT) lymphoma.

» **Human herpes virus 8 (HHV-8):** The virus is spread during sex, through blood or saliva, or from an infected mother to her baby during birth. The virus can cause Kaposi's sarcoma. The virus is also known as Kaposi's sarcoma-associated herpesvirus (KSHV).

>> **Human T-cell lymphoma virus 1 (HTLV-1):** HTLV-1 is transmitted primarily through infected bodily fluids including blood, breast milk, and semen. Risk factors include unprotected sex, injection drug use and transplantation of tissue, blood and blood products. HTLV-1 can cause a type of cancer called adult T-cell leukemia/lymphoma (ATL) in around 1 in 20 people with infection.

Searching for Sources of Epidemiologic Data

Epidemiologists use primary and secondary data for calculating rates and conducting research. Collecting primary data is expensive and time-consuming, but it's often essential to obtain quality and unbiased data. Secondary data obtained from reliable sources is easy-to-get and can be used for quality research too. Here are some examples of commonly used secondary sources of health-related data:

>> Agency for Toxic Substances and Disease Registry (ATSDR)

>> Cancer Registry

>> Centers for Disease Control and Prevention (CDC)

>> Environment Protection Agency (EPA)

>> Johns Hopkins Coronavirus Resource Center

>> National Center for Health Statistics

>> Population Census Records

>> Public Health Department

>> Vital Statistics

>> World Health Organization (WHO)

Here I discuss a few of them in greater detail.

From the Centers for Disease Control and Prevention (CDC)

CDC (www.cdc.gov/) collects data from state, local, and territorial health departments. This data is de-identified to protect individual privacy. The National Center for Health Statistics (NCHS) at the CDC maintains and updates data and provides users with quick and easy access to the wide range of health information and survey data.

From the National Center for Health Statistics (NCHS)

As the nation's principal health statistics agency, the National Center for Health Statistics (NCHS) (www.cdc.gov/nchs/index.htm) compiles statistics on many diseases. It maintains a data visualization gallery for birth, death, and some provisional data (such as infant mortality, neonatal mortality, and post-neonatal mortality). You can generate charts on the indicators that you want. For example, if you want data for teen birth rate for females aged 15–19 years, just select those indicators.

Secondly, NCHS provides updated information on Covid-19. You can select data that covers the whole United States or data at the state or county level. Other data available includes age and sex, race and Hispanic origin, and place of death from Covid-19, comorbidities, and other conditions.

Third, if you click on Health, United States, you can explore data by topic. For example, if you click on health risk factors, you can filter by topics, such as asthma, cancer, cigarette smoking, fertility, healthcare access, and so on (listed alphabetically).

From the World Health Organization (WHO)

For an epidemiology student or a professional, this is one of the most resourceful websites. The WHO website (www.who.int) includes data for the following categories: health topics, countries, newsroom, emergencies, data, and About WHO. If you want to know a particular disease, go to health topics, which are listed from A to Z. You'll get fact sheets, pictures, publications, Q&As, and tools and toolkits.

From census data

The U.S. Census Bureau maintains a website (https://data.census.gov/cedsci/) for data about U.S. people, places, and the economy. You can access tables for population by state. The populations are again categorized by one of multiple races, age, and sex, demographic and housing, income, selected economic characteristics, poverty status, and many more.

For example, you're conducting a study on senior citizens. When you click on population 65 years and over in the Unites States, you get statistics on many variables such as total population, sex and age, median age, race (one or multiple), population in the household and the percentages based on the relationship, household by type, marital status, educational attainment, responsibility for grandchildren under 18 years, veteran status, disability status, and many more.

From the Vital Statistics System

The CDC maintains the National Vital Statistics System (NVSS) website (www.cdc.gov/nchs/nvss/index.htm), which provides a link to reporting guidelines for CDC data on Covid-19. If you're interested in health disparities in Covid-19 deaths, you can find information on the following:

>> Race and Hispanic origin

>> Race and Hispanic origin and age

>> Urban/rural status

>> Social vulnerability index

>> County-level data on race and Hispanic origin

>> Education

NVSS provides the most complete data on births and deaths in the United States. The data is categorized by births, deaths, fetal deaths, linked birth/infant death, life expectancy, and marriages and divorces. For example, if you want to know about life expectancy, you can get the latest reports and a quick link for data visualizations.

Chapter 3

Exploring the Development of Epidemiological Thinking

The historical development epidemiology dates back to 400 B.C. when Hippocrates described diseases in terms of climate, season, and the quality of water in his legendary treatise *Airs, Waters, and Places*. However, only since World War II has the science experienced a rapid expansion. I'm not a historian nor are my intentions to write a comprehensive history of epidemiology. In this chapter I highlight several historical figures who made significant contributions to the evolution of epidemiologic thinking and studies that are considered landmarks in the development of the discipline.

Meeting Hippocrates — the First Epidemiologist

Hippocrates (460 B.C.–370 B.C.), referred to as the Father of Medicine, is also recognized as the first epidemiologist in history. The Hippocratic School emphasized the clinical doctrines of observation and documentation. These doctrines dictate that physicians record their findings and their medicinal methods in a very clear and objective manner so that these records may be passed down and other physicians can use them. To Hippocrates medicine is indebted to the art of clinical inspection and observation. He began to categorize illnesses as acute, chronic, endemic, and epidemic. In his book *On Epidemics*, he advised doctors to note specific symptoms and what they observed on a day-to-day basis. By doing this, they could describe a natural history of an illness.

An especially important contribution of Hippocrates is The Hippocratic Oath, a fundamental document on the ethics of medical practice. Here I delve deeper into his contribution to epidemiology.

Observing "airs, waters, and places"

In his book *Airs, Waters, and Places*, Hippocrates referred to what is now the basis of epidemiologic investigation. He described the distribution of disease in terms of time, space, and person. He studied the distribution of diseases according to season, climate, age, individual body-build, habits, activity level of the people, and their mode of life. He introduced the idea that disease might be associated with the physical environment.

Relating diseases to polluted water

Hippocrates described how marshy, standing, and stagnant water in the summer becomes unhealthy, and how frosty, cold, and turbid water in the winter is conducive to the buildup of phlegm, coughing, and sore throats. He also described physical features of people who become malnourished after drinking polluted water: "Those who drink it have always large, stiff spleens, and hard, thin, hot stomachs, while their shoulders, collarbones, and faces are emaciated."

Tackling the Miasma Theory

The *miasma theory* explained that diseases were caused by the presence in the air of a *miasma*, a poisonous vapor in which were suspended particles of decaying matter (*miasmata*). These sections explain what you need to know about this theory that originated in the fourth or fifth century B.C.

Believing in bad air

One example of the miasma theory was the case of malaria. Malaria is so named — from the Italian *mala* (which means *bad*) and *aria* (which means *air*) and is evidence of its suspected miasmic origins. Marcus Vitruvius Pollio (80–70 B.C. to 15 B.C.), a Roman author, architect, and engineer, in his *Ten Books on Architecture*, warns against various kinds of bad air — marshy air, pestilential air, and unhealthy vapors. The most famous Roman physician Claudius Galen (129–199 A.D.) believed that disease resulted from an internal imbalance of the four humors: air (blood), fire (yellow bile), earth (black bile), and water (phlegm).

In the 1850s, miasma was used to explain the spread of cholera in London and in Paris. Other diseases then considered linked to bad air (miasma) included the Black Death of plague, chlamydia infections, cold, influenza, heat strokes, malaria, and dysentery. The proponents of the miasma theory included Florence Nightingale, William Farr, and Thomas S. Smith.

The Indians invented *paan*, a paste from the *gambier* plant that was believed to help prevent miasma and was considered as the first anti-miasmatic application.

Getting benefits from a misconception

The miasma theory was subsequently proven wrong. However, what people gained most out of the misconception of the miasma theory is that they started working to improve environmental conditions in order to stop the spread of infection.

REMEMBER

In 19th-century England the miasma theory made sense to the sanitary reformers. Edwin Chadwick mentioned, "All smell is disease." The theory led to sanitation improvements, such as preventing the reflux of noxious air from sewers back into houses by implementing separate drainage systems in sanitation designs. By improving housing, sanitation, and general cleanliness, levels of disease decreased.

Examining Contributions to Medicine and Public Health – Thomas Sydenham

Thomas Sydenham (1624–1689) is considered the English Hippocrates because he elaborated on the Hippocratic idea of epidemics. He studied variations in epidemics of different diseases with respect to age, season, and year. One of his contributions to modern medicine is that he classified fever into three levels: continued, intermittent, and sporadic. Modern medicine still recognizes the former two types of fever.

Contrary to other physicians of his time, Sydenham, who is often referred to as the founder of clinical medicine and epidemiology as it's known today, recognized the importance of physical exercise, diet, and fresh air as part of treatment. His many important contributions in epidemiology and medicine include the following:

>> The study of epidemics

>> The identification of the link between fleas and typhus fever

>> The study of natural history of disease

>> Sydenham chorea, also referred to as St. Vitus dance, a neurological symptom of rheumatic fever in children

Using Concepts of Environmental Epidemiology — Noah Webster

Noah Webster Jr. (1758–1843), published a booklet on global warming titled *Are Our Winters Getting Warmer?* For his contributions in the investigation of epidemics and in relating environmental factors for diseases, Webster is honored as the "Father of Epidemiology and Public Health in America."

Webster's contribution to epidemiology is remarkable — he studied epidemics of influenza, yellow fever, and scarlet fever, and demonstrated that epidemics were related to certain environmental factors that affected a large group of populations.

The Germ Theory — Washing Hands Is Essential

The germ theory of disease emerged in the second half of the 1800s and gradually replaced the miasma theory (refer to the section, "Tackling the Miasma Theory," earlier in this chapter). The germ theory gained momentum after the discovery of the microscope. Until the 15th century scientists such as Hieronymous Francastorius believed in the theory of contagion. Among the pioneers of the germ theory include Edward Jenner, Louis Pasteur, and Robert Koch, who I discuss here.

THE INVENTION OF THE MICROSCOPE AND MICROBES

The discovery of the microscope made a revolutionary change in epidemiology. The prevailing germ theory of the 18th century was spotlighted when microbes or germs were seen under a microscope.

The first microscope dates back to 1590 in Middelburg, Netherlands. In 1644 a microscope magnified the interior structure of living tissue when Marcelo Malpighi in Italy analyzed biological structures beginning with the lungs. The discovery of red blood cells and spermatozoa under the microscope made the instrument a popular technique in science. Antonie van Leeuwenhoek discovered microorganisms on October 9, 1676, and his contributions changed the history of medicine and the epidemiologic theory of disease causation.

Over the next few centuries microscopes advanced. In 1893 August Köhler developed a key technique for sample illumination, Köhler illumination, which is central to modern light microscopy. In the early 1900s a significant alternative to light microscopy was developed, using electrons rather than light to generate the image. Ernst Ruska started developing the first electron microscope in 1931, which was a transmission electron microscope (TEM). In 1935, Max Knoll developed the scanning electron microscope.

The most recent development in light microscopy is the use of the fluorescence microscopy technique in biological science and medicine. During the last decades of the 20th century, particularly in the post-genomic era, many techniques for fluorescent labeling of cellular structures have been developed. The main advancements include the small chemical staining of cellular structures, (for example diamidino-2-phenylindole (DAPI) to label deoxyribonucleic acid (DNA)), which is a self-replicating material present in nearly all living organisms as the main constituent of chromosomes.

Hieronymous Fracastorius

Hieronymous Fracastorius (1478–1553), an Italian poet, scholar, and physician, believed that disease was transmitted from one person to another by particles too small to be seen. Calling this transmission process *contagion* in 1546, he hypothesized that "minute particles" could be transmitted from one person to another.

He described three types of contagion:

>> Direct person-to-person contagion

>> Contagion transmitted through *fomes* (clothing or other objects, later known as *fomites*)

>> Contagion at a distance

The concept of contagion was later evolved to the germ theory. About 40 years after his death, the discovery of the microscope made it possible for scientists to view these minute particles, or microorganisms.

Edward Jenner

Edward Jenner (1749–1823), an English rural physician, observed that when a person had cowpox, the same person wouldn't get smallpox if exposed to it. Smallpox, now eradicated from the world, was once a deadly disease characterized by chills, high fever, body ache, and eruption of pimples that blister and form pockmarks. Jenner exposed a dairymaid who was exposed with a mild case of cowpox in her youth to smallpox by cutting her arm and rubbing her wound with some of the infectious "grease" (pus and fluid obtained from the lesion). The dairymaid didn't become ill. Exposure to cowpox made her immune to smallpox. With this knowledge, Jenner invented a vaccine against smallpox, and it eventually helped to eradicate smallpox from the world.

Louis Pasteur

Louis Pasteur (1822–1895), a French chemist and microbiologist, was one of the most important founders of medical microbiology. Pasteur is well-known in the field of epidemiology and medical science for inventing the bacteria-killing process called *pasteurization*. Pasteur also discovered vaccines against anthrax and rabies through his research on weakening microbes.

Robert Koch

Robert Heinrich Herman Koch (1843–1910) is considered to be the founder of modern bacteriology. Koch, together with his teacher Friedrich Gustav Jacob Henle, developed the theory known as *Henle-Koch postulates* for the causation of infectious diseases. The postulates state that to be a cause of disease, the infectious agent must be able to be isolated from all cases of a disease, grown in culture media in a laboratory, and when introduced into a susceptible host, cause the disease in suitable conditions. Similarly, the infectious agent must be able to be isolated from these new cases and grown in culture. These postulates made a remarkable revolution in the field of microbiology and became the standard for the isolation of disease agents in the laboratory.

In 1882, Koch discovered the tubercle bacillus with the use of special culturing and staining methods. He and his team also discovered the bacteria *Vibrio cholera*. Another important contribution in epidemiology is that he established how waterborne epidemics occur and how they can be prevented by proper water purification. For all his contributions in microbiology, Koch was awarded the Nobel Prize in 1905.

FLORENCE NIGHTINGALE — THE LADY WITH THE LAMP

Florence Nightingale (1820–1910), the founder of modern nursing, was the pioneer who made nursing a respectable profession and who improved the sanitary conditions in England. She worked day and night in the Crimean War caring tirelessly for wounded soldiers. *The Times* immortalized her as the "Lady with the Lamp" after her habit of making solitary rounds at night. Nightingale advocated that nurses should be trained in science and emphasized cleanliness and an innate empathy of nurses for their patients. In 1860, Nightingale laid the foundation of professional nursing with the establishment of her nursing school at St Thomas Hospital in London, the first secular nursing school in the world, now part of King's College London.

Her social reforms include improving healthcare for all sections of British society, improving healthcare, advocating for better hunger relief in India, helping to abolish laws regulating prostitution that were overly harsh to women, and expanding the acceptable forms of female participation in the workforce. In addition, Nightingale contributed to the development of order and method within the hospital's statistical records. She developed applied statistical methods to display data that provided an organized and improved way of learning medical and surgical procedures. In 1858, she became a Fellow of the Royal Statistical Society, and in 1874 she became an honorary member of the American Statistical Association.

Working on Workers' Diseases — Bernardino Ramazzini

Bernardino Ramazzini (1633–1714), an Italian physician, became interested in practical problems in medicine and in public health. Ramazzini investigated complaints of blindness of cesspool workers and found that continuous work in the poor environment caused their blindness. The event with the cesspool workers turned his interest to other workers' health.

In his book *The Diseases of Workers*, he explained that disease among workers arose from two common causes:

>> The inhalation of noxious vapors and very fine particles

>> Violent and irregular motions and unnatural body posture

Ramazzini described diseases associated with occupation, such as lead poisoning among pottery glazers and mercury poisoning among mirror makers, goldsmiths, and others. He documented lung disease due to inhaling fine dust particles among mill workers, bakers, starch makers, tobacco workers, and those who processed wool, flax, hemp, cotton, and silk. He also described diseases as a result of physical and mechanical strain on the body that cause varicose veins, nerve pain, hernia, and other health problems. His major achievement in occupational health is that he recommended safety measures and the use of protective clothing to prevent workplace injuries.

The Birth of Vital Statistics: No Labor Pains Involved

As you know from your studies in epidemiology, statistics is a very important discipline in public health. Here, I give you an idea how the concept of statistics was first developed in England.

John Graunt

John Graunt (1620–1674), an English statistician, is generally considered to be the founder of *demography,* the study of human populations. Graunt developed a systematic recording of deaths, called the *Bill of Mortality* that commenced in London in 1603; he summarized mortality data and developed a better understanding of disease and their causes of death. He classified deaths into acute (sudden onset) and chronic (long lasting). He identified variations in death according to age, sex, residence, and season.

Based on his works, he wrote the book *Natural and Political Observations Made Upon the Bills of Mortality* in 1662. Perhaps his most important innovation was the life table, which presented mortality in terms of survivorship. Using only two rates of survivorship (to ages 6 and to 76), he predicted the percentage of people that would live to each successive age and their life expectancy year by year.

William Farr

Willian Farr (1807–1883) made many important advances in epidemiology during the mid-1800s. Upon being appointed registrar general in England, Farr further advanced the ideas of Graunt and developed a modern vital statistics system. He replaced the concept of political arithmetic with a new term, *statistics*. Farr emphasized the importance of accuracy and completeness of data. He sought to establish the determinants of public health and used data to form hypotheses about the cause of a disease. He applied this knowledge to the prevention and control of disease.

REMEMBER

Another important contribution of Farr in epidemiology was the concept of *multifactorial causal theory* of chronic diseases, which states that multiple risk factors contribute to chronic diseases (refer to Chapter 16 for more information). He devised a classification system for the cause of death, which provided the foundation for the modern *International Classification of Diseases*. He also invented the method of *standardized mortality rate*, an important analysis technique used in statistics to standardize the observed death rate of a population (find more information in Chapter 10).

Examining the Start of Epidemiology and Public Health in the United States

The *American Journal of Public Health* and the *Nation's Health* attempted to compile a list of the great pioneers of public health in America. The report, published in 1953, included 11 major categories and 30 separate divisions of public health and listed men and women who had been active in each of these fields. This section details some of the contributions of selected public health specialists and epidemiologists in the United States, including Wade Frost, Alice Hamilton, William Sedgwick, Lemuel Shattuck, Stephen Smith, Lillian Wald, and Benjamin Waterhouse. Table 3-1 identifies some others who made significant contributions.

TABLE 3-1 Pioneers of Public Health in America, 1610–1925

Name	Specific Areas of Contributions
Josephine Baker, 1874–1945	Child health protection as a function of municipal government
Hermann M. Biggs, 1859–1923	State and municipal health administration, tuberculosis control, health education
John S. Billings, 1839–1913	Epidemiologist, vital statistician, cofounder, National Board of Health, librarian, hospital administration
Charles V. Chapin, 1856–1941	Communicable disease control, municipal health administration
Daniel Drake, 1785–1852	Epidemiology of malaria in the United States
Dorothea Dix, 1802–1887	State and national responsibility for care of persons with mental illness
Oliver Wendell Holmes Sr. 1809–1894	Author of the essay "Contagiousness of Puerperal Fever"
George M. Kober, 1850–1931	Industrial medicine, exponent of housing, a teacher of public health in medical colleges
William H. Park, 1863–1939	Communicable disease control, diphtheria immunization, diagnostic laboratories
Walter Reed, 1851–1902	Discoverer of transmission of yellow fever by mosquito
Howard T. Ricketts, 1871–1910	Pioneer work in virus disease, etiology, epidemiology, and control of Rocky Mountain spotted fever
Milton J. Rosenau, 1869–1946	Teacher of preventive medicine and public health, epidemiologist, milk sanitation
Theobold Smith, 1859–1934	Immunologist, bacteriologist, tuberculosis control, founded state biological products laboratory
George M. Sternberg, 1838–1915	Diagnostic laboratories, bacteriology, malaria, yellow fever, national health administration
Charles W. Stiles, 1867–1941	Discovered hookworm disease in the South and lead development of rural sanitation in America
Victor C. Vaughan, 1851–1929	Pioneer in immunology, epidemiology, and sanitation, public health teacher
William H. Welch, 1850–1934	Public health statesman, bacteriologist, public health teacher
John M. Woodworth, 1837–1879	Organized Marine Hospital Service in 1872, which became U.S. Public Health Service

Wade Hampton Frost

Wade H. Frost (1880–1938) was the first resident lecturer at the Johns Hopkins School of Hygiene and Public Health and later a professor of epidemiology, establishing epidemiology as a science in the United States. He understood the importance of transmission in poliomyelitis — knowledge that prepared the ground for the worldwide campaign against that disease; the first to understand the cyclical nature of influenza and the epidemiology of diphtheria and tuberculosis; the first to develop the historical cohort approach and undertake longitudinal cohort analyses; and the first to design life tables for expressing data in person-years.

In 1933, he came up with the concept of the *index case* (also known as the *primary case*), which refers to the first case identified in an epidemic. Chapter 14 discusses primary and secondary cases in more detail. For his contribution in epidemiology, Frost is often considered to be the Father of Modern Epidemiology.

Alice Hamilton

Alice Hamilton (1869–1970) was a physician, scientist, humanitarian, and undisputed leader in the social reform movement of the 20th century. She is known in the history of public health as a pioneer of occupational medicine and industrial hygiene in the United States. She is best recognized for her scientific investigations of carbon monoxide poisoning in steelworkers, mercury poisoning in hatters, and dead fingers syndrome among laborers using jackhammers. In 1919, Dr. Hamilton was appointed assistant professor of industrial medicine at Harvard Medical School, the first woman to be on the faculty of Harvard University.

In 1908, she published an article on industrial diseases in relation to women's employment. In 1943, she published an autobiography, *Exploring the Dangerous Trades*, in which she described vividly "the unprotected, helpless state of workingmen."

William Sedgwick

William Thompson Sedgwick (1855–1921) was a teacher, epidemiologist, sanitarian, and a key figure in shaping public health in the United States. He is considered the Father of the Modern Public Health Movement in the United States. In 1883, Sedgwick was appointed to the faculty at the Massachusetts Institute of Technology (MIT). In 1902, he published the groundbreaking book, *Principles of Sanitary Science and the Public Health*, which was a compilation of his lectures at MIT. He was one of three founders of the joint MIT-Harvard School of Public Health in 1913, which was the first formal academic program designed to train public health professionals.

Lemuel Shattuck

Lemuel Shattuck (1793–1859), a teacher, sociologist, and statistician, was the chair of a legislative committee to study sanitation and public health in Massachusetts. In 1850, he published the first report on sanitation and public health, in which he suggested several reforms and needs for the public health program for the next century. One of his suggestions was to ensure that epidemiologic investigations and preventive and control measures for diseases be established in an organized and structured manner.

His report emphasized the need for establishing the following:

>> State and local boards of health

>> School health programs

>> Organized efforts to collect and analyze vital statistics

>> Sanitary inspections

>> Medical education on sanitation and disease prevention

Based on his report, boards of health were established, with state departments of health and local public health departments soon to follow. In 1902, the United States Public Health Service was founded. In 1906, the Pure Food and Drug Act was passed, and standards for water analysis were adopted. In 1913, the method of pasteurization of milk was established.

Stephen Smith

Stephen Smith (1823–1922) was an American surgeon, attorney, and a pioneer in public health. He was also a pioneer of sanitary reforms in New York City. In 1866, Smith led the establishment of the Metropolitan Board of Health in New York City, the first such public health agency in the United States. He founded the American Public Health Association (APHA) in 1872. APHA is now the oldest and most diverse organization of public health professionals in the world and continues to protect the nation through preventive health services and activities.

Lillian Wald

Lillian D. Wald (1867–1940) was an American nurse, humanitarian, and author. She was known for her contributions to human rights and was the founder of American community nursing. She graduated from the New York Hospital Training School for Nurses in 1891 and then took courses at the Woman's Medical College. By 1893, she started to teach a home class on nursing for poor immigrant families on New York City's Lower East Side.

Shortly thereafter, she began to care for sick Lower East Side residents as a visiting nurse. Around that time she coined the term *public health nurse* to describe nurses whose work is integrated into the public community. Wald founded the Henry Street Settlement, which eventually expanded into the Visiting Nurse Service of New York. She advocated for nursing in public schools, and her ideas led the New York Board of Health to organize the first public nursing system in the world. She was the first president of the National Organization for Public Health Nursing.

Benjamin Waterhouse

Benjamin Waterhouse (1753–1846) was a physician and co-founder and professor at the Harvard Medical School. He's most well known for being the first doctor to test the smallpox vaccine in the United States. On July 4, 1800, Waterhouse obtained a sample of cowpox matter — a thread soaked with cowpox lymph and placed in a sealed glass vial. Four days later, Waterhouse vaccinated his children and his servants. Subsequently, the children were experimentally inoculated with smallpox and found to be immune.

Developing public health institutes

A $25,000 donation from businessman Samuel Zemurray instituted the first School of Public Health and Tropical Medicine at Tulane University in 1912. The Welch–Rose Report of 1915 (that outlined plans for an "Institute of Hygiene") has been viewed as the basis for the critical movement in the history of the institutional schism between public health and medicine because it led to the establishment of schools of public health supported by the Rockefeller Foundation. The Johns Hopkins School of Hygiene and Public Health founded in 1916 became the first degree-granting institution for research and training for public health in the United States. By 1922, schools of public health were established at Columbia, Harvard, and Yale.

TYPHOID MARY — THE REVITALIZATION OF PUBLIC HEALTH IN THE UNITED STATES

In the 19th century when public health was in its rudimentary stage in the United States, people didn't know much about spreading an infection from one person to another as a result of a lack of cleanliness and hygienic practice. Mary Mallon was presumed to have infected about 51 persons with typhoid fever during the course of her career as a cook, simply because she probably didn't know the importance of hand

(continued)

(continued)

washing and didn't practice it. Scientists now know that the germ of typhoid fever, *Salmonella typhi*, can stay in the gall bladder for a long time, and humans can serve as chronic carriers and spread the disease to others.

After immigrating to the United States from Ireland, Mallon started a job as a cook in Mamaroneck, New York in 1900. Within two weeks of her employment, residents started coming down with typhoid fever. In 1901 she moved to Manhattan where she infected members of the family she served and one died. She then moved to an employment with a lawyer where seven out of eight family members developed typhoid fever. She moved to Long Island, where within two weeks ten out of eleven family members were hospitalized with typhoid fever. She changed her employment again, and three more households she served got the disease. In 1906, Mallon worked for a banker, and six of eleven members of his family came down with typhoid fever.

One of the victims of typhoid fever hired a researcher George Soper to investigate the case. Soper found that all cases were related to the description of a cook, about 40 years old, unmarried, and Irish. After each case, the woman left the area leaving no forwarding address. Soper traced her to a household in a Park Avenue penthouse, where two people had an active disease due to typhoid fever and one had died. Soper asked Mallon to submit urine and stool samples for examination, but she refused. Eventually, the New York City Health Department forced her to quarantine. Mallon got much media attention, and the famous *Journal of American Medical Association* published an article in 1908 calling her *Typhoid Mary*. Cultures of her urine and stools, taken forcibly with the help of prison matrons, revealed that her gallbladder was swarming with typhoid bacteria *Salmonella typhi*. Upon a signed agreement that she would change her job and take adequate hygienic precautions, she was released.

After being released, Mallon worked as a laundress for a short time. Soon she went back to her profession as a cook after changing her name to Mary Brown. For the next five years, she was employed in a number of kitchens with outbreaks of typhoid following her. Public health authorities again traced her and quarantined her on March 27, 1915. Mallon remained confined for the rest of her life. Her story helped public health authorities investigate and learn how typhoid fever can be spread by a chronic carrier who remained symptomless throughout her life. It also helped revitalize the importance of public health practices in the United States.

Reforming Public Health in England

Here I describe how the health conditions of Europeans deteriorated rapidly with the rapid growth of population after the Industrial Revolution. I discuss the foundation of sanitary reforms in England and the development of public health programs in England.

Deteriorating health after the Industrial Revolution

As the Industrial Revolution developed in England, the health and welfare of workers deteriorated. From about 1750 the population of England increased rapidly, and with this increase came a heightened awareness of the large numbers of infant deaths and of the unhealthy conditions in prisons and in mental institutions. Between 1801 and 1841 the population of London doubled; that of Leeds nearly tripled. With such growth there also came rising death rates. Between 1831 and 1844, the death rate increased in Birmingham from 14.6 to 27.2 per thousand; in Bristol, from 16.9 to 31.0 per thousand; and in Liverpool, from 21.0 to 34.8 per thousand. These figures were the result of an increase in the urban population that far exceeded available housing and of the subsequent development of conditions that led to widespread disease and poor health.

Moving toward sanitary reforms

England first experienced the negative health effects of the Industrial Revolution. As a result, in the 19th century a movement started toward sanitary reform that finally led to the establishment of public health institutions. Movements to improve sanitation occurred simultaneously in several European countries.

The Poor Law Commission, created in 1834, explored the problems of community health and suggested means for solving them. Its report, in 1838, argued that "the expenditures necessary to the adoption and maintenance of measures of prevention would ultimately amount to less than the cost of the disease now constantly engendered." Sanitary surveys proved that a relationship existed between communicable disease and the filth in the environment, and the report said that safeguarding public health is the province of the engineer rather than of the physician.

The Public Health Act of 1848 established a General Board of Health to furnish guidance and aid in sanitary matters to local authorities, whose earlier efforts had been impeded by lack of a central authority. The board had authority to establish local boards of health and to investigate sanitary conditions in particular districts. Since this time several public health acts have been passed to regulate sewage and refuse disposal, the housing of animals, the water supply, the prevention and control of disease, the registration and inspection of private nursing homes and hospitals, the notification of births, and the provision of maternity and child welfare services.

SIR EDWIN CHADWICK'S WORK WITH THE POOR

Sir Edwin Chadwick (1800–1890) is recognized as the Father of Public Health Reform in England for his work to reform the Poor Laws and improve sanitary conditions and public health during the era of Queen Victoria. Chadwick began to make improvements with sanitary and health conditions of England in 1832. Chadwick and Nassau William Senior drafted the famous report of 1834 recommending the reform of the old Poor Law. The new Poor Law ensured that the poor were housed in workhouses, clothed, and fed. Children who entered the workhouse would receive some schooling. In return for this care, all workhouse people would have to work for several hours each day. However, some people, such as Richard Oastler, spoke out against the new Poor Law, calling the workhouses "Prisons for the Poor."

Chadwick's second biggest achievement in public health was the improvement of water and sanitation systems in England. In 1837 and 1838 the cities had typhoid epidemics, and the government appointed him to start an enquiry into the sanitation of the major cities. In 1842 Chadwick, assisted by Dr. Thomas Southwood Smith, published his landmark report, "The Sanitary Conditions of the Labouring Population." The report stated that there was an urgent need to improve their living conditions and that the lack of public health directly related to their lifestyle.

Looking At Modern Epidemiology

Modern epidemiology encompasses the range of acute and infectious causes of disease to multifactorial causes of chronic and noninfectious diseases. Epidemiology has expanded its scope in other branches of medicine, such as occupational medicine, nutrition, and environmental health. Some newer branches of epidemiology include field epidemiology; injury epidemiology; and molecular and genetic epidemiology (the following sections focus on two of these areas). Another new direction of epidemiologic research involves the study of determinants at the biological and societal level.

John Snow (1813–1858) is recognized as the Father of Modern and Field Epidemiology and was one of the advocates of the germ theory. His legendary research on the 1854 cholera epidemic in London's Golden Square along with several other milestone findings in epidemiology are described in Chapter 4.

Global warming in the 21st century poses more challenges for epidemiologists because of the increase of vector-borne diseases, some other infectious diseases, chronic diseases including cancers, and natural calamities such as cyclone and tsunami. The recent pandemics of HIV/AIDS and Covid-19 also have posed an enormous burden to global health. Now, global health is an important field of public health in many institutions.

Field epidemiology

Training programs in field epidemiology prepare epidemiologists for detecting and responding to health threats and disease outbreaks at a local level thus preventing them from spreading.

Field epidemiologists must be specially trained to deal with unexpected, sometimes urgent problems that demand immediate solutions. For example, Disease Control in Humanitarian Emergencies (DCE) provides technical and operational field epidemiological support in outbreak investigation and response; surveillance of early warning alert and response in acute emergencies; and surveillance of reviews, surveys, program monitoring, and evaluation.

For example, field epidemiologists helped in the polio eradication activities in India in 2007–2010 and guinea worm eradication in Northern Uganda in 2009.

Molecular and genetic epidemiology

The mapping of the human genome and the tremendous advances in molecular biology will make advances in the epidemiological research of disease identification. Modern epidemiologists find themselves equipped with several new techniques to identify biological markers of exposure and search for the biologic basis for responses.

Molecular epidemiology refers to techniques of molecular biology applied in epidemiologic studies. One use of molecular epidemiology is the study of tumor markers to identify potentially heterogeneous subsets of breast cancer.

Meanwhile, genetic epidemiology studies the hereditary bases for disease. For example, genetic epidemiology investigates the genomic link of breast cancer and ovarian cancer, sickle cell disease, cystic fibrosis, thalassemia, and many more.

Chapter **4**

Eyeing the Milestones in Public Health

The achievements in public health are a long history. Humans have observed several diseases over thousands of years, but epidemiologists have only discovered the real causes of those diseases in the recent past.

This chapter describes the discovery of some of those diseases. I examine how scientists debunked many misbeliefs about how diseases — like scurvy, pellagra, cholera, and others — were transmitted. Furthermore, I present some real-life data from the 1918 influenza pandemic that took several million lives in the world. I also discuss how a large pandemic of smallpox was eradicated and how smoking cigarettes was found to be a cause of lung cancer and many other cancers.

Finding the Treatment of Scurvy — James Lind

Scurvy is an age-old disease. Hippocrates (460 B.C.–370 B.C.) and the Egyptians identified scurvy as early as 1550 B.C. The disease killed more than two million sailors between the time of Christopher Columbus's transatlantic voyage and the rise of steam engines in the mid-19th century. The disease was so common that governments and shipowners anticipated about 50 percent of the people would die in a long-term voyage.

James Lind (1716–1794), a British physician and surgeon, is recognized as the founder of naval hygiene in England. As surgeon of the *HMS Salisbury*, he observed in March 1747 thousands of cases of scurvy, typhus, and dysentery that caused the death of soldiers on board during long voyages. In the history of modern medicine, Lind usually receives credit for being the investigator of the first controlled clinical trial, conducted 275 years ago while working as the ship surgeon. In fact, Clinical Trials Day is held on May 20 every year to commemorate the day he began the trial.

As a result of Lind's early studies, scientists now know that scurvy is a severe form of vitamin C deficiency. A person's body needs vitamin C to produce *collagen* (the tissue that connects muscles and bones and forms skin), to heal wounds, to support the immune system, and to help in many other internal systems. The tissue loses collagen due to vitamin C deficiency, which causes body tissue to become spongy and having bleeding.

Enquiring into the diet

People observed that sailors in long voyages were dying from a deadly but yet an unknown disease. The earliest symptoms of scurvy included lethargy and body weakness, which can be so debilitating that the person is unable to get out of bed. That symptom made people once believe that laziness was a cause of the disease. The patient also suffers aching joints, swelling of the arms and legs, and skin bruising at the slightest touch. As the disease progresses, the patient's gums become spongy and bleed easily and teeth fall out. Old wounds open and bleed, and mucus membranes bleed. Internal organ bleedings cause death.

At that time, the prevailing assumptions surrounded around several unhealthy living conditions, such as cold and moist weather, dirty water, and poor diet in association with the disease. Through Lind's observation of the living conditions, the weather, and the food that sailors consumed during the voyage, he was convinced that "the calamity (of the disease) can be removed only by change of diet."

Examining Lind's experiment

After eight weeks at sea, scurvy began to take toll on the crew, so Lind decided to conduct his dietary experiment. In addition to the regular daily diet common to all the people on board, he prescribed six dietary regimens given to 12 people in his study, having two in each group:

>> Two people each received a quart of cider a day.

>> Two people received 25 drops of elixir of vitriol (a mixture of diluted sulfuric acid and alcohol) three times a day on an empty stomach.

>> Two people were given two spoonful of vinegar three times a day upon an empty stomach.

>> Two people were given a half pint of seawater daily.

>> Two people had a nutmeg-sized paste of garlic, mustard seed, horse-radish, balsam of Peru, and gum myrrh three times a day.

>> Two people daily consumed two oranges and one lemon each.

As a result of the treatments, he wrote in his 1753 historical work *A Treatise of the Scurvy* that the two people who received oranges and lemon had marked recovery from scurvy symptoms, even though the oranges and lemons ran out after six days. One of them "was fit for duty on the sixth day." The two people who took oranges and lemon "best recovered of any of his symptoms and was appointed nurse to the rest of the sick."

Although Lind's experiment suggested that oranges and lemons were a cure for scurvy, he conceived that scurvy wasn't a disease of dietary deficiency. After this historical discovery, it took 42 years before the admiralty issued seamen with regular doses of lemon juice. Vitamin C wasn't discovered for more than 130 years after Lind's death.

Discovering Sources of Cholera in London's Golden Square — John Snow

Hippocrates and Galen described an illness that may well have been cholera. Since antiquity numerous cholera-like maladies have affected populations in the Delta plains of the River Ganges. Gaspar Correa (also known as Gaspar India), a Portuguese historian and the author of *Legendary India*, gave one of the first detailed descriptions of an epidemic of "*moryxy*" in 1543, which is supposed to be an epidemic of cholera.

Cholera became a disease of global importance because of a deadly outbreak that occurred in Jessore (then India, now a district in Bangladesh) in 1817. The outbreak spread in the form of an epidemic throughout most parts of India and affected Burma (now Myanmar) and Ceylon (now Sri Lanka). It eventually turned into a pandemic, devastating 100,000 people in Java and Indonesia and causing 18,000 deaths in a three-week period in the Philippines.

A second pandemic of cholera reached Europe and the Americas in 1829. The third pandemic of cholera erupted in India in 1852 and traversed through Persia (Iran) to Europe, the United States, and the rest of world. This pandemic of cholera is considered the most deadly, causing 23,000 deaths in Great Britain alone in 1854.

Cholera broke out in the Golden Square near Broad Street (now Broadwick Street) in London's Soho District in 1854 and is considered the third pandemic. This epidemic took 616 lives in a ten-day period. John Snow (1813–1858), an English physician who is widely viewed as the Father of Contemporary Epidemiology, compared the cholera outbreak in two regions of the city:

>> One receiving sewage-contaminated water

>> The other receiving relatively clean water

Here I discuss how John Snow ruled out a prevailing *miasma* (or bad air) theory as a cause of cholera and showed that contaminated water is the real source of the disease.

Questioning the miasma theory

Most scientists including physicians at that time believed in Galen's miasma theory of disease transmission, which referred to the belief that a disease like cholera was transmitted by a noxious form of bad air (refer to Chapter 3 for more specifics about this theory).

Snow was skeptical of the then-dominant miasma theory. Through his research he showed that environmental factors such as contaminated water could transmit an infectious disease like cholera. He first published his theory in an essay — *On the Mode of Communication of Cholera* — in which he correctly suggested that cholera is transmitted by the fecal-oral route. In 1855, he further proposed that the structure of the cholera-causing agent was that of a cell.

Suspecting a hand pump

Snow believed that sewage dumped into rivers and cesspools near town wells could contaminate water supplies and cause cholera outbreaks in London's Golden Square. As a doctor working in Soho, he immediately started to investigate the

1854 outbreak, and in an attempt to prove his theory, he began by talking to local residents and started to suspect that the source of the outbreak was the public water pump on Broad Street. He used information from the local hospital and public records and asked residents if they had consumed water from the pump.

Mapping cases and deaths

Snow made the determination by creating a data set correlating mortality (death) rates with street addresses. Using this information he was able to create a dot map to illustrate the cluster of cases around a single water pump. A *dot map* is a geographic distribution of cases/deaths of a disease. A dot map is also useful for tracing causes of infection and exposure — refer to Chapters 7 and 20 for more information about geographic information system (GIS) where scientists use a dot map.

Within 250 yards of the spot where Cambridge Street joins Broad Street, Snow identified approximately 500 cholera deaths in ten days. The investigation pinpointed the source of the cholera epidemic as the Broad Street water pump, which drew water from underground sources of heavily contaminated areas. Researchers later discovered that the public well from which the pump drew water was dug only a few feet from a cesspit. A cloth diaper of a baby, who had contracted cholera from another source, had been washed in this cesspit and was the point source of the outbreak.

Snow's investigation also identified cholera death cases by residence and by the two water companies that supplied the homes: the Southwark and Vauxhall Company and the Lambeth Company. The Southwark and Vauxhall Company relied on its water intakes from a part of the Thames River that was relatively heavily populated with sewage compared to the Lambeth Company that drew its water from a less populated upstream part of the Thames.

By using a *2x2 contingency table* (a table showing the distribution of one variable in a row and another variable in a column), epidemiologists can easily analyze the association between variables — refer to Chapters 14, 15, and 17 for more information about mathematical calculations using a contingency table. Snow showed the differences in cholera deaths for a seven-week period in homes supplied by each of the two water supply companies. Table 4-1 is possibly the most famous presentation of an epidemic investigation data using a 2x2 contingency table in epidemiology.

TABLE 4-1 **Cholera Deaths from Two Water Supplies in Soho, London over Seven Weeks, 1854**

Water Supply Company	No. of Houses	No. of Deaths	Deaths per 10,000 Houses
Southwark and Vauxhall	40,046	1,263	315
Lambeth	26,107	98	37
Rest of London	256,423	1,422	59

Snow showed that the number of cholera deaths were about 13 times higher for the Southwark and Vauxhall Company (1,263) compared to the Lambeth Company (98), and the corresponding death rates from cholera were 8.5 times higher — 315 for the Southwark and Vauxhall Company versus 37 for the Lambeth Company per 10,000 households.

Removing the handle

On September 7, 1854, Snow took his findings to local officials and convinced them to take the handle off the pump, making it impossible to draw water from it. Today this action would be considered an *intervention* in an experimental study. Shortly after the handle was removed, the outbreak ended with no additional deaths from the epidemic. Snow's experiment on disease transmission helped determine that the cholera epidemic in London's Golden Square wasn't related to the miasma theory, but rather contaminated water transmitted the disease.

Some critiques, however, pointed out that the cases of cholera in Golden Square were already decreasing as a result of the natural course of the epidemic. In an analysis of the available data, one author showed that one to two people died from August 1 to 30 and four died on August 31. The death toll suddenly reached 72 on September 1, and the peak of deaths (127) and the number of fatal attacks (128) were on September 2, 1854. The pump handle was removed and the pump closed on September 8, which is about eight to nine days after the suspected start of the epidemic (or at least from the point of increase in the number of deaths). Henry Whitehead, in the article entitled, "Remarks on the Outbreak of Cholera in Broad Street, Golden Square, London," published in 2014, suspected that the decline of the epidemic probably wasn't a result of the removal of the pump handle itself but rather a natural course of the disease.

MORE BREAKTHROUGHS ABOUT CHOLERA

Scientists continued making more advancements in understanding the cause of cholera. As I describe in Chapter 3, the discovery and advancement of the microscope helped scientists identify cells, which led to Louis Pasteur revolutionizing medical knowledge with the introduction of the germ theory of disease transmission.

During an 1854 outbreak of cholera in Florence, Italy, an Italian physician Filippo Pacini, performed autopsies of patients who died of cholera and conducted histological examinations of the intestinal mucosa. He discovered a typical comma-shaped bacillus that he described as a *Vibrio*. He published his report "Microscopical Observations and Pathological Deductions on Cholera" in which he described the organism and its relation to the cholera disease. After his discovery, Robert Koch in India identified the bacteria independently in 1883. A German physician Richard Friedrich Johannes Pfeiffer renamed it as *Vibrio cholerae* in 1896.

Uncovering Causes of Pellagra — Joseph Goldberger

Pellagra is a systemic disease caused by a severe deficiency of niacin (vitamin B-3) or tryptophan or by a defect in the metabolic conversion of tryptophan to niacin. The disease is manifested by the three Ds:

>> Dementia (or loss of memory or mental disorders)

>> Diarrhea (gastrointestinal disorder)

>> Dermatitis (erythema of skin)

Starting with sore tongue and gastrointestinal disturbances, the disease progresses until patients display severe skin lesions and neurological symptoms with many patients eventually dying. Scientists now know that the most typical cause of primary pellagra is the inadequate dietary intake of the specific vitamin B (niacin or tryptophan). However, Joseph Goldberger was the first to disprove some of the misconceptions about the cause of the disease through experimental studies, which the following sections discuss.

LOOKING AT THE HISTORY OF PELLAGRA

Don Gaspar Casal first identified pellagra among Spanish peasants in 1735. At that time, the disease was known as *mal de rosa*. Casal claimed that *mal de rosa* was caused by food. However, for nearly two centuries a group of people believed that the disease was due to poisons in Indian corn. In 1905, another scientist known as Louis Sambon introduced a new theory that pellagra is an insect-bite disease, similar to malaria, yellow fever, and sleeping sickness.

Pellagra reached epidemic proportion in the United States in the early 20th century. In 1912, approximately 12,000 South Carolina pellagra patients died out of the 30,000 total cases reported. In 1914, a commission, called the Thompson-McFadden Commission, sought to find the cause of the pellagra epidemic. The Commission Report concluded that pellagra is an infectious disease, which is communicable from person to person, but the cause of the transmission is unknown. Although there were incidences throughout the country, pellagra was particularly rampant among impoverished Southern sharecroppers and textile mill workers, leading many medical experts to conclude that it was an infectious disease caused by poor hygiene. Others believed it was hereditary.

Evidence for the cause of the disease was inconclusive. Between 1907 and 1940, approximately three million Americans contracted pellagra and 100,000 of them died. The cases and deaths were escalating in the South.

Doctors in Spartanburg, South Carolina, were deeply concerned about pellagra. In the early 1910s, Spartanburg County physicians Dr. H. R. Black, Dr. James L. Jefferies, and Dr. William Smith urged the Thompson-McFadden Pellagra Commission, a private effort funded by two Pennsylvania philanthropists, to visit Spartanburg to study the problem. By 1914, alarmed by the rising rates of pellagra, the U.S. Public Health Service created the Spartanburg General Hospital to research causes and treatments for pellagra.

Suggesting pellagra not communicable

As pellagra became alarmingly prevalent in southern parts of the United States, particularly in prisoners and orphanages, a worried Congress asked the Surgeon General to investigate the disease, and the U.S. Public Health Service appointed one of its eminent epidemiologists, Joseph Goldberger, in 1914 to lead the investigation. Goldberger was highly regarded as an infectious disease specialist and a top epidemiologist for his earlier work on yellow fever, typhus, and diphtheria, but he lacked much experience in dealing with cases of pellagra. He started visiting orphanages, mental hospitals, prisons, and hospitals throughout the South for cases with pellagra.

Goldberger's theory on pellagra contradicted common-held medical opinions. His own observations of patients convinced him that germs don't cause pellagra, and the disease isn't communicable. After thorough investigations, Goldberger made two important observations:

>> The caregivers of pellagra patients never contracted pellagra. As a result, he was almost certain that pellagra isn't contagious.

>> Orphans 6 to 12 years old overwhelmingly suffered from pellagra. This observation led him to believe that pellagra was probably of dietary origin because orphans under age 6 received a large quantity of milk and orphans over age 12 obtained a better supply of meat.

Connecting pellagra with poverty and helping with diet

Goldberger connected the dots between the disease and the dietary deficiency with poverty. People in the South were historically poor, and the economy was dependent on the labor-intensive production of cotton. He observed the food habits of the poverty-driven areas — most people likely to get pellagra had a corn-based diet with a lack of fresh vegetables, meat, or milk — but he couldn't isolate anything in the food that caused pellagra.

His next move: a food intervention study. He requested food shipments from D.C. be sent and fed to children in two Mississippi orphanages and to inmates at the Georgia State Asylum. The pellagra patients were fed a diet of fresh meat, milk, and vegetables instead of a corn-based diet. The results were dramatic:

>> All the patients recovered and didn't have any recurrences.

>> Those who didn't have pellagra but ate the new diet didn't contract the disease.

Those findings convinced him the importance of this healthy diet in not only curing pellagra but also preventing it. Goldberger made an immediate conclusion that "pellagra may be prevented by appropriate diet without alteration in the environment, hygienic or sanitary."

He then developed an experimental study among Mississippi prisoners. With the cooperation of Mississippi's progressive governor, Earl Brewer, Goldberger experimented on 11 healthy volunteer prisoners at the Rankin State Prison Farm in 1915. Offered pardons in return for their participation, the volunteers ate a corn-based diet. Six of the 11 showed pellagra rashes after five months. Expert dermatologists made the actual diagnoses of pellagra to avoid the appearance of a conflict of interest on Goldberger's part.

To persuade his critics that pellagra was dietary and not communicable, in April 1916 he injected five cubic centimeters of a pellagra-infected person's blood into the arm of his assistant, Dr. George Wheeler. Wheeler then shot six centimeters of such blood into Goldberger. They then swabbed out the secretions of a pellagra patient's nose and throat and rubbed them into their own noses and throats. They swallowed capsules containing scabs of a pellagra patient's rashes. Neither Goldberger nor Wheeler got pellagra. This experiment definitely proves that pellagra isn't contagious.

Describing the 1918 Influenza Pandemic

This influenza pandemic of 1918–19, also called the Spanish influenza pandemic or Spanish flu, is the most severe influenza outbreak of the 20th century in terms of the total numbers of deaths. It started in 1918, and people in the military were the first affected by it during the spring of 1918 with epidemiologic studies and lay reports identifying the first outbreak at Camp Funston (now Fort Riley) in Kansas. Caused by an H1N1 virus with genes of avian origin, the pandemic was the most devastating pandemic other than the more recent Covid-19 pandemic.

These sections analyze the archived data obtained from the 1918–1919 influenza pandemic and discuss how the pandemic was controlled.

Gathering mortality data of the pandemic

The pandemic resulted in an estimated 25 million deaths, and according to some researchers, it caused as many as 40 to 50 million deaths worldwide. The number of deaths due to the pandemic in the United States alone was approximately 675,000. The highest death toll of the influenza pandemic occurred in October 1918 (see Figure 4-1).

Just in October 1918, a total of 289,399 people died: of them, 117,255 deaths from influenza, 63,532 deaths from pneumonia, and 198,612 deaths from other causes, resulting in an average 9,335 deaths per day in this month. The peak of the epidemic lasted from October 2018 to March 2019, which caused 291,811 deaths out of the total of 318,403 deaths (92 percent).

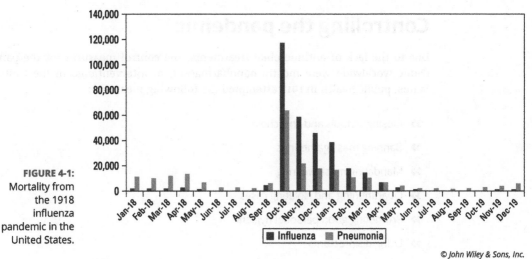

© John Wiley & Sons, Inc.

FIGURE 4-1:
Mortality from the 1918 influenza pandemic in the United States.

The death rates were highest among:

» Children younger than 5

» Adults 20 to 40 years of age

» Senior citizens 65 years and older

Here are the main reasons for the high mortality:

» **Lack of immunity:** The people didn't have any immunity from the disease. Now people have developed immunity over time from getting infections and through vaccines.

» **No vaccine:** There wasn't a flu vaccine. Now a flu vaccine is available and is given every year.

» **No available treatments:** There were no treatments available for the disease. Now there are a few FDA-approved anti-viral medicines available to treat severe flu cases, including

  • *oseltamivir* (trade name Tamiflu)

  • *zanamivir* (trade name Relenza)

  • *peramivir* (trade name Rapivab)

  • *baloxavir* (trade name Xofluza)

» **Cause of death:** Victims of the 1918 influenza pandemic mostly died from secondary bacterial pneumonia.

Controlling the pandemic

Due to the lack of antimicrobial treatments, the control measures for the pandemic worldwide were mostly nonpharmaceutical interventions. In the United States, public health in 1918 attempted the following measures:

>> Closing schools and churches

>> Banning mass gatherings

>> Mandating mask wearing

>> Quarantining and isolating cases

>> Promoting good personal hygiene

>> Using disinfectants

A research article published in 2007 by Martin Bootsma and Neil Ferguson showed that early and effective interventions had the most effective impact in reducing the transmission rates of the 1918 influenza pandemic by up to 30 to 50 percent in certain U.S. cities, such as San Francisco, St. Louis, Milwaukee, and Kansas City.

Eradicating Smallpox

Wiping out smallpox has been one of the major achievements of public health — thanks to the success of the worldwide vaccination programs! Edward Jenner, considered the founder of vaccinology in the world, helped create the first smallpox vaccine in 1798 (refer to Chapter 3 for more about Jenner and his work).

TECHNICAL STUFF

The most vivid description of the disease from pre-modern times is in the ninth century book written by a Persian physician, Muhammad Ibn Zakariya ar-Razi, also known as Rhazes. He differentiated smallpox symptoms from measles and chickenpox.

Smallpox has appeared in many pandemics, including some of the deadliest:

>> **Japan:** The Japanese smallpox epidemic killed as many as one-third of Japanese population in 735–737.

>> **Russia:** Smallpox appeared as a major killer disease in the 18th century, when every seventh child born in Russia died of smallpox.

>> **Europe:** It killed an estimated 400,000 people each year in Europe in the late 18th century.

>> **India:** In 1849, 13 percent of the people in Calcutta (now Kolkata) died of smallpox.

>> **During the Franco-Prussian War:** The biggest pandemic of smallpox was from 1870–1874 where the war triggered the pandemic that claimed 500,000 lives.

The last natural outbreak of smallpox occurred in the United States in 1949, and the last known natural case of smallpox was in Somalia in 1977. The World Health Assembly declared smallpox eradicated in 1980, which was almost two centuries after Jenner suggested that vaccination could eliminate smallpox.

Finding Smoking as a Cause of Lung Cancer

Cigarettes cause about 1.5 million deaths from lung cancer per year, a number that will rise to nearly 2 million per year by the 2030s. According to the 2004 U.S. Surgeon General report, "The Health Consequences of Smoking," sufficient evidence infers that the relationship between smoking and cancers is causal. In other words, smoking causes multiple kinds of cancer.

A number of organs develop cancer from the chemicals found in smoking. These organs include lung, larynx, oral cavity, pharynx, esophagus, pancreas, bladder, kidney, cervix, and stomach.

Every time a person smokes cigarettes, cigars, pipes, and any tobacco products, those chemicals enter the bloodstream, which then carries the chemicals to all parts of the body. Furthermore, many of these chemicals can damage a person's DNA, the blueprint of life. DNA controls how the body makes new cells and directs each kind of cell to do what it's supposed to do. Damaged DNA can make cells grow differently from normal. These unusual cells can turn into cancer.

The link between smoking and lung cancer was found as early as in the 1940s. Scientists conducted experimental studies in the 1950s and found strong evidence that chemicals in cigarettes can cause cancer in mice. Much research, thereafter, including epidemiologic studies, animal experiments, chemical analysis, and cellular pathology, provided substantial evidence that convincingly established the link between smoking with lung cancer and many other cancers.

Here, I narrate a few earlier studies on smoking and lung cancer and identify the chemicals in cigarettes that cause cancer.

Looking at early studies

Two landmark epidemiologic studies published in 1950 are often credited with the discovery that smoking causes lung cancer. However, several case studies in the 1930s contributed early evidence that most patients with lung cancer smoked heavily. In 1939, one case-control study conducted by F. H. Mueller showed a stronger association of smoking in 86 men with lung cancer compared with men who didn't have lung cancer but admitted to having other diseases.

Three other case-control studies published in the 1950s consistently provided similar evidence. Papers continued to be published on the link between smoking and lung cancer.

In the 1950s two large studies, with clearly defined categories of smoking, showed the deadly effects of smoking. They are as follows:

>> A study published by Ernest Wynder and Evarts Graham in May 1950 was based on 684 patients with proved lung cancer (bronchogenic carcinoma). The investigators personally interviewed 634 of them, sent a mailed survey to 33, and the remaining 17 cases were reported by one person who had direct contacts with the patients. Lung biopsy results confirmed the diagnosis. The authors concluded that "excessive and prolonged use of tobacco, especially cigarettes, seems to be an important factor in the induction of bronchogenic carcinoma (lung cancer)."

>> The second study, entitled "Smoking and Carcinoma of the Lung: Preliminary Report," was published by Richard Doll and Austin Bradford Hill in September 1950 in the *British Medical Journal,* one of the most prestigious journals in medical science. Hill later suggested The Hill's Criteria for the causal theory of a disease (see Chapter 16 for more about this theory).

Between 1922 and 1947, the annual number of deaths from lung cancer increased roughly 15-fold in England and Wales. This study put forth two main causes: environmental pollution and the rise in tobacco smoking. They studied 709 cases with lung carcinoma (lung cancer) and a similar number of controls that had diseases other than cancer and classified them into two groups: smokers and nonsmokers and also by the amount they smoked. The authors concluded that "there is a real association between carcinoma of lung and smoking."

Recognizing what chemicals in cigarette cause cancers

Tobacco smoke contains many chemicals that are harmful to the human body. Even if someone isn't a smoker, being near to a smoker means they're inhaling the same air that contains the harmful chemicals. So the nonsmoker is affected by the air they're breathing — called passive smoking, also called secondhand smoking.

Among the 250 known harmful chemicals in tobacco smoke, at least 70 can cause cancer. Some of the cancer-causing chemicals include the following:

>> **Acetaldehyde:** Also referred to as *ethanol* — a colorless chemical

>> **Aromatic amines:** In addition to tobacco smoke, also in industrial and manufacturing plants, commercial hair dyes, and diesel exhaust

>> **Arsenic:** Can cause many health problems including cancer

>> **Benzene:** Also found in gasoline

>> **Beryllium:** A toxic metal

>> **Butadiene:** A hazardous gas

>> **Cadmium:** A toxic metal

>> **Chromium:** A metallic element

>> **Ethylene oxide:** Also found in antifreeze, textiles, detergents, adhesives, and pharmaceuticals

>> **Formaldehyde:** Used to preserve dead bodies

>> **Nickel:** A metallic element

>> **Polonium-210:** A radioactive chemical element

>> **Polycyclic aromatic hydrocarbons (PAHs):** A class of chemicals that occur naturally in coal, crude oil, and gasoline

>> **Tobacco-specific nitrosamines:** Formed when tobacco leaves are grown, cured, aged, and processed

>> **Vinyl chloride:** Used to make pipes

Of these chemicals, the most studied is polycyclic aromatic hydrocarbons (PAHs). They're produced when organic matter, such as a tobacco leaf, is burned. PAH is found in chimney sweeps, car exhausts, coal tar, and charred meat. When PAH enters the body, it becomes a powerful DNA disruptor, producing mutations that can lead to cancer.

Here are two additional chemical toxins found in cigarettes:

>> **Nicotine:** The addictive chemical that produces the effects in the brain that people seek when smoking

>> **Hydrogen cyanide:** A poison that can kill a person in a matter of seconds

Feeling the Beat of the Framingham Heart Study

The Framingham Heart Study (FHS) is a major breakthrough in research that provided substantial insight into the epidemiology of cardiovascular disease and its risk factors. In the world of epidemiology, the FHS has attained iconic status, both as a model of the cohort study and as a result of its scientific successes.

The origin of the study is closely linked with the premature death of President Franklin D. Roosevelt from hypertensive heart disease and stroke in 1945. The FHS, first launched as a longitudinal cohort study by enrolling its first participant on October 11, 1948, started with 5,209 men and women between the ages of 30 and 62 from the town of Framingham, Massachusetts. For the first round the participants had extensive physical examinations and lifestyle interviews that the researchers later analyzed for common patterns related to cardiovascular disease development. Since the initial round, the participants continued to return to the study approximately every two to six years to give researchers a detailed medical history and to get physical exams and laboratory tests.

In 1971, the study enrolled a second generation — 5,124 of the original participants' adult children and their spouses — to participate in similar examinations. In April 2002, the study entered a new phase: the enrollment of a third generation of participants, the grandchildren of the original cohort.

Over the years, the FHS has become a successful, multigenerational study that analyzes family patterns of cardiovascular and other diseases, while gathering more genetic information from the two generations that followed the original study participants. The FHS also has expanded to include diverse populations so that risk factors in these different groups can be understood. The study mapped the relations of coronary heart disease (also known as heart disease) to factors such as blood cholesterol, blood pressure, and cigarette smoking. Much of the now-common knowledge concerning heart disease, such as the effects of sex, race, diet, exercise, and common medications such as aspirin, is based on this study.

USING FLUORIDE IN WATER TO REDUCE TOOTH DECAY

Oral health in the United States is much better today than it was many years ago because of the introduction of the water fluoridation program. Grand Rapids, Michigan, became the first U.S. city to fluoridate its public water supply in 1945. Five years later, when the schoolchildren of Grand Rapids were found to have significantly fewer cavities than children from surrounding communities, other Michigan cities also began fluoridating and soon achieved similar results. Within a few years, cities and towns across the United States were fluoridating their water.

Water fluoridation is one of the greatest public health measures of all time. Fluoride in water strengthens tooth enamel and prevents cavities, tooth decay, and tooth loss. Today more people drink fluoridated water in the United States than the rest of the world combined.

Currently, about 378 million people worldwide receive artificially fluoridated water in about 25 countries, including Argentina, Australia, Brazil, Canada, Chile, Egypt, Guatemala, Israel, Ireland, Malaysia, New Zealand, Singapore, Spain, the United Kingdom, the United States, and Vietnam. Among the Asian countries, Singapore was the first to institute a water fluoridation program in 1956 that covers 100 percent of the population.

On the other hand, only a fraction of Nigerians receive water from waterworks, so water fluoridation affects very few people there. A 2009 study found that about 21 percent of water sources naturally contain fluoride to the recommended range of 0.3–0.6 ppm. About 62 percent have fluoride below this range.

South Africa's Health Department recommends adding fluoridation chemicals to drinking water in some areas. It also advises the removal of fluoride from drinking water where the fluoride content is too high.

The association between fluoride in drinking water and the reduction of tooth decay was first documented in the 1930s in communities with naturally occurring fluoride. Dr. Frederick McKay and Dr. Henry Trendley Dean established a standard of one part of fluoride per million gallons of water for reducing tooth decay while avoiding discoloration. The water fluoridation programs have several advantages including its effectiveness for everyone, ease of delivery, safety, equity, and low cost.

(continued)

(continued)

However, too much fluoride in water can cause harm to the body; it can result in dental fluorosis or mottled enamel and discoloration of the teeth. An excess of fluoride also causes skeletal fluorosis, arthritis, bone damage, osteoporosis, muscular damage, fatigue, and joint-related problems. More than 50 population-based studies have looked at the potential link between water fluoride levels and cancer. Most of these studies haven't found a strong link to cancer. Excessive amounts of fluoride can be due to natural occurrence or industrial contaminations like in many areas in China. However, domestic water in Hong Kong has been fluoridated since 1961. Water fluoridation isn't practiced in India. Due to naturally occurring fluoride, both skeletal and dental fluorosis have been endemic in India for at least 20 states. The government of India has been obligated to install fluoride removal plants to reduce fluoride levels from industrial waste and mineral deposits.

Chapter **5**

Recognizing Diseases and Controlling Them

D isease agents survive in the environment and find ways to get into the human body through different vehicles, such as food, water, air, or soil, or carried by arthropod (or invertebrate) vectors, such as mosquitoes, ticks, mites, or other parasites. Diseases are also transmitted human-to-human by direct methods, such as through hands, kissing, body fluids, or sexual contact.

As an epidemiologist, you need to know the different methods of disease transmission and find out the weakest point where you can hit to break the chain of transmission. This chapter gives you an overview of different routes of disease transmission and ways of controlling diseases.

Identifying the Modes of Transmission

People live in an environment where germs can infect them by two general modes of transmission:

>> **Direct transmission:** This method occurs when direct physical contact with an agent infects an individual. For example, the mucous membranes of sex organs transmit sexually transmitted infections (STIs), direct bites of an

infected animal transmit rabies, and the ingestion of infected food transmits food poisoning due to *salmonella* (or other germs).

>> **Indirect transmission:** This mode occurs when some intermediate vehicle, item, or process carries an agent and infects a susceptible host. For example, water, fecal materials, or flies transmit diarrheal diseases; dust particles and droplets transmit respiratory diseases; and mosquitoes, fleas, or ticks transmit *vector-borne* illnesses (diseases that are transmitted by an insect or other arthropods (invertebrate vectors).

REMEMBER

Diseases are often transmitted via five common pathways. Remember the following five Fs:

>> **Feces:** Many diseases are transmitted by the fecal contamination of food or water. Common examples are diarrheal diseases, typhoid or enteric fever, hepatitis A, and salmonella infection.

>> **Fingers:** People carry germs in their fingers. A good example is shigellosis (or blood dysentery), which can be easily transmitted from one person to another by touching a person's contaminated hands and fingers by a simple handshake.

>> **Flies:** House flies carry germs from feces and contaminated food to another food. House flies are known to carry at least 65 diseases, such as typhoid fever, shigellosis, poliomyelitis, cholera, and others.

>> **Fomites:** *Fomites* are inanimate items, such as a towel, handkerchief, paper, pen, glass, and so on. For example, adenovirus can spread through fomites.

>> **Food:** Food is a common source of diseases. Food can be contaminated in different ways:

- Infected water contaminates food.
- If food isn't properly refrigerated, it can spoil and cause diseases to occur.
- Food can be mixed with inferior substances (called *adulterated*) and poisoned. The presence of toxins or chemicals in adulterated food can cause serious illnesses. For example, turmeric is a plant root, which is used in power form in cooking. In a study, turmeric roots were reported to turn yellow from lead paints, which can cause lead poisoning.

Eyeing the Chain of Infection: Can You Break It?

Epidemiologists try to discover how to stop the process of disease transmission and how to prevent an infection. The *chain of infection*, sometimes referred to as the *chain of disease transmission*, is a model used to understand how infections are able to spread. Refer to Figure 5-1 for an example of the chain that shows some elements or steps in disease transmission.

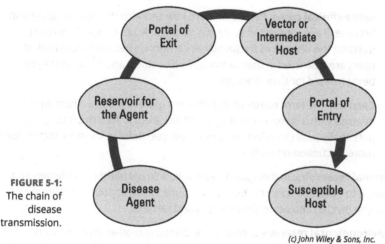

FIGURE 5-1:
The chain of disease transmission.

(c) John Wiley & Sons, Inc.

For any particular disease that you want to control, find answers to some common questions, such as:

» Where does the disease agent (or the germ) live, multiply, and survive?

» How is the agent carried from one person to another?

» Is there any intermediate host for the agent?

» What is the route of exit of the agent from an infected person?

» What is the route of entry of the agent to a susceptible host?

» How can you improve resistance or defense in the human body (or the host) against the infection?

The following sections elaborate on the elements of the chain of infection so that you have a better idea of each of the steps of disease transmission.

Classifying reservoirs

The *reservoir* is the usual habitat in which an infecting agent lives, multiplies, and propagates a disease. Examples of reservoirs are feces, decaying organic matter, and food that are conducive to the growth of agents. Reservoirs are classified as the following forms:

>> **Human reservoirs:** In this type of reservoir, infecting agents or microbes use the human body for their survival, growth, and multiplication, and then they find an opportunity to pass on to other people. Here are the two types of human reservoirs:

- **Acute clinical cases:** People who are infected with the disease agent and become ill are considered *acute clinical cases*. Acute clinical cases can't transmit the disease as frequently as carriers do because acute clinical cases are restricted in their activities and contacts and because they're being treated for their illnesses.

- **Carriers:** The term *carrier* of an infection refers to a human host who is infected with a disease, but they aren't sick from it. As a result they can potentially pass the infection to other people. Refer to the next section for more discussion on carriers.

>> **Animal reservoirs:** In this type of reservoir, animals harbor a pathogen and pass it to other animals or humans. The same is true for human reservoirs: They're divided into acute clinical cases and carriers.

>> **Environmental reservoirs:** Water, soil, plants, and other environmental sources may serve as the reservoirs of infection for many diseases.

Some examples of environmental reservoirs include the following:

REAL LIFE EXAMPLE

- **Soil:** *Clostridium tetani*, the agent that causes tetanus, is widely distributed in cultivated soil and in the gut of humans and animals. *Bacillus anthracis* is the agent of anthrax, which produces spores. Spores of anthrax may remain viable in contaminated soil for many years and infect people.

- **Water and plants:** *Vibrio cholera*, the germ that causes cholera, survives and multiplies in aquatic plants and water.

Discovering what carriers are

People who aren't sick but harbor the disease agent are called *carriers*. Carriers may present more risk for disease transmission than acute clinical cases because their contacts are unaware of their infection and the illness doesn't restrict their activities. The following sections discuss several types of carriers.

Inapparent infections

People with *inapparent infections* (also known as *subclinical cases*) don't show any clinical illnesses, but they're able to transmit their infection to others. Epidemiologists also refer to them as *healthy carriers.*

For example, epidemiologists make some assumptions:

>> For every case of cholera found in a clinic or a hospital, there are about 5 to 10 individuals with inapparent infections (or asymptomatic people) of the disease in the community.

>> For each child under the age of 5 having jaundice due to hepatitis A infection, there are ten inapparent cases.

>> Of every 100 individuals infected with the poliomyelitis virus, only one becomes paralyzed, four others will have a mild illness, and 95 out of the 100 will have no symptoms at all.

Convalescent carriers

People are called *convalescent carriers* if they harbor a pathogen and spread the disease during the period of recovery. For instance, patients with *Salmonella* infection may excrete the bacteria in feces for several weeks and sometimes even for a year or more. Inadequate treatment with antibiotics may prolong the convalescent carrier phase.

Chronic carriers

An individual who harbors and transmits an infectious agent for an extended period without showing any signs of the disease is called a *chronic carrier.* For example, about 5 to 10 percent of individuals with hepatitis B infection may progress to a chronic carrier state. About 15 to 40 percent of people who develop chronic carrier state may develop cirrhosis and end-stage liver disease.

Incubatory carriers

People who are going to become ill but begin transmitting their infection before their symptoms start are *incubatory carriers.* Examples include a person infected with measles who begins to shed the virus in nasal and throat secretions a day or two before any cold symptoms or rash are noticeable. Many other diseases also have an incubatory carrier phase. Most notably, HIV infection may be present for years before the person develops any symptoms.

Recognizing a susceptible host

Individuals who are likely to develop a disease after exposure to the infectious agent are called *susceptible hosts*. *Immunity* refers to the resistance of an individual to diseases. An individual is susceptible to disease due to several reasons, including the following:

>> Genetic makeup

>> Inadequate or no vaccinations

>> Low level of immunity

>> Personal habits, such as alcohol intake, smoking, and lack of exercise

>> Poor hygienic practice

>> Poor nutrition

>> Poor sanitation

>> Pregnancy

>> Unsafe drinking water

REMEMBER

The human body has natural defense mechanisms that protect against many infections, including

>> Skin

>> Mucous membranes

>> Gastric acidity

>> *Cilia* (hairlike structures) in the respiratory tract

>> Cough reflex, which means when something accidentally enters through the throat and the person starts coughing

>> Sneezing reflex, which is when something enters through the nose and the person starts sneezing

Focusing on the portals of exit

A *portal of exit* is the site from where microorganisms leave the host to enter another susceptible host to cause disease or infection. The microorganism enters a susceptible host through six major portals:

>> **Respiratory tract:** The *respiratory tract* is the air pathway consisting of nasal orifices, trachea, bronchi, and lungs. A microorganism may leave the reservoir

through the nose or mouth when someone sneezes or coughs. The upper respiratory tract consisting of the nose, trachea, and bronchi acts as the portal of exit for respiratory diseases such as the common cold, influenza, tuberculosis, and so on.

>> **Alimentary tract:** This tract is the pathway that food and its products take, starting from the mouth and moving through the esophagus, stomach, small intestine, large intestine, and the anal canal. Diarrheal diseases exit through the alimentary tract.

>> **Genitourinary tract:** This pathway consists of the urinary tract, starting with the kidneys, ureters, urinary bladder, and urethra (the urinary passage) and the genital organs (testis, seminal vesicles, prostate, and penis in case of males, and vagina, uterus, fallopian tubes, and ovaries in females). Sexually transmitted infections exit via the genitourinary tract.

>> **Conjunctiva:** The *conjunctiva* is the outer lining of the eyes. It acts as a physical barrier to protect the eyeball from injuries and infections.

>> **Transplacental:** This term refers to mother to child transmission. Many conditions, including HIV infection, herpes infection, rubella, cytomegalovirus infection, and syphilis are transmitted through the transplacental route.

>> **Skin:** The skin acts as the largest physical barrier covering the body. *Staph* infection is a common infection that causes a boil, which is a pocket of pus. If a boil breaks open, it drains pus and the agent exits from skin.

Examining the Natural History of Disease

The *natural history of disease* refers to the life history of a disease process if no medical interventions are taken. The natural course of a disease starts from the point of infection, or more technically, the introduction of the causative agent to an individual. Some diseases get cured in a few days without having any treatments. These types of disease are called *self-limiting diseases.*

On the other hand, some diseases progress to produce symptoms, some short-term or long-term complications, disabilities, or death. The natural course of a disease depends on preventive or therapeutic measures, the nature of the infecting agent, the host's resistance, environmental factors, and a number of other factors.

The following sections describe the properties of an infectious agent that are responsible for causing an infection, disease, and the complications of the disease. The process from an infection to the disease to the disease complications including recovery or death involves several stages that I also discuss here.

Describing the nature of infectious diseases

In the case of infectious diseases, three terms describe the nature of the agent:

» **Infectivity:** It's the ability of the agent to produce an infection. Remember, all infections don't cause a disease.

» **Pathogenicity:** It's the potential capacity of certain agents to cause a disease. For example, the common cold is highly pathogenic whereas poliomyelitis is less pathogenic.

» **Virulence:** It's the capacity of an agent to cause severe illnesses or death. For instance, the Ebola virus causes severe hemorrhagic fever in primates, resulting in mortality rates of up to 100 percent, making it an extremely virulent agent.

Here are a few examples of diseases with different levels of pathogenicity and virulence. In the case of hepatitis A, many people remain asymptomatic and few develop a severe infection, whereas when people are infected with hepatitis B, the infection may lead to complications of chronic hepatitis, cirrhosis of liver, and *hepatocellular carcinoma* (or liver cancer).

Measles is a highly infectious disease, meaning that it can be easily transmitted from one person to another. In most cases, patients recover from measles after 5 to 7 days without any complications. However, a few people have complications, such as pneumonia and encephalitis (brain swelling) following a measles infection. Rabies is another highly pathogenic disease and can be almost 100 percent fatal.

Passing through the stages

A disease passes through four stages: from the point that an infecting agent enters someone's body and ends after recovery, disability, or death of the individual. The following sections explain these four stages of the natural history of a disease (refer to Figure 5-2).

Stage of susceptibility

At this stage, the natural history of disease starts as soon as a person's body is exposed to an infecting agent. After the exposure, the agent multiplies in a sufficient amount, overpowers the body's immune system, and produces the disease process in the person who's susceptible to the disease.

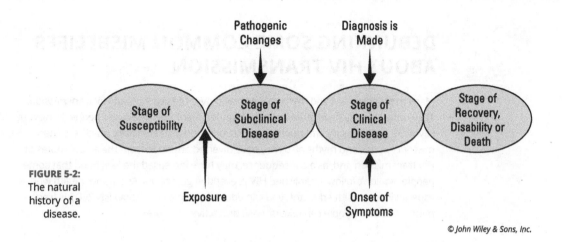

FIGURE 5-2: The natural history of a disease.

© John Wiley & Sons, Inc.

Stage of subclinical disease

The time between infection and the appearance of symptoms is known as the stage of subclinical disease. Two terms you need to know:

>> **Incubation period:** In case of infectious diseases, this stage is called the *incubation period*.

>> **Induction period:** For chronic disease this stage is called the *induction period*, also referred to as the *latency period*.

This stage may vary from a few hours to as long as a few years. For instance, in case of cholera, the incubation period is only a few hours to three days, whereas the period varies from 9 months to several years from the time of getting HIV infection until the development of AIDS. Screening programs during this period identify the disease at an early stage so that interventions can reduce the burden of the clinical stage and/or decrease disability and prevent death.

Stage of clinical disease

Clinical symptoms are manifested during this stage. In addition, most diagnoses are made at this stage.

Stage of recovery, disability, or death

This is the final stage of the natural history of a disease. People either recover from a disease or have complications leading to disability or death. Depending on the availability of treatment and advances of science, some diseases are easily treatable now. For example, syphilis can be cured 100 percent by the use of penicillin. However, recovery from a disease also depends on virulence of the pathogen, drug resistance of the pathogen, host resistance or immunity, nutrition, and other factors.

DEBUNKING SOME COMMON MISBELIEFS ABOUT HIV TRANSMISSION

Many misconceptions and myths have spread over the years about HIV transmission. They unfortunately have often led to unfounded fears, stigma against people living with HIV/AIDS, unnecessary and punitive restrictions, and discriminatory practices. These misconceptions and myths also may have diverted attention from the actual routes of HIV transmission and, as a consequence, may have increased the likelihood that some people wouldn't follow established HIV prevention guidelines. As a public health worker, especially as a health educator, you can educate people about how HIV/AIDS is transmitted and how people can take disease protective measures.

Here are some common myths debunked:

Myth: HIV can be transmitted through casual contact.

Truth: HIV can't be transmitted through casual, everyday contact, such as shaking hands or sharing eating utensils, even when people are living in close quarters because the virus can't survive outside the body for a long time; body fluids aren't transferred during a casual contact; and only certain body fluids, such as blood and genital secretions, can transmit the virus.

Myth: HIV can be transmitted through insect bites.

Truth: Studies conducted by the Centers for Disease Control and Prevention (CDC) and others have shown no evidence of HIV transmission through bloodsucking or biting insects, including mosquitoes, flies, ticks, and fleas. When a mosquito transmits a disease agent from one person to another, the infectious agent must remain alive inside the mosquito until the transfer is completed. Mosquitoes that ingest HIV-infected blood digest that blood within one to two days and completely destroy any virus particles that could potentially produce a new infection.

Myth: In the United States, donating blood or receiving donated blood is risky.

Truth: With new, advanced tests, the risk of transmitting HIV through a blood transfusion is 1 in 1.5 million. If you're at risk for getting and spreading HIV, then you shouldn't give blood. When people volunteer to donate blood, they must answer a number of questions about their health and risk factors for disease. According to the Food and Drug Administration (FDA), you're at risk if:

- You're a male who has had sex with another male since 1977, even once.

- You've ever used a needle, even once, to take any illegal drugs or steroids.

- You've taken clotting factor concentrates for a bleeding disorder such as hemophilia.

- You've ever had a positive test for HIV or AIDS antibody or antigen.

- You have AIDS or one of its symptoms.

- You've had sex with any person previously described in the last 12 months.

- You've been given money or drugs for sex since 1977.

The FDA maintains a website about facts on HIV/AIDS, which is frequently updated. You may visit the website at www.fda.gov/consumers/minority-health-and-health-equity-resources/human-immunodeficiency-virus-hiv.

Myth: Pets and other animals can carry HIV and transmit it to people.

Truth: Humans are the only animals that can harbor HIV. Some animals do carry viruses similar to HIV that cause immune deficiency in their own species. For example, cats can get feline immunodeficiency virus (FIV) and some monkeys can get simian immunodeficiency virus (SIV). However, neither FIV nor SIV can be transmitted to people. Similarly, people can't transmit HIV to their pets. An exception to this rule is chimpanzees that have been infected with HIV for research purposes. Contact with their blood could infect the researchers who work with them.

Myth: HIV can be transmitted through contact with saliva, tears, or sweat.

Truth: HIV has been found in saliva and tears in extremely low quantities in some AIDS patients. Understand that just finding a small amount of HIV in a body fluid doesn't necessarily mean that body fluid can transmit HIV. As for sweat, HIV hasn't been recovered from the sweat of HIV-infected persons. Contact with saliva, tears, or sweat has never been shown to result in transmission of HIV.

Listing Common Notifiable Diseases

Notifiable diseases are those that can cause serious morbidity or mortality and can spread to individuals, causing a considerable public health problem. The list of notifiable diseases varies from state to state, based on the priority of interventions. Here is a list of most common notifiable diseases in the United States:

>> **Chlamydia:** A sexually transmitted infection that affects men and women.

>> **Influenza A and B:** They cause flu.

- » **Staph infection:** It causes skin infection; can be serious or life-threatening.

- » *E. coli* **infection:** Can cause diarrhea or urinary infection.

- » **Herpes Simplex 1 (HSV-1):** Causes most oral herpes, also referred to as fever blisters or cold sores. It can be spread to genital areas through oral sex.

- » **Herpes Simplex 2 (HSV-2):** Causes most genital herpes.

- » **Shigella** *spp.*: Causes blood dysentery (also called shigellosis).

- » **Syphilis:** A sexually transmitted infection.

- » **Gonorrhea:** A sexually transmitted infection.

- » **Norovirus:** Highly contagious, it's one of the causes of food poisoning or stomach flu.

- » *Salmonella:* A person can get this bacteria from eating raw or uncooked food.

- » **Hepatitis C:** This infection is spread via contact with infected blood.

- » **HIV:** This virus is spread through unprotected sex or contact with infected blood.

For further information about notifiable diseases, check out www.cdc.gov/mmwr/preview/mmwrhtml/mm6217md.htm.

Controlling Waterborne Diseases

Waterborne diseases are any illness caused by drinking water contaminated by human or animal feces that contain pathogenic microorganisms. The lack of safe drinking water throughout the world is the main culprit behind waterborne diseases that cause one child to die every 20 seconds from a water-related disease.

Although certain diseases aren't directly caused by contaminated water, they're caused by vectors (such as mosquitoes, ticks, and so on) that live and multiply in contaminated water. The latter diseases are called *water-related diseases*. These following sections identify the different waterborne diseases and how epidemiologists work to prevent these types of diseases.

Naming common waterborne diseases

Some waterborne diseases pose a health risk to a large number of people in a short period of time, causing epidemics of diarrheal diseases, which occur due to climatic changes, seasonal factors, and changes in the person's immunity. Such epidemics of diarrheal diseases are commonly caused due to cholera and blood dysentery:

>> Cholera epidemics happen in the winter months and during and after monsoons. They also occur after a natural disaster such as a flood or a cyclone.

>> Blood dysentery epidemics occur in dry seasons when water in many developing countries is scarcer. Blood dysentery is easily spread from one person to another due to the lack of proper hand washing practices.

The following lists the waterborne diseases that affect the world's population:

>> **Diarrheal diseases:** Diarrhea remains the second leading cause of death among children under 5 globally. It kills more young children than AIDS, malaria, and measles combined. The following is a list of common diarrheal diseases:

- **Cholera:** A bacterial disease that occurs mostly in older children and adults. It causes profuse watery diarrhea and vomiting, resulting in dehydration (or loss of fluid and electrolytes).

- *E. coli* **infection:** Another bacterial infection that causes watery diarrhea.

- **Rotavirus diarrhea:** This is the most common viral diarrhea affecting children.

- **Diarrhea due to *Campylobacter:*** This bacterial disease causes watery or dysenteric stools.

- **Giardiasis:** The parasite *Giardia lamblia* causes this diarrhea. This disease is also a parasitic infection.

>> **Parasitic infections:** Many parasites such as round worm, hook worm, whip worm, cryptosporidium, and so on are transmitted by water. Refer to the section, "Identifying common parasitic infections," later in this chapter for specifics about parasitic infections.

>> **Mosquito-borne diseases:** The following are diseases that are transmitted by mosquitoes:

- **Malaria:** Several malarial parasites known as *Plasmodium* cause the disease. The type of mosquito that transmits the disease is called the female *Anopheles*. Symptoms include high fever with chills and rigors.

- **Dengue fever:** Four dengue fever viruses, known as DEN 1-4, are transmitted by *Aedes* mosquitoes. The disease causes high fever and severe joint pain. Because of extreme joint pain, the disease is also called *break-bone fever*.

- **Japanese encephalitis:** Bites of infected *Culex* mosquitoes cause this viral disease. *Encephalitis* means inflammation of the brain.

>> **Diseases due to heavy metal poisoning:** Some heavy metals, such as lead and arsenic, can be transmitted through water and other vehicles (refer to the later section, "Identifying Diseases Caused by Heavy Metals" for more information):

- **Arsenic poisoning:** Arsenic in toxic form is transmitted mainly by contaminated water. It causes skin lesions, cancers, and many other symptoms.

- **Lead poisoning:** Lead can enter the human body through water, air, soil, and food. This heavy metal poisoning affects mostly small children, resulting in physical, mental, and developmental problems.

>> **Miscellaneous water-related diseases:** Some other water-related diseases include the following:

- **Enteric fever:** *Salmonella enteritidis* causes this bacterial disease.

- **Hepatitis:** Hepatitis viruses cause this viral disease. A common symptom is jaundice.

- **Scabies:** A mite called *Sarcoptes scabiei* causes this very contagious skin disease. Scabies is a condition of very itchy skin caused by tiny mites that burrow into the skin. Scabies mites spread by close contact with someone who has scabies.

Taking steps in controlling waterborne diseases

The best measure in controlling waterborne diseases is to ensure the public uses clean and quality water. Several parameters are used for measuring the quality of water, and they fall under these two categories:

>> **Chemical/physical parameters:** They include heavy metals, trace organic compounds, total suspended solids (TSS), and cloudiness.

>> **Microbiological parameters:** They include *coliform* bacteria, *E. coli*, and specific pathogenic species of bacteria (such as cholera-causing *Vibrio cholerae*), viruses, and protozoan parasites that may be present in water.

Water treatment plants purify water by filtrating it in large scale. People also use some other methods such as utilizing hand-pump tube wells or suction wells, desalinating coastal areas, treating rainwater, and using oxidation, coagulation, sorption, nanofiltration, and reverse osmosis techniques for the removal of physical, chemical, and microbiological contaminants from the water.

Tackling Problems of Airborne Infections

Airborne diseases are spread when droplets of pathogens are expelled into the air due to coughing, sneezing, or talking. Airborne transmission occurs typically when droplets (most commonly mucous droplets) remain suspended in the air as *aerosols* (very small droplets) or mixed with dust particles, and then inhaled. The following sections examine common airborne infections and their prevention.

Recognizing common airborne infections

The following airborne diseases require respiratory precautions:

>> Chickenpox

>> Herpes zoster

>> *Hemophilus influenza*

>> Measles (rubeola)

>> Meningitis

>> Mumps

>> Pertussis (whooping cough)

>> Rubella (German measles)

>> Tuberculosis

Controlling airborne infections

Exposure to a patient or animal with an airborne disease doesn't guarantee contracting the disease. The changes in host immunity and the amount of particles suspended in the air that a person is exposed to make a difference in causing an airborne infection in your body.

TIP

Here are ways to help prevent airborne diseases:

>> Using a surgical mask to cover the nose and mouth

>> Washing hands

>> Using appropriate hand disinfectant

» Getting regular immunizations

» Limiting time spent in outdoor activities

» Staying away from sick people and social distancing

Curving Vector-Borne Diseases

Vector-borne diseases are infections transmitted by the bite of infected arthropod species, such as mosquitoes, ticks, sandflies, and blackflies. Arthropod vectors are cold-blooded and thus especially sensitive to climatic factors. However, climate is only one of many other factors influencing vector distribution. Other factors include habitat destruction, land use, pesticide application, and human density. These sections mention the common vector-borne diseases and the best ways to prevent them.

Listing common vector-borne diseases

Vector-borne infectious diseases, such as malaria, dengue fever, yellow fever, and the plague, cause a significant occurrence of the global infectious disease burden; indeed, nearly half of the world's population is infected with at least one type of vector-borne pathogens.

Here are a few vector-borne diseases:

» **Dengue fever:** The World Health Organization (WHO) currently estimates between 50 to 100 million dengue infections worldwide every year.

» **Kala-azar or leishmaniosis:** Leishmaniosis is a disease spread by the bite of the female sandfly. Leishmaniasis can be found in India, Mexico, and South America.

» **Lyme disease:** A new study suggests that an estimated 15 percent of the world's population has been infected with Lyme disease — of them, approximately 30,000 cases occur annually in the United States.

» **Malaria:** The disease is more common in Sub-Saharan Africa, Asia, Latin America, and to a lesser extent in Middle East.

» **Plague:** The bacteria *Yersinia pestis* causes plague. Rodents, such as rats, carry the disease, and their fleas spread it. Plague can still be found in Africa, Asia, and South America.

>> **Rocky Mountain spotted fever (RMSF):** Ticks cause this disease that afflicts more than 4,000 U.S. cases each year, including some that result in death. Most cases of RMSF occur in the southeastern and south central United States.

>> **West Nile virus infection:** Mosquitoes carry the highest amounts of virus in the early fall, which is why the rate of the disease increases in late August to early September.

>> **Yellow fever:** This disease is common in South America and in Sub-Saharan Africa.

Finding ways to combat vector-borne diseases

Vector-borne diseases are among the most complex of all infectious diseases to prevent and control. Not only is predicting the habits of mosquitoes, ticks, and fleas difficult, but most vector-borne viruses or bacteria infect animals as well as humans.

TIP

Here are some strategies to control vector-borne diseases:

>> **Environmental management:** This includes reducing or eliminating vector breeding grounds.

>> **Biological control:** This strategy uses bacterial larvicides (that kills larvae) and larvivorous fish that eat vector larvae.

>> **Chemical control:** This includes indoor residual spraying, space spraying, and using chemical larvicides and adulticides (that kill adult mosquitoes).

>> **Personal protection and preventive measures:** This strategy utilizes insecticide-treated nets and repellants, uses long sleeve shirts, reduces outdoor activities, and so on.

Limiting Parasitic Infections

Diseases due to parasites are widespread in Africa, southern Asia, and Central and South America, especially among children. Here I list common parasitic infections and their control measures.

Identifying common parasitic infections

Parasites that reside in a person's intestinal cavity are called *intestinal parasites.* However, they may also harbor in a person's blood, lymphatic system, or other parts. Although parasitic diseases are common in tropical countries, some parasites are found worldwide, even in cooler climates and in wealthier nations, including the United States.

Some common parasites are as follows:

>> **Cryptosporidiosis:** This parasitic disease is more common in immunocompromised patients (patients with malnutrition or HIV/AIDS).

>> **Hookworm:** A common helminthic infection is hookworm or *Ankylostoma duodenale* infection. It's a leading cause of anemia and protein malnutrition. The largest numbers of cases occur in impoverished rural areas of Sub-Saharan Africa, Latin America, and Southeast Asia.

>> **Malaria:** Of all parasitic diseases, malaria causes the most deaths globally. I also list this disease under mosquito-borne diseases earlier in this chapter because it's carried by mosquitoes.

>> **Onchocerciasis:** Also known as *river blindness,* this disease infects 26 million people living near the rivers and fast-moving streams of Sub-Saharan Africa.

>> **Pinworm:** Pinworm or *Enterobius vermicularis* is another common helminthic infection affecting small children. Pinworm causes itchiness around the anus, especially at night.

>> **Roundworm:** The intestinal roundworm, called *Ascaris lumbricoides,* is the most common parasite infecting 1 billion people around the world.

>> **Scabies**: Scabies can spread by close contact, sharing towels, bed sheets, and other personal belongings. See the section, "Naming common waterborne diseases," earlier in this chapter for more information.

>> **Schistosomiasis:** Schistosomiasis, also known as *bilharzia* or *snail fever,* is a parasitic disease carried by freshwater snails. It affects more than 200 million people worldwide.

Taking steps to control parasitic infections

The two most important strategies in controlling parasitic diseases are to provide safe drinking water and sanitary disposal of excrement because parasites are transmitted through the fecal-oral route.

TIP

Keep in mind these other ways to prevent and control parasitic infections:

>> **Avoiding contact:** The most obvious way is to steer clear, either of the parasite or of the infected person, particularly with scabies, including not having sex.

>> **Proper hand washing:** Stringent hand washing is essential in controlling scabies because mites can live under fingernails or in the fine crevices of the cuticles.

>> **Using insecticides:** Although insecticides are used in Africa, resistance is one of the biggest threats to sustainable malaria control. Control of *Anopheles* mosquitoes relies mainly on the use of bed nets soaked with the chemical, *pyrethroid*.

>> **Washing bedding:** If a person is living with an infected person, make sure to wash bedding in very hot temperatures. Alternately dry-clean items to help kill existing mites.

>> **Wearing shoes:** The hookworm larva enters the human body from contaminated soil by penetrating the skin. To avoid hookworm infection, a person should wear shoes in areas where hookworms are common.

Controlling Sexually Transmitted Infections

In the United States about 19 million new infections of sexually transmitted infections (STIs) occur each year. These infections affect men and women of all backgrounds and economic levels, although almost half of new infections are among young people ages 15 to 24. The following sections point out some widespread STIs and the best ways to prevent them.

Listing common STIs

The term *sexually transmitted infection (STI)* is preferred compared to *sexually transmitted disease (STD)* because a person may be infected and may potentially infect others without having a disease.

STIs are infections that are spread primarily through person-to-person contact by means of human sexual behavior, including vaginal intercourse, oral sex, and anal sex. Several STIs, in particular HIV and syphilis, can also be transmitted from mother to child during pregnancy, childbirth, and breastfeeding, and through blood products and tissue transfer. More than 30 different bacteria, viruses, and parasites are sexually transmissible.

Here are the most common ones along with a few symptoms:

>> **Bacterial vaginosis:** Most women have no symptoms. Common symptoms include vaginal itching, pain when urinating, and discharge with a fishy odor.

>> **Chancroid**: The bacteria *Haemophilus ducreyi* causes chancroid. Chancroid is a risk factor for contracting HIV because both the diseases are associated with the common risks of exposure.

>> **Chlamydia:** Most women have no symptoms. Women with symptoms may have abnormal vaginal discharge, burning when urinating, bleeding between periods, lower abdominal pain, low back pain, and pain during sex. Men's symptoms include pain when urinating; white, cloudy or watery discharge from the tip of the penis; burning or itching urinary passage; and pain in the testicles.

>> **Genital herpes:** Some people may have no symptoms. Common symptoms include small red bumps, blisters, or open sores on the penis, vagina, or mouth; vaginal discharge; fever; pain when urinating; and itching, burning, or swollen glands in the genital area.

>> **Gonorrhea:** Symptoms are often mild, but most people have no symptoms. They include pain or burning when urinating, yellowish and sometimes bloody vaginal discharge, bleeding between periods, pain during sex, heavy bleeding during periods, and pus-like discharge from the penis.

>> **Hepatitis B infection:** Some people have no symptoms. People with symptoms may have low-grade fever, tiredness, loss of appetite, upset stomach or vomiting, dark-colored urine, and *jaundice* (skin and whites of eyes turning yellow).

>> **Human immunodeficiency virus (HIV) infection and AIDS:** Some people may have no symptoms for ten years or more. About half of people with HIV get flu-like symptoms about three to six weeks after becoming infected.

>> **Human papillomavirus (HPV):** Some women have no symptoms. Women with symptoms may have visible warts in the genital area, including the thighs. Warts sometimes are cauliflower-shaped growths. Most men don't have any symptoms. Men can develop cancer of the penis. Cancer of the rectum, mouth and throat occur in both men and women.

>> **Pelvic inflammatory disease (PID):** PID refers to infection of the uterus (womb), fallopian tubes (tubes that carry eggs from the ovaries to the uterus), and other reproductive organs.

>> **Syphilis:** Syphilis progresses in stages. Symptoms of the primary stage are a single, painless sore appearing 10 to 90 days after infection. It can appear in the genital area, mouth, or other parts of the body. The sore goes away on its own.

If the infection isn't treated, it moves to the secondary stage. This stage starts three to six weeks after the sore appears. Symptoms of the secondary stage are skin rashes with rough, red or reddish-brown spots on the hands and feet that usually don't itch and clear on their own, fever, sore throat and swollen glands, patchy hair loss, weight loss, and tiredness.

>> **Trichomoniasis:** Sometimes called *trich,* this infection is due to a protozoan parasite called *Trichomonas vaginalis*. Many women don't have any symptoms. Symptoms usually appear 5 to 28 days after exposure and can include yellow, green, or gray vaginal discharge (often foamy) with a strong odor; discomfort during sex and when urinating; and itching or discomfort in the genital area.

Carrying out control measures for STIs

A person can lower their risk of getting an STI with the following tips. These measures work best when used together. No single strategy can protect you from every single type of STI:

>> **Condom use:** Use of condoms is important in all types of sexual contact, even if intercourse doesn't take place. They need to be used from the very start to the very end of each sex act and with every sex partner.

Some methods of birth control, such as birth control pills, shots, implants, or diaphragms, don't protect against STIs. Condom use should be practiced every time and by all sexual partners to protect you from STIs.

WARNING

>> **Communication:** Sex partner(s) need to regularly discuss STIs and what precautions they will take before having sex.

>> **Doctor's advice:** A person's doctor and sex partner(s) need to be informed about any STIs.

>> **Regular testing:** Receiving regular STI testing at a county health department or a family doctor is also important in diminishing the chances of spreading STIs. The patient can discuss how often they need to be retested based on their sexual history. The sooner an STI is found, the easier it is to treat.

>> **Illicit drugs and alcohol:** Avoiding illegal drug use and/or excessive drinking of alcohol is important. These activities can lead to diminished inhibitions, which can lead to poor decisions.

>> **Abstinence:** The surest way to keep from getting any STI is to practice total abstinence, which means not having vaginal, oral, or anal sex. However, some STIs, such as genital herpes, can be spread without having intercourse.

>> **Monogamy:** This means having sex with one sexual partner and no one else. Having a sexual relationship with one partner who has been tested for STIs and isn't infected is another way to lower risk of infection.

>> **Taking PrEP:** Pre-exposure prophylaxis (or PrEP) can reduce the risk of getting HIV from sex in about 99 percent of cases when used as prescribed by your doctor. It can also reduce the risk of getting HIV from injection drug use by more than 70 percent. Condom use is still important for protection against other STIs.

Dealing With Emerging Infectious Diseases

An *emerging infectious disease* (EID) is an infectious disease whose incidence has increased in the recent past or could increase in the near future. Several factors of a disease make it an emerging infection, including

>> The disease is caused by a new strain or species of a pathogen, for example, SARS and AIDS.

>> The disease is spread to a new population or area, such as West Nile disease and Lyme disease.

>> An old disease may emerge in a more virulent form, affecting a larger group of people, such as the plague and influenza.

>> Strains of a known disease may develop a resistance to common antimicrobials — for instance, Methicillin-resistant *Staphylococcus aureus* (MRSA) infection, multi-drug resistant tuberculosis, and so on.

These sections look at the prevalent emerging infections and the preventions that epidemiologists use to avoid these infections.

Finding common emerging infections

The World Health Organization (WHO) and the Centers for Disease Control and Prevention (CDC) have described more than 100 emerging infectious diseases that affect humans. The most common are listed here:

>> **AIDS:** Refer to the section, "Listing common STIs," earlier in this chapter for more information.

>> **Anthrax:** *Bacillus anthracis* can cause three different kinds of disease: cutaneous anthrax, intestinal anthrax, and pulmonary anthrax.

>> **Botulism:** *Clostridium botulinum* causes several nerve toxins:

- Foodborne botulism is caused by eating foods that contain botulism toxins.

  - Infant botulism results from consuming spores of the bacteria that then grow in the intestines and produce the toxins.

    - Wound botulism is caused by toxins produced in wounds infected with the botulism bacteria.

>> **Chagas disease:** This potentially chronic, fatal disease currently affects 12 million people throughout Mexico and Central and South America. The protozoan parasite *Trypanosoma cruzi* causes it.

>> **Creutzfeldt-Jakob disease:** Prions are infectious agents composed of protein, which causes abnormal folding and damage of the brain and death. Prions are thought to be responsible for scrapie, mad cow disease, and chronic wasting disease of animals and Creutzfeldt-Jakob disease (CJD) in humans.

>> **Chikungunya:** *Chikungunya* is a virus that can be transmitted to humans by mosquitoes. Outbreaks of Chikungunya were reported mostly from Africa and Southeast Asia in 2005–2006. In 2013 it appeared in the Western hemisphere. Since then, 46 countries from the Americas reported more than 1.7 million suspected cases.

>> **Dengue fever:** A re-emergence of dengue fever and the more fatal dengue hemorrhagic fever (DHF) were reported in Bangladesh in 2000, with more than 5,000 cases.

>> **Hanta virus infection:** Hanta viruses are carried primarily by rodents and can infect humans who breathe contaminated dust after disturbing or cleaning rodent droppings or nests, or who live or work in rodent-infested settings. The major diseases caused by Hanta viruses are hantavirus pulmonary syndrome (HPS) and hemorrhagic fever with renal syndrome (HFRS).

>> **Lyme disease:** Borrelia burgdorferi causes Lyme disease by being transmitted between mammals and the black-legged tick, *Ixodes scapularis*. The most common early symptoms of Lyme disease in humans are rash, flu-like symptoms, chills, headache, and fatigue. Later symptoms may include joint pain, headache, facial paralysis, myocarditis (inflammation of the heart muscle), and heart block.

>> **Nipah virus:** Several outbreaks of *Nipah* virus encephalitis have been reported in Bangladesh since 1999. Bats carrying the *Nipah* virus cause the disease. People are infected with the virus after drinking sap from palm trees that the bats have infected.

>> **Plague:** This is another old disease that has seen a re-emergence. In the United States, plague presently occurs as scattered cases in rural areas, with an average of 10 to 15 persons each year. If not treated with antibiotics, the bacteria can invade the bloodstream and produce potentially fatal septicemia and lung infection.

>> **SARS:** Severe acute respiratory syndrome (SARS) is a disease caused by infection with a coronavirus. It's spread by close person-to-person contact, particularly by respiratory droplets or when a person touches a surface or object contaminated with infectious droplets and then touches their mouth, nose, or eyes. During 2002–2003, a major epidemic caused more than 8,000 cases and more than 750 deaths, mostly in China, Taiwan, Singapore, Vietnam, and the Philippines.

>> **Tuberculosis:** Cases of tuberculosis increased in patients with AIDS.

>> *Vibrio cholera* **0139:** A new toxigenic strain of *Vibrio*, known as *Vibrio cholera* 0139, emerged during 1992–1993 causing epidemics in the Indian subcontinent and some other countries.

>> **West Nile disease:** The disease was first documented in the United States in New York City during an epidemic in August 1999. A total of 5,674 cases and 286 deaths were reported to the CDC in 2012.

Controlling emerging infections

Recognizing EIDs in a timely fashion is important to reduce morbidity and mortality from the disease. Also, an EID requires continuous monitoring of the disease, known as *surveillance* (refer to Chapter 13) for an early detection of such health problems so that they may be promptly investigated and controlled before they become a public health crisis.

As with many issues of health, education is a vital part of the battle against the spread of infectious diseases. By knowing what threats are posed by EIDs and by changing behavior, the risk can be reduced. Although a healthy immune system is the best defense, basic hygiene, such as proper hand washing and cleaning the kitchen and bathroom, can help defend against harmful microorganisms.

Identifying Diseases Caused by Heavy Metals

Heavy metals and chemicals from industrial and agricultural discharges pollute the environment and can cause several illnesses. Some of these chemicals include lead, arsenic, mercury, chromium, and so on. Toxicity due to heavy metals can result in damaged or reduced mental and central nervous function, lower energy levels, and damage to blood composition, kidneys, liver, lungs, and other vital organs. Long-term exposure may result in slowly progressing physical, muscular, and neurological degenerative processes. Repeated long-term contact with some metals (or their compounds) may cause cancer.

Chronic arsenic poisoning, *arsenicosis,* can increase the risk of several health hazards, including skin lesions, cancers, restrictive pulmonary disease, peripheral vascular disease (blackfoot disease), gangrene, hypertension, non-cirrhotic portal fibrosis, ischemic heart disease, and diabetes mellitus. However, arsenic poisoning can be prevented by getting drinking water free of arsenic.

REAL LIFE EXAMPLE

Cases have been reported from mass scale poisoning due to chemicals all over the world. Here is one case study of arsenic poisoning in Bangladesh that was especially alarming. About 30 percent of 10 million shallow tubewells (hand pumps) were highly contaminated. Shallow tubewells are metallic or plastic pipes vertically set into the ground for the purpose of suction lifting of underground water. In fact, almost half of the Bangladesh populations were exposed to the risk of arsenic poisoning. Chronic arsenic exposure increases the risk of skin cancer, diabetes, heart disease, liver toxicity, and other conditions.

2

Understanding Disease Causation

Be familiar with the epidemiologic triangle — the acute disease model of disease causation.

Examine how biological agents, the human host and intermediary hosts, and environmental factors interplay with each other in creating an imbalance for causing a disease.

Find how the association of person factors such as age, sex, and occupation, and place of living affect overall health and act as potential risk factors of diseases.

Define epidemiologic transition and explore reasons for the changing pattern of diseases from acute and infectious diseases to chronic and noncommunicable diseases in the United States and many other developed countries.

Understand demographic transition and the four stages of demographic transition due to the changes in birth rates, death rates, and migration.

Compare population growth patterns in selected countries and identify the top ten countries with the largest proportions of senior citizens.

Figure out how to estimate the future population of a country.

Know how to calculate important rates for a population.

Chapter **6**

Tackling the Epidemiologic Triangle

I n order to understand a disease, you need to answer the following fundamental questions to identify what's needed for a disease to occur:

» What causes the disease?

» What makes some people more susceptible to a disease and some people spared of contracting the disease?

» What factors in the environment favor the disease-causing agent survival and transmit the disease to humans?

An American pathologist, Theobald Smith, in his book, *Parasitism and Disease*, clearly articulated how an interaction happens among three factors — the agent, the host, and the environment — and that these three factors interplay with each other in causing a disease or an event (such as accident or suicide) in humans. Collectively, they're called the *epidemiologic triangle* or the *epidemiologic triad*.

This chapter looks more closely at these three factors of the epidemiologic triangle for an acute disease model and a chronic disease model. I explain how climate changes affect health, and I examine four vector-borne diseases that are mostly affected by climate changes.

Scrutinizing an Acute Disease Model

The epidemiologic triangle, first introduced as a traditional model for infectious diseases, is the simplest model (Figure 6-1a) of all models that look at what causes an acute and infectious disease.

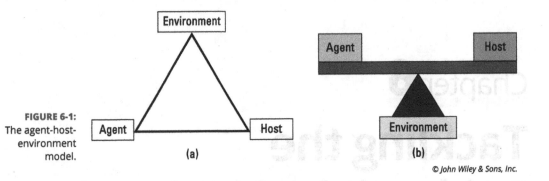

© John Wiley & Sons, Inc.

FIGURE 6-1: The agent-host-environment model.

Here are the parts of the triangle:

>> **Agent:** The cause of the disease

>> **Susceptible host:** Either humans or animals who are victims of the disease

>> **Environment:** Where both the agent and the host live and interplay

A suitable environment also helps the agent to grow and multiply, and in a favorable situation, the agent enters the host to cause a disease. In other words, the environment keep the balance. The environment factor works like a fulcrum of the balance between the agent on one side and the host on the other side, as shown in Figure 6-1b.

If the balance between the agent and the host goes down on one side, the other side gets an upper hand. For example, if the host (the human body) gets weaker due to the loss of host immunity or host resistance, the agent gets easy access to the human body. On the other hand, if the human body grows resistance like getting a vaccine and by practicing a healthy lifestyle, then the agent fails to attack the person.

The following sections take a closer look at the three parts of the triangle.

Examining agent factors

In an infectious disease model, an agent is a bacteria, virus, parasite, or fungus. Agents are infectious because they can spread from one person to another. However, some don't infect people directly; they're transmitted from one infected person to another through a vehicle, such as drinking contaminated water or through the bites of an insect, such as a mosquito.

Table 6-1 provides a list of agents that cause human diseases.

TABLE 6-1   Type of Agents and the Diseases Caused by Agents

Type of Agent	Agent Name	Diseases
Bacteria		
	Streptococcus	Sore throat
	Pneumococcus	Pneumonia
	Vibrio choleriae	Cholera
	Mycobacterium tuberculosis	Tuberculosis
Virus		
	Rhinovirus	Common cold
	Coronavirus SARS-CoV-2	Covid-19
	Influenza viruses	Flu
	Rotavirus	Diarrhea
	Human papilloma virus (HPV)	Genital warts
	Human immunodeficiency virus (HIV)	AIDS
Parasite		
	Necator americanus	Hook worm disease
	Ascaris lumbricoides	Round worm disease
	Plasmodium spp.	Malaria
Fungus		
	Trichophyton	Athlete's foot
	Cryptococcus	Lung infection in people with weakened immune system
	Histoplasma	Lung infection in people with weakened immune system

Considering host factors

Although humans are natural hosts of diseases, certain diseases actually have more than one host. For example, the parasitic life cycle of *Plasmodium*, the agent for malaria, involves two hosts:

>> **Mosquitoes:** The sexual cycle of the parasite is completed in mosquitoes, and mosquitoes are the primary host.

>> **Humans:** The asexual cycle of the parasite is completed in humans, and humans are the secondary host.

The agent can live in a second host other than mosquitoes. For example, In the case of schistosomiasis, humans are the primary host, and snails are an intermediate host.

The factors that can protect a host from contracting a disease include getting vaccines and eating healthier. Treatment, such as taking antibiotics for the disease, can also break the disease transmission cycle because antibiotics can kill the agent.

Looking at environment factors

Both agents and hosts (such as humans) live within the environment. Therefore, the environment is a key player in the chain of infection. Many natural elements in the environment such as heat, cold, humidity, noise, and others affect people's health and the growth and survival of an agent. For instance, public health officials can help by minimizing or destroying the growth and multiplication of mosquitoes by removing their breeding places (stagnant water).

Inspecting a Chronic Disease Model

The epidemiologic triangle later was extended as a framework for understanding chronic and noninfectious diseases. In a chronic disease model, the concept of agents and environment is much wider. Heart disease, diabetes, cancer, and asthma are chronic diseases. No single agent causes any of these chronic diseases. The causative agents are referred to as *risk factors* for chronic conditions.

However, some infectious agents, such as bacteria or a virus, can also be involved in causing some chronic diseases, if the infection is left untreated or poorly treated. Here are some examples of infectious agents that can cause chronic diseases:

>> *Streptococcus pyogens* (also commonly called *Strep throat*) is a bacterial infection that causes sore throat. If not treated or poorly treated, the throat infection can affect a person's heart and can increase the risk of rheumatic heart disease.

>> *Human papillomavirus (HPV)* infection can cause many cancers including cancer of the cervix (the mouth of the uterus), vulva, vagina, penis, or anus. A screening test is the best option to prevent such cancers (Chapter 15 describes more details about screening tests).

REMEMBER

In case of a chronic disease, the conventional agent-host-environment model can be modified to add more factors. Consider the following and refer to Figure 6-2:

>> **Agent factors:** A number of factors, including obesity, high blood pressure, high cholesterol, unhealthy diet, and an infection of *Streptococcus pyogens* (in the case of rheumatic heart disease) can cause heart disease.

>> **Host factors:** Host factors for heart disease are also many: genetics, older age, gender, family history of heart disease, and personal habits such as smoking, heavy drinking, and not exercising.

>> **Environmental hazards:** They weigh heavily in causing heart disease. Air pollution from dust, smoke, and particulate matters in the air, indoor pollution due to secondhand smoke, traffic, noise pollution, excessive heat, and heavy metals such as arsenic and lead in water are important contributory factors that cause heart disease.

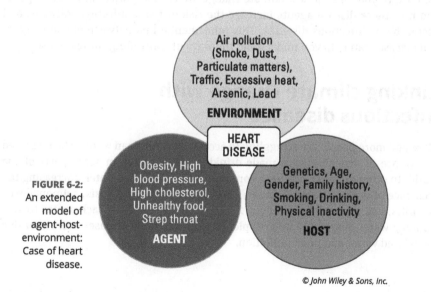

FIGURE 6-2: An extended model of agent-host-environment: Case of heart disease.

© John Wiley & Sons, Inc.

Understanding How Climate Change Can Affect Health

Climate is a part of environmental factors that can affect a person's health. Global warming has impacted the planet in many respects. The following are three significant areas where the rising temperatures are affecting people's health:

>> **Food production and global agriculture:** The incidence of drought and floods have increased, significantly impacting global agriculture and food production. The result: rising rates of food insecurity and malnutrition.

>> **Unhealthy air:** Approximately nine out of ten people worldwide breathe unhealthy air. Because of increased air pollution, diseases such as lung cancer, asthma, and heart disease are also increasing. Thirteen people die every minute from diseases directly linked to air pollution. Between 2030 and 2050, climate change is expected to cause approximately 250,000 additional climate-related deaths every year globally from malnutrition, malaria, diarrhea, and heat stroke.

>> **People's mental health:** The trauma related to extreme climate is affecting people's mental health worldwide. Due to unstable and severe weather, the most vulnerable people — children, adolescents, and the elderly — are victims of more stress, anxiety, and depression. The direct damage cost to health is estimated to be between $2 to 4 billion per year by 2030.

Here I give you an idea how climate change affects the growth of disease agents and how these disease agents increase the risk of many infectious diseases and vector-borne infectious diseases. This fundamental link between climate, agent, and diseases can help you understand the ways of controlling these diseases.

Linking climate change with infectious diseases

More and more people are struggling to access safe and clean water. The increased occurrence of droughts have made drinking water scarce in some parts of the world. In other areas, floods have contaminated the surface water, increasing the incidence of water-related diseases, such as diarrhea, shigellosis, salmonellosis, hepatitis, and typhoid fever. About 2 billion people currently lack access to safe drinking water. About 829,000 people die from diarrheal diseases every year due to polluted water and poor sanitation.

Finding vector-borne diseases related to climate change

The numbers of mosquitoes, flies, and ticks increase with warmer temperatures and larger amounts of precipitation. Temperature determines the rate at which insects develop into adults, the frequency of their blood feeding, the rate at which they get disease pathogens, and the rate at which the pathogens develop inside the vectors (such as mosquitoes).

In medical terms, a *vector* is a living organism that transmits an infectious agent from an infected animal or a human to another animal or a human. Vectors frequently are insects, such as mosquitoes, ticks, flies, fleas, and lice. Because the vectors lack a thermostatic mechanism, their body temperature is highly sensitive and influenced by the ambient temperature.

As temperature rise, mosquitoes spread diseases faster than they do during cooler temperatures. If global warming continues to rise, an additional 4.7 billion people could be at risk of vector-borne diseases like malaria, dengue fever, and others by 2070.

REMEMBER

Infectious diseases that involve either mechanical means (such as soil) or a biological vector (mosquitoes, ticks, flies, flies, or lice) for transmission from one person to another are highly sensitive to the climate conditions. Several vector-borne diseases that are susceptible to climate change include malaria, West Nile fever, dengue fever, and Chikungunya, which I discuss in the following sections. Here are a couple other diseases also affected by climate change:

>> **Leishmaniasis:** The *Leishmania* protozoan parasite causes leishmaniasis (also) referred to as or *Kala Azar*). It's the result of a bite from a sandfly. Symptoms include high fever, difficulty breathing, diarrhea, vomiting, and weight loss. It has two forms: cutaneous and visceral. The visceral form is more severe.

>> **Crimean-Congo hemorrhagic fever:** First identified in Crimea, the cause of this severe viral disease was discovered in Congo. Ticks are the vectors or carriers of this disease. Symptoms include high fever, back pain, joint pain, stomachache, vomiting, red eyes, and red spots on the palate. Death rate from the disease is between 15 to 75 percent.

Managing malaria

Approximately 85 countries are prevalent of having malaria, of which 95 percent of the burden occurs in the African region. According to the World Health Organization (WHO) report, there were 241 million cases and 627 thousand deaths due to malaria in 2020 compared to 227 million cases and 558 thousand deaths in 2019.

That means a 6 percent increase in the number of cases and 12 percent increase in deaths from malaria from 2019 to 2020.

Four common species of the *Plasmodium* parasite cause malaria:

>> *Plasmodium vivax*

>> *Plasmodium falciparum*

>> *Plasmodium malariae*

>> *Plasmodium ovale*

P. vivax and *P. falciparum* are the most common malarial parasites, and *P. falciparum* is the most dangerous type. The vector of malaria is the female anopheles mosquito.

SEEING THE EFFECT OF CLIMATE CHANGE ON MALARIA

The humid and warm climate in African countries and in Asia creates perfect conditions for the proliferation of malaria's vector mosquitoes. With record-breaking heat waves and changing rainfall patterns there is an increased risk of mosquito-borne diseases such as malaria. The recent UN climate report projects vector-borne diseases in Africa, such as malaria and dengue, may double by 2050 and triple by another 30 years in 2080.

DIAGNOSING MALARIA

Classical symptoms of malaria are high fever with chills, sweating, body ache, and severe shivering. The fever often goes away and then comes back every other day. Long-standing malaria enlarges the liver and the spleen.

A severe form of malaria, called *cerebral malaria* (or the brain-affecting malaria) occurs from *P. falciparum*. This disease may show other serious symptoms, including abnormal behavior, impaired consciousness or coma, seizures, and other neurological abnormalities. If the patient does a blood test, they may have severe anemia (low hemoglobin level) and low blood sugar level. A blood test can also detect the malarial parasite.

Controlling and preventing malaria

Malaria, a mosquito-borne disease, is very endemic in African countries and in Southeast Asia. Many countries have programs to control malaria and reduce malaria transmission to a level where it's no longer a public health problem. The choice of interventions depends on the malaria transmission level in the area.

Here are the four components for controlling malaria:

» **Chemical control:** Chemical insecticides are used to kill the mosquitoes such as by fogging.

» **Source reduction:** By removing containers with water or used car tires from the yard where mosquitos can reproduce.

» **Environmental control**: Eliminate the breeding places by altering the environment and making it unfavorable for mosquitoes to breed. Use chemicals (*larvicides*) to kill mosquito larvae and mosquito fish that eat mosquito larvae.

» **Personal protective measures:** Use a physical barrier to avoid getting mosquito bites.

When you're working in public health, if you or someone else plans to travel to a malaria-affected country, do the following:

• Get good advice on malaria prevention with oral antimalarial medicine before you depart for your holiday. Visit your local doctor four to six weeks before travelling into a malaria area.

• Take the oral antimalarial pills on the same day each week — weekly or at the same time of the day if daily. Continue prophylaxis for four weeks after your return.

• Apply insect repellent to exposed skin. The recommended repellents contain 20 to 35 percent diethyl-meta-toluamide (DEET).

• Wear long-sleeved clothing, trousers, and socks if you're outdoors during your visit.

• Sleep under a mosquito-proof net.

• Make sure windows and doors have screens.

• Close windows and doors at night unless they're screened.

The essential components of malaria intervention are as follows:

» **Case management:** It includes the diagnosis and treatment of malaria.

» **The use of insecticide-treated nets:** Refer to the earlier bullet about taking personal protective measures.

» **Intermittent preventive treatment of malaria for pregnant women:** Malaria infection during pregnancy can have adverse effects on both the mother and fetus, including maternal anemia, fetal loss, premature delivery, intrauterine growth retardation, and delivery of low birth-weight infants. All pregnant women in malaria-affected areas are given a curative dose of an effective antimalarial drug whether or not they're infected with the malaria parasite.

>> **Indoor residual spraying:** The mosquito vectors rest inside houses after taking a blood meal. That's the best time when indoor residual spraying with insecticides can kill these mosquitoes.

>> **Chemoprophylaxis:** It's a method of using a medicine before, during, and after you visit a malaria-prone area. Here are two medicines:

- *Doxycyline* can prevent malaria, especially in areas with chloroquine or multidrug resistant *P. falciparum*. This medicine is taken once daily beginning 1 to 2 days before travel, while in the malaria-endemic area, and for 4 weeks after leaving the area.

- *Mefloquine* is another medicine, which is taken weekly for 2 weeks before travel, during the duration of travel, and for 4 weeks after return.

West Nile disease: Not going west

The name *West Nile disease* came from the West Nile Virus (WNV), which was first isolated in a woman in the West Nile district of Uganda in 1937. The virus was also identified in birds in the Nile delta region in 1953.

The bite of an infected mosquito of the *Culex* species transmits the virus. WNV is also transmitted to birds and many other animals such as bats, horses, cats, dogs, squirrels, rabbits, and alligators in the same manner. However, no evidence suggests that a person can get the disease from live or dead infected birds, animals, or from contacts with another person.

CONNECTING WEST NILE WITH CLIMATE CHANGE

WNV cases are clustered (almost 90 percent) from July through September. High humidity isn't necessary for West Nile disease outbreaks. Many episodes of WNV disease occur during or after drought, when mosquitoes and birds are brought together in close proximity to the available water sources, facilitating transmission.

Under experimental conditions, scientists performed viral transmission of the WNV strain, which was responsible for the West Nile disease in the United States. The scientists found that the transmission was more efficient under higher-than-normal temperatures.

In another study of 16,298 cases of WNV disease reported to the CDC from 2001 to 2005, scientists found that warmer temperatures and heavy precipitation increased the incidence of the disease significantly in North America.

KNOWING SYMPTOMS AND PREVENTING WEST NILE DISEASE

The disease symptoms include high fever, severe headache, nausea, vomiting, chills, muscle pain, and muscle stiffness. A blood test may show a rising level of antibodies to WNV in an infected person. The antibody is detectable 3 to 8 days after onset of the illness and generally persists for 30 to 90 days. Viral cultures can be done on blood, the spinal fluid, and tissue specimens.

No vaccine is available for West Nile disease. The best way to prevent it is to protect oneself from mosquito bites (refer to the section, "Controlling and preventing malaria," earlier in this chapter). Many of those precautions apply when preventing West Nile disease.

Dealing with dengue

Dengue is another mosquito-borne viral disease. (The virus is an arbovirus, and the vector is an *Aedes Aegypti* mosquito.) More than 125 countries are known to be dengue endemic. That means the disease is found in those countries most of the time. The prevalence of dengue has increased more than nine-fold over the last two decades, from 505,430 cases in 2000 to more than 5.2 million in 2019. Each year, an estimated 21,000 people die from dengue.

LINKING DENGUE WITH CLIMATE CHANGE

Dengue season peaks during the time of high humidity and temperature. Scientists have found that in Mexico, dengue increased by 600 percent from 2001 to 2007. The cases increased by 2.6 percent for every 1°C (33.8 °F) increase in weekly maximum temperatures, and by 1.9 percent for every 1 cm increase in weekly precipitation.

IDENTIFYING AND PREVENTING DENGUE

Symptoms of dengue vary from mild to severe:

» **Mild cases:** Symptoms include fever, cold, cough, headache, pain behind the eyes, red eyes, muscle and joint pain, and skin rash. The rash usually appears as the fever subsides and it lasts for 2 to 4 days. Rashes appear in small patches, and they become scaly and itchy. On a blood test, the platelet counts gradually decrease, which at a certain level cause bleeding.

» **Severe cases:** The critical type of the disease is *dengue hemorrhagic fever (DHF)*, where bleeding is so severe that the patient needs blood (or platelet) transfusion. Because of profuse bleeding and decreased blood pressure, the patient can develop a more severe condition, known as *dengue shock syndrome (DSS)*.

Dengue has no specific treatment. A patient needs bed rest, fluids to prevent dehydration, and acetaminophen to control a fever.

WARNING

A patient shouldn't take aspirin, aspirin-containing drugs, and other nonsteroidal anti-inflammatory drugs (NSAIDs), such as ibuprofen and naproxen, to control fever due to dengue. These medicines increase blood loss because they have anti-coagulant properties, meaning they prevent blood clotting.

REMEMBER

To prevent dengue, follow the 4 Ss:

>> Search and destroy mosquito breeding places.

>> Secure self-protection from mosquito bites, as I discuss in the section, "Controlling and preventing malaria," earlier in this chapter.

>> Seek early treatment when signs and symptoms of dengue occur.

>> Say yes to fogging to control mosquitoes.

Challenging Chikungunya

Chikungunya is a viral disease transmitted to humans by the infected *Aedes* mosquito — the same that transmits dengue (see the previous section). As of August 2022, a total of 229,029 cases and 41 deaths have been reported worldwide. The majority of cases (88 percent) have been reported from Brazil. In the United States, most cases are among travelers visiting or returning from affected areas in Asia, Africa, or the Indian Ocean. In 2014, only 12 confirmed cases in the United States were locally acquired, meaning that they weren't brought from another place.

RELATING CHIKUNGUNYA WITH CLIMATE CHANGE

As drought and heavy rainfall events increase, the number of people infected also goes up because of the proliferation of the vector mosquitoes. Scientists have projected that the disease will steadily increase in the Gulf Coast, southern Florida, Cuba, the Yucatan peninsula, Sinaloa, and across much of the Central America.

CONTROLLING CHIKUNGUNYA

No specific antiviral treatment is available for Chikungunya. Treatment of symptoms include rest, fluid intake, and the use of fever medicines. As I discuss in the earlier section, "Identifying and preventing dengue," a person shouldn't take any NSAID for Chikungunya treatment. Reducing mosquito populations and using personal protection against mosquito bites remain the only measures for control and prevention.

Chapter **7**

Inspecting Descriptive Epidemiology: Person, Place, and Time

I n *descriptive epidemiology*, you collect, organize, summarize, and analyze data according to the person, place, and time. These three characteristics of a disease provide important information about who's affected, where the disease occurs, and when it occurs (what time of the year). If someone refers to *epidemiologic variables*, they mean the three variables of person, place, and time. With these variables, you can also identify populations that are at a greater risk of the disease being investigated.

REMEMBER

As an epidemiologist, you need to be a good observer, listener, and narrator. In many instances, epidemiology resembles detective work because your job is to find out the unknown causes of a disease. By analyzing these three variables, you can come up with a hypothesis about the cause of the disease. Then you can conduct another epidemiological study to test the hypothesis with analytical epidemiology (refer to Chapter 2 and Chapter 17 for more information). *Analytical epidemiology* attempts to determine the cause or risk factors of a health outcome.

This chapter delves deeper into descriptive epidemiology and discusses the three variables of person, place, and time factors and explains why each is important.

Knowing Person Factors

With *person* factors, you're trying to know who is getting the disease. Epidemiologists describe a disease in terms of age, gender, race/ethnicity, occupation, income, education, and so on. The following sections examine the important areas of interest on the person level.

REAL LIFE EXAMPLE

HOW DESCRIPTIVE AND ANALYTICAL EPIDEMIOLOGY WORK

An 8-year-old boy succumbed to death on January 22, 2013, and his father was critically ill and admitted in an intensive care unit of a hospital in Dhaka, Bangladesh. The family drank raw date sap brought from a village on January 11, 2013, and fell ill six days later. Drinking raw date or palm sap in the morning is an old practice, especially in winter months in rural Bangladesh. Why did this child die and what caused his father's illness? Descriptive and analytical epidemiology can help answer those questions.

First, epidemiologists described the incidence and nature of the disease among the affected people. By analyzing the descriptive statistics, epidemiologists came up with some testable hypotheses based on discovering the cause of the outbreak. The first part of their investigation was descriptive in nature and the second part analytical.

They followed the families who received the date sap from the same source and discovered that one person from the same village supplied 100 bottles of sap to families in Dhaka, and many of those families were sick. By using infrared cameras, the investigators found that the fruit bats that perch on the jars put up on trees to collect the sap also urinate in the jars. These bats carried a virus called the *Nipah virus*, which investigators determined was the cause of the disease. Since 2001, when the disease due to *Nipah virus* first broke out as an unknown disease, the virus has killed 136 of its 176 victims in 21 districts across Bangladesh.

Investigators discovered that the virus can be destroyed at 70°C (158°F) temperature. They advised the people that they shouldn't drink raw sap. They also found that people can largely prevent the spread of the disease from one person to another if the people in close contact with the infected person follow hand washing.

Age — More than just a number

Age is one of the most important variables to study because many diseases are determined by age. If you know a person's age, you can narrow down your focus about the possible causes of the symptoms. Some diseases occur mainly in younger age groups because either the infant or child's immune system isn't fully developed and/or a small dose of infection can easily affect people when they're young.

For example, here are some diseases that affect mostly younger children:

>> **Measles:** Worldwide about 134,200 children die from measles each year. The disease is easily transmitted from one person to another.

>> **Pneumonia:** Although pneumonia affects all age groups, the highest rate of pneumonia caused by *pneumococcal* infection occurs in young children and in the elderly population.

>> **Diarrhea:** Diarrhea caused by the rotavirus infection is common in young children less than 2 years of age.

The incidence of some diseases increases with age because of several factors, such as personal habit, exercise, diet, stress, exposure to the environmental pollution, and so on. For example, heart disease, blood pressure, stroke, and cancer are diseases of people older than 50. Table 7-1 lists some diseases that are common at different age groups.

TABLE 7-1   ## Diseases and Age Groups at Risk

Disease	Who Are at a Higher Risk (Age in Years)
Rotavirus diarrhea	Children younger than 2.
Measles	Children younger than 5.
Mumps	Children aged 5 to 9.
Chickenpox	Children younger than 10.
Whooping cough	Infants younger than 6 months old before they're adequately vaccinated.
Heart disease	Women after menopause and men after 50.
Hypertension	No age limit — men often develop it between 35 and 55, and women often develop hypertension after menopause.
Diabetes mellitus	Type 2 diabetes is common in people older than 40; the risk increases with age.
Osteoporosis	Type 1 osteoporosis is common in women after menopause. Senile osteoporosis or type 2 osteoporosis occurs mostly after 75.

Gender — Battle of the sexes

Gender is another significant area of interest when you look at the cause of a disease. Certain diseases are more common among women than men and *vice versa*. For example, breast cancer is more common among women. Until age 45, men are more likely to have high blood pressure. Here I focus on some reasons why gender is relevant.

Looking at how cultural gender differences play a role

The distinct roles and behaviors of men and women in a given culture give rise to gender differences. In most countries, females live longer than males. In fact, life expectancy is one of the most important indicators of a nation's health. *Life expectancy* means the average period that a person is expected to live. Table 7-2 shows a list of life expectancy at birth in different countries in 2022.

TABLE 7-2   **Estimated Life Expectancy at Birth (in Years) by Gender in 2022**

Country	Male	Female	Total Population
Five countries having high life expectancy			
Monaco	85.4	93.1	89.2
Japan	83.2	90.1	86.5
Singapore	83.8	89.4	86.5
Macao	81.7	87.7	84.7
San Marino	81.0	86.4	83.6
Five countries having low life expectancy			
Gabon	52.5	53.2	52.8
Guinea-Bissau	50.6	54.9	52.7
Chad	51.1	53.8	52.4
South Africa	53.3	51.0	52.1
Namibia	51.5	49.6	50.6

Public health measures are credited with much of the recent increases in life expectancy. For example, during the early 1600s in England, life expectancy was only about 35 years, largely because two-thirds of all children died before the age of 4. In the United States, the life expectancy for the total population increased by almost ten years, from 69.7 years in 1960 to 79.4 years in 2015. This increase can be attributed largely to advances in public health. However, the life expectancy in the United States declined by 1.5 years from 2019 to 2020 — the greatest decrease happened among White Americans, which could be related to increased death tolls at the early stage of the Covid-19 pandemic when no effective vaccines were yet available.

Recognizing the differences in genders

Overall, women tend to have a lower death rate at a given age. Although epidemiologists don't have many answers to why a gender gap exists in life expectancy or why women live longer than men, they do focus mostly on a biologic cause. Furthermore, men generally are more risk takers and prone to unintentional injuries. Men tend to smoke and drink more often and in a heavier amount than women in many societies. Men are also more exposed to extraneous conditions because of the nature of their jobs.

Sometimes hormonal difference between men and women can contribute to the difference in some disease occurrences, which can help women in some instances and hurt them in others. For example, women are less vulnerable to heart disease than men before age 55; however, after menopause when the female sex hormone estrogen begins to decline, women's rate of heart disease kicks in.

Some diseases tend to affect women more, perhaps because of those hormonal differences. In addition to mood swings, sleep disorders, migraines, irregular periods, hot flashes, and weight changes, women also face the following ailments at a higher level than men because of hormones:

>> **Osteoporosis:** With this degenerative bone disease women lose bone mass much more quickly in the years immediately after menopause than they do at any other time in their lives.

>> **Asthma:** The disease is more life threatening in women than in men. Scientists aren't exactly sure why, but they believe that it has to do with hormones. Until puberty, more boys than girls develop this condition. However, after puberty the girls develop the condition more than boys.

Although women do generally live longer than men, women still face issues, such as differences in food distribution and level of healthcare that affect their overall life expectancy. In certain societies in developing countries, males get preferential share of intra-family food distribution, meaning that they get better nutritious foods compared to females.

My research group studied why girls died more often than boys due to the same illness in an intensive care unit (ICU) of a diarrheal disease hospital in Bangladesh. We found that males were admitted at a higher proportion than females at that hospital. Also, the time between the onset of illness and hospital admission was longer among females than their male counterparts, suggesting preferential healthcare for males in that society.

Race/ethnicity — Inequalities exist

Epidemiologists have observed racial disparity with several diseases and health events. *Racial disparity in health* refers to inequalities in disease conditions and deaths and the quantity and quality of healthcare by racial and ethnic differentials. For example, the incidence of prostate cancer is four times more likely in Black men than White men. Breast cancer incidence is more common among White females; however, more Black women die of breast cancer than White women.

These racial and ethnic disparities in disease incidence are more likely due to differences in the following:

>> **Access to healthcare:** Low-income and minority populations often suffer from a lack of access to regular healthcare and preventive services due to lack of health insurance, lack of transportation, or their inability to meet out-of-pocket expenses.

>> **Socioeconomic status:** Because of poor economic conditions, people are reluctant to seek healthcare unless the condition is more severe and often complicated. Some other social determinants such as low educational attainment, and lack of access to healthy food may also determine health disparities.

>> **Discrimination in healthcare:** Healthcare providers usually treat everybody equally; however, there are situations where factors such as *unconscious bias* (also called *implicit bias*), combined with lack of healthcare, poor patient-provider communication, and poor education may result in discrimination associated with race, body size, and gender.

>> **Exposure to environmental pollutants:** Poor living conditions are likely to be contaminated with environmental pollutants. Unsanitary housing conditions, lack of electricity, improper disposal of garbage, overcrowding, and a number of other adverse environmental conditions prevail in a growing number of blighted areas in big cities in developing countries. These unhealthy living conditions invite diseases.

>> **Personal habits:** People of underserved communities and minorities are more likely to practice unhealthy lifestyles. *Personal habits*, such as smoking, drinking, and lack of exercise are preventable causes of heart disease, stroke, and many cancers. Drinking and not wearing seatbelts are causes of unintentional injuries and death among adolescents.

Occupation — A person's job matters

A distinct area of public health called *occupational medicine* or *industrial hygiene* has emerged because a large number of diseases occur in association with occupation. People's working conditions, long work hours, unprotected clothing, and stress can trigger unhealthy work environments and invite diseases.

TECHNICAL STUFF

Several lung diseases occur due to exposure to dusts from industries. These diseases are referred to as *pneumoconiosis* with the Greek words *pneumon* referring to *lung* and *konis* meaning *dust*. Pneumoconiosis is a group of lung diseases caused by the inhalation of dusts. Only microscopic sized dust particles, about $1/5,000$ of an inch or smaller, can easily pass through the respiratory system and lodge into the tiniest air sacs called *alveoli* and develop an inflammatory process in the lung.

The following list includes common occupational lung diseases due to inhalation of dusts:

>> **Asbestosis:** This disease occurs due to the inhalation of asbestos fiber dust.

>> **Bagassosis:** This disease occurs due to the inhalation of sugarcane fiber dust.

>> **Berylliosis:** This disease occurs due to the inhalation of beryllium dust.

>> **Byssinosis:** This disease occurs due to the inhalation of cotton dust.

>> **Siderosis:** This disease occurs due to the inhalation of iron dust.

>> **Silicosis:** This disease occurs due to the inhalation of silica or sand dust, also known as *grinder's disease*.

Many other diseases occur as a result of working conditions, including coal miners' disease, Meniere's syndrome, carpel tunnel syndrome, tennis elbow, farmer's lung, wool slaughter's disease, and Raynaud's syndrome. The following sections provide some details on a few of them.

Coal miners' disease

People who work in jobs where they're exposed to coal dust get a chronic lung condition called *progressive fibrosis of the lung* or more commonly *coal miners' disease.* Inhaled coal dusts settle deep in their lungs and harden the lung tissue. As the lungs harden, breathing becomes more difficult and worsens over time. The lungs become black due to deposition of carbon. This disease doesn't have a treatment or cure. Several complications worsen the condition as the disease progresses including heart failure, respiratory failure, tuberculosis, and lung cancer.

Meniere's disease

Meniere's disease affects the middle ear, causing hearing defect, vertigo, *tinnitus* (buzzing in the ear), and loss of hearing due to excessive noise pollution or other causes. People who operate machinery that produces excessive noise without using any noise protectors can develop the symptoms. In patients with Meniere's disease, hearing tests usually indicate a sensory type of hearing loss in the affected ear. Some medication, surgery, and dietary changes can help control or improve the symptoms.

Carpal tunnel syndrome

Carpal tunnel syndrome is a condition in which pressure on the *median nerve,* the nerve in the wrist that supplies feeling and movement to parts of the hand, can lead to numbness, tingling, weakness, or muscle damage in the hand and fingers. Many people develop this syndrome by making the same hand and wrist motion over and over. Some occupations, such as typing, repeating movement of hands, playing an instrument, or playing sports, may cause carpal tunnel syndrome. In addition, using hand tools that vibrate may cause the syndrome.

Farmer's lung

In villages, farmers store hay and paddy straw in their yard or in their fields for months for the use as animal fodder. This hay and straw can grow mold. After inhaling the mold and dust from hay and other agricultural products, farmers get an allergic reaction in the lung, called *hypersensitivity pneumonitis* or *farmer's lung.* Common symptoms for farmer's lung include chronic cough, tiredness, or depression.

Income — Money makes the world go 'round

Income and occupation are often interrelated. However, income can also be an independent risk factor for a disease or a health condition because low-income people are often victims of adverse health behaviors such as tobacco use, alcohol consumption, and lack of physical exercise. The rate of suicide, depression, and other psychological illnesses are more common among people coming from low-income families. Low-income populations often live in poor living conditions.

My research team had some personal experience in dealing with data on lead poisoning. In our study of lead poisoning in children in Mississippi, we observed that the rate of lead poisoning was significantly higher among people from lower income families who lived in houses built before the 1950s.

Education — Knowledge is power

A better education is directly related with better healthcare and a higher quality of life. Scientists have convincingly demonstrated that a mother's education influences her child's health. National surveys and censuses conducted in developing countries have shown maternal education level to be a strong and consistent predictor of reduced child mortality and morbidity, as these three studies demonstrate:

>> In Uganda, infants whose mothers had a secondary education were at least 50 percent less likely to miss scheduled vaccinations compared to those infants whose mothers only had a primary education.

>> In Ethiopia, children with mothers who have a secondary education have survival rates twice as high as children with mothers with only a primary education.

>> In Bangladesh, my research team's study effectively showed that the nutritional status of a child improved when mothers had knowledge of food and nutrition and provided a healthy diet for the child.

Focusing on Place Factors

By knowing the relationship of diseases with place, you can demonstrate the physical conditions that favor transmission of the disease. *Place* means the geographic location of a country, state, or region, the housing, the workplace, the school, and the physical environment. It's important to know the proximity of homes to the risk factors and housing conditions that may increase the risk. For example, if a house is located near an industry that discharges obnoxious smells in the air, people living in the area may get adverse health conditions. These sections examine a couple ways that epidemiologists use place to determine how a disease agent is distributed in a locality and how the physical conditions favor disease transmission.

Spot mapping

Spot mapping, also referred to as *hot-spot analysis*, helps police identify high-crime areas, types of crimes being committed, and the best way to detect crimes. Similarly, spot mapping of diseases and associated risk factors can help epidemiologists identify areas to target resources and who should intervene for a possible benefit.

REMEMBER

As an epidemiologist, you should know applications of spot mapping to identify areas where certain health conditions, diseases, or deaths are prevailing. You may suggest interventions more effectively if you know which localities are more important to target. You may use a special tool called a geographic information system (GIS) to put information on a map (see the next section for more details).

Place may be important in diagnosing malaria because it occurs more frequently in some parts of the world, especially in African countries. One of my friends developed high fever with chills and rigor immediately after he returned from Nigeria. After careful examination and a blood test, he was found to be positive for *Falciparum malariae*, an organism that causes a serious type of malaria.

Spot mapping the cases of malaria in the world can help in identifying areas at risk of malaria. Figure 7-1 shows countries where malaria is more commonly found. You can see that all cases of malaria are limited to Africa, south of the Sahara Desert, central and southeastern Asia, eastern Asia and Oceania, and Central and South America.

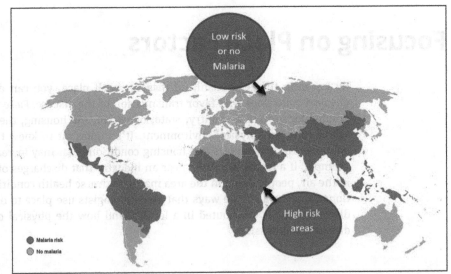

FIGURE 7-1: A map showing countries where malaria is prevalent.

© Amal Mitra

Using GIS

GIS is an excellent technology for the collection, storage, analysis, manipulation, and presentation of a geographical location. Epidemiologists use this technology a lot to learn about a disease. For example, they often get help from a GIS specialist to spot map the location of cases or deaths from a disease to correlate an environmental factor, such as the amount of an air pollutant with a disease or event or sometimes to monitor a real-time pattern of a disease in relation to its environmental conditions.

GIS consists of three things:

>> **Database:** First, you use a spreadsheet (for example, Excel) to store data about the important variables.

>> **Map information:** You need a map of the locality in which to plot the data.

>> **A computer-based link between them:** You need a mechanism (such as GIS) by which you can link the computer-based data with the map.

REAL LIFE EXAMPLE

My research team collected data on incidences of lead poisoning and locations of older houses in Mississippi and attempted to find out if people living in older houses are likely to have more children with high levels of lead in their blood. As expected, we found a good correlation between the two. We used GIS to display the data. In Figure 7-2, you can see that Forrest and Oktibbeha counties had the most number of children with high blood lead levels. High lead levels can lead to physical and neurological damages. At the time blood lead levels greater than or equal to 5 µg/dL were considered high. However, now blood levels greater than or equal to 3.5 µg/dL are considered high. Using this mapping, we provided health education programs for people in targeted areas where lead poisoning cases were higher.

To use the map, check the bottom left legend for the blood levels of lead (BLL), and then check what areas in the map are marked darker than others. The darker areas (or counties) on the map are at higher risk of having children with lead poisoning.

CONSIDERING A GIS SPECIALIST DEGREE?

In epidemiology, a geographic information system (GIS) specialist is very demanding. Epidemiologists and GIS specialists work hand-in-hand to assess a community's health needs, to find out risk factors for a disease, and to examine the effect of an intervention. Becoming a GIS specialist is a good career choice. You can also be an epidemiologist and a GIS specialist at the same time.

(continued)

(continued)

A number of college programs and private agencies offer a degree, certificate programs, or short courses on GIS. Graduate certificate and master's degree seekers should look for a hands-on approach in project-oriented courses that provide students with a better understanding of how to plan, implement, and execute a GIS project. You can also take some free training courses from ESRI (makers of the GIS software) by visiting www.esri.com/training/.

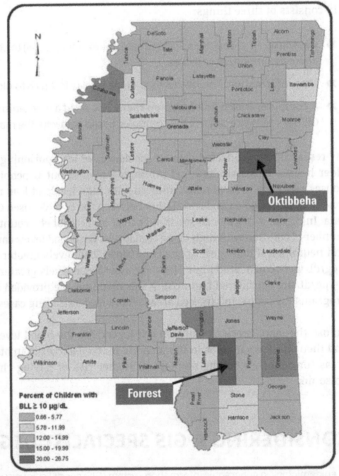

FIGURE 7-2:
A GIS map showing percentage of children with high blood levels of lead in Mississippi.

Percent of Children with
BLL ≥ 10 µg/dL
- 0.66 - 5.77
- 5.78 - 11.99
- 12.00 - 14.99
- 15.00 - 19.99
- 20.00 - 26.75

© Amal Mitra

Checking Time Factors

Diseases fluctuate over time. Some disease incidences change in a short period of time, which epidemiologists can monitor by the seasonal pattern of diseases. Some diseases appear every few years in a cyclic pattern. By knowing when diseases occur, epidemiologists can better predict a disease well ahead of time and can get ready to fight it. These sections identify various terms used to delineate the extent of a disease in an area over time and explain them with some real-life examples.

Defining endemic diseases

Endemic diseases refer to the constant presence or usual prevalence of diseases or infectious agents within a given geographic area or population group. Examples of endemic diseases include diarrheal diseases and respiratory infections in Bangladesh; common cold incidences in most countries during winter; and malaria in African, Asian, Latin American, and Middle Eastern countries. Some of the diseases can be endemic in some parts of a country, such as goiter, which is endemic in northern Bangladesh.

REMEMBER

By identifying the endemic nature of diseases in a locality, you can find out an outbreak of the disease based on the number of cases over time.

Finding sporadic diseases

Cases are *sporadic* if the number of a disease or an event is scattered in time and small in number. For instance, snakes can be active almost any time of the year in the south, such as Mississippi. Most snakebites occur when weather warms in the spring until about the month of October. Epidemiologists call this a *seasonal pattern.* However, if you hear about two cases of snakebites in the month of January or February in some parts of the country, it would be considered sporadic in nature.

Because many vaccines almost eradicated several diseases, cases of tetanus, diphtheria, and rabies are considered examples of sporadic disease in the United States.

Discovering epidemics

An *epidemic* is an unusual increase in the number of cases of an infectious disease that already exists in a certain region or population. You can't use a unique number to constitute an epidemic. It depends upon the endemic nature of the disease, which means how many cases you normally see in a particular place at a particular time. For example, in Bangladesh where cholera is common throughout the year, several cases of cholera occurring in a single day may be considered endemic, whereas only two or three cases of cholera in New York City may constitute an epidemic.

REMEMBER

Here are two types of epidemics:

» **Common source epidemic:** A *common source epidemic*, also referred to as a *point source epidemic*, occurs when a group of people is exposed to a single common source of infection at a single place and time. John Snow's study of cholera epidemic in London in 1854 is a classic example (see Chapter 4). He demonstrated that the people who drank contaminated water from London's Broad Street pump got cholera, and consequently the removal of the handle of the water pump led to the cessation of the epidemic. Figure 7-3 shows the curve of the epidemic.

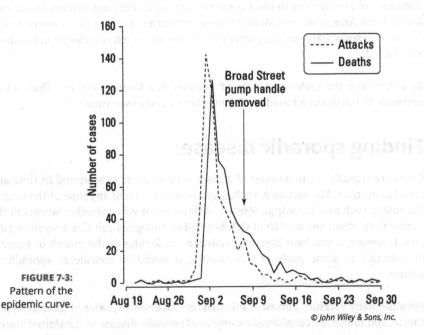

FIGURE 7-3:
Pattern of the epidemic curve.

© John Wiley & Sons, Inc.

TECHNICAL STUFF

A waterborne outbreak, such as cholera outbreak that's spread through a contaminated community water supply, is a common source outbreak. The epidemic curve of a common source outbreak shows a tight temporal clustering, with a sharp upslope and a gentler down slope (as you can see in Figure 7-3).

>> **Propagated source of epidemic:** A *propagated epidemic* occurs when an infection is spread from person to person, either directly or via a vector. An example of a propagated source epidemic is an outbreak of hepatitis B virus infection. Figure 7-4 shows a propagated source epidemic curve — the curve gradually increases, with a peak in about 25 days, and then falls rapidly thereafter.

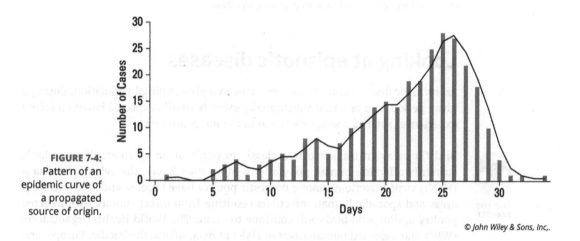

FIGURE 7-4:
Pattern of an epidemic curve of a propagated source of origin.

© John Wiley & Sons, Inc,.

Considering pandemics

A *pandemic* refers to an epidemic that encompasses the boundary of a country and affects several countries or regions at a given time. Here are examples of some pandemics:

>> **Covid-19:** The pandemic that started in 2019 has affected more than 225 countries and territories. As of mid-January 2023, about 671.5 million cases and 6.7 million deaths have occurred worldwide. The United States alone has had more than 103.5 million cases and 1.1 million deaths.

>> **HIV/AIDS:** Nearly every country in the world has been affected, with more than 38 million people currently living with HIV.

>> **Cholera:** This pandemic has affected humans for at least a millennium and persists as a major cause of illness and death in the developing world.

>> **Influenza:** In 1918, influenza infected 500 million people across the world, killing 50 to 100 million.

Influenza A viruses continuously undergo antigenic evolution. They do so by two main mechanisms:

- *Antigenic drift* causes regular influenza epidemics.

- *Antigenic shift* is the cause of occasional global outbreaks of influenza (pandemics). Antigenic shift is the process by which two or more different strains of a virus, or strains of two or more different viruses, combine to form a new subtype that's more virulent.

Looking at epizootic diseases

An *epizootic* disease appears as new cases in a given animal population, during a given period, at a rate that substantially exceeds what's expected based on recent experience (such as a sharp elevation in the incidence rate).

REAL LIFE EXAMPLE

Bird flu or avian influenza is a classic example of an epizootic disease that's currently affecting human populations. More than likely, the avian influenza A (H5N1) virus infections among domestic poultry have become endemic in certain areas and sporadic human infections resulting from direct contact with infected poultry and/or wild birds will continue to occur. The World Health Organization (WHO) has reported human cases of H5N1 in Asia, Africa, the Pacific, Europe, and the Near East. Indonesia and Vietnam have reported the highest number of H5N1 cases to date. Overall mortality in reported H5N1 cases is approximately 60 percent. The majority of cases have occurred among children and adults younger than 40 years old. Studies have documented the most significant risk factors for human H5N1 infection to be direct contact with sick or dead poultry or wild birds or visiting a live poultry market.

Changing patterns by seasonality

Diseases differ by season. For example, viral infections, such as the common cold, influenza, chickenpox, allergic rhinitis, bronchial asthma, and pneumonia, are common during the winter. Acute symptoms of chronic obstructive pulmonary disease (COPD) manifest during winter months. The cases of cholera are more pronounced in winter months. On the other hand, food poisoning is typically more common in the hot summer months because hot and humid weather creates an ideal condition for bacterial growth, leading to food contamination.

Differentiating between outbreak and cluster

Epidemiologists can differentiate between two types of diseases and determine whether the diseases are acute in nature and infectious and whether the diseases are noninfectious and noncommunicable. Epidemiologists use the following classifications:

» **Outbreak:** This term in epidemiology describes an occurrence of a disease greater than usual. The outbreak may affect a small and localized group or impact thousands of people across an entire continent. Outbreaks may also refer to *epidemics,* which affect a region in a country or a group of countries. Outbreaks usually refer to diseases due to infectious agents. For example, an unusual number of cases of foodborne gastroenteritis (due to an infectious agent) from eating in a restaurant is an outbreak.

» **Cluster:** This term refers to chronic diseases such as stroke and heart disease that occur near the same time in a given place. If you find a situation where several cases of suicide happened in a shorter period of time, you may call it a cluster of suicide.

Chapter **8**

Viewing Disease Patterns

The search for the leading causes of human diseases and the leading causes of deaths goes back to antiquity. Almost all countries in the world have enjoyed more than a century of nearly uninterrupted rise in longevity. For example, a baby born in the United States in 1900 could hope to live on an average 46 years (for males) to 48 years (for females). After 100 years, in 2000, a baby in the United States can expect to live approximately 77 years. Have you thought about the reasons behind it happened? This chapter explains the reasons.

When you hear a child in India died of cholera, you probably aren't surprised because cholera is common in India. However, if you hear news that two cases of cholera were found in Mississippi because of a disrupted water system for more than a week and that people have been warned against drinking from the supply water, you'd be panicky. That's because you don't expect cholera to reemerge in any parts of the United States at this time. This chapter also examines what diseases scientists have conquered and what contributions public health and medical science have made toward controlling deaths and advancing life expectancy of the people.

Defining the Epidemiologic Transition

The history of diseases tells you how diseases evolved over time, what factors contributed to the changes in disease pattern, and how those changes affect human life and longevity. With the invention of modern medicine and people's lifestyle changes, the disease pattern and major causes of deaths have changed.

In general, chronic and noncommunicable diseases and conditions have replaced acute and infectious diseases as the major causes of morbidity and mortality in contemporary developed nations. Also, the overall death rate from all causes declined drastically and life expectancy increased over the past 100 years. These changes in disease pattern and mortality and the corresponding increase in life expectancy are called the *epidemiologic transition.*

For example, in the United States, the overall death rate has declined from 745.2 per 100,000 population in 1990 to 715.2 per 100,000 population in 2019. However, because of the Covid-19 pandemic, the overall death rate in the United States increased to 1,027.0 per 100,000 population in 2022.

The life expectancy at birth increased dramatically from 46.6 years in 1900 to 79.9 years in 2020. Again, because of Covid-19–related deaths, the life expectancy dropped to 79.05 in 2022.

The following sections discuss changes in disease pattern in the United States and in developing countries and analyze possible factors for such changes.

Seeing how leading causes of death have changed

Public health came into shape in the second half of the 19th century in the United States. In the early 1900s, public health developments were rudimentary. Healthcare was virtually unregulated and health insurance nonexistent. Infectious diseases, such as pneumonia, tuberculosis, and diarrhea were the three top killer diseases, accounting to 54 percent of all deaths in 1900 (refer to Figure 8-1a).

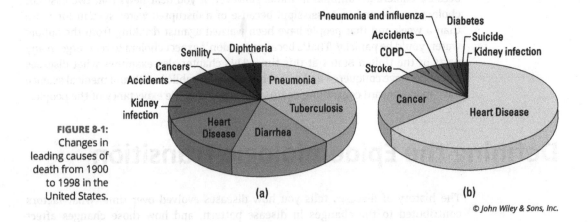

FIGURE 8-1: Changes in leading causes of death from 1900 to 1998 in the United States.

(a)   (b)

© John Wiley & Sons, Inc.

Heart disease occupied the fourth position in 1900, whereas if you look at the 1998 graph (refer to Figure 8-1b), heart disease was at the top position in the causes of death. Cancer and stroke deaths followed heart disease. You may also find that infectious diseases, such as pneumonia and influenza, are almost at the bottom of the top list of deaths in 1998.

However, the situation changed dramatically after Covid-19 appeared in 2019 and became a pandemic in 2020. According to the top 10 causes of death in the United States in 2022, Covid-19 occupies the third position, after heart disease and cancer. Here are the leading causes of death in 2022 (they're listed based on the number of annual deaths, with heart disease causing the highest number of deaths of all):

>> Heart disease

>> Cancer

>> Covid-19

>> Accidents

>> Stroke

>> Chronic obstructive pulmonary diseases, such as chronic bronchitis and emphysema

>> Alzheimer's disease

>> Diabetes

>> Influenza and pneumonia

>> Kidney disease (nephritis, nephrotic syndrome, and nephrosis)

This list shows that the majority of the causes of deaths are due to chronic diseases, except Covid-19, accidents, influenza and pneumonia, and kidney disease.

Considering causes of death in the world

According to the World Health Organization list of leading causes of death globally in 2019, noncommunicable diseases have taken over the lead. Only three infectious diseases out of the top ten causes of deaths are pneumonia, neonatal conditions, and diarrhea around the world. Covid-19 didn't yet appear as one of the major causes of death in 2019.

The major three diseases causing one-third of all deaths are heart disease (16 percent), stroke (11 percent), and COPD (6 percent). Here is a list of the top 10 killer diseases in the world in 2019:

- » Heart disease
- » Stroke
- » COPD
- » Pneumonia
- » Neonatal conditions
- » Lung cancer
- » Alzheimer's disease
- » Diarrhea
- » Diabetes
- » Kidney disease

Transitioning stages in some developing countries

The transition from infectious diseases to chronic and noncommunicable diseases has been slower in developing countries compared to that in the developed nations. Infectious diseases are still rampant in most developing countries. For example, the leading causes of death in Bangladesh, India, and nearly all African countries are still mostly due to infectious diseases. Table 8-1 compares the top ten killer diseases in Bangladesh, India, and Nigeria in 2000.

Among the three countries mentioned, the case of Nigeria is most striking — the top seven are infectious diseases. In both Bangladesh and India, a few chronic diseases, such as heart disease, stroke, and COPD, occupy the list.

TABLE 8-1: Top Ten Killer Diseases in Selected Developing Countries

Bangladesh	India	Nigeria
Neonatal conditions (mostly infections)	Diarrhea	Neonatal conditions (mostly infections)
Tuberculosis	Neonatal conditions (mostly infections)	Diarrhea
Stroke	Heart disease	Malaria

Bangladesh	India	Nigeria
Diarrhea	Pneumonia	Measles
Pneumonia	COPD	Pneumonia
Heart disease	Tuberculosis	Tuberculosis
COPD	Stroke	HIV/AIDS
Cirrhosis of liver	Cirrhosis of liver	Stroke
Drowning	Asthma	Heart disease
Measles	Suicide	Accidents

Grasping Why Epidemiologic Transition Happens

Advances in medical science and public health get the credit for the decline in infectious diseases and overall mortality and thereby the increase in life expectancy of people around the globe. As I discuss in the section, "Defining the Epidemiologic Transition," earlier in this chapter, some of the major achievements of health science have greatly reduced many infectious diseases and also prevented or eradicated some diseases.

Here are some of the specific public health measures that were pivotal in the containment of infectious disease:

>> **The discovery of antibiotics:** Since the discovery of penicillin in 1928, the treatment with antibiotics had greatly reduced the number of deaths from acute infections.

>> **The discovery and use of vaccines:** Vaccines have eradicated some diseases like smallpox. A number of other diseases, such as diphtheria, whooping cough, tetanus, and measles, have been greatly reduced. Polio is close to being eradicated due to the effectiveness of the polio vaccine around the world. (Chapter 12 discusses vaccines in greater detail.)

>> **Improved sanitation:** Many communicable diseases, such as helminthic infections, shigellosis, and others, enter the human body through the fecal-oral route. Proper sanitation can control such diseases.

>> **Safe drinking water:** Safe drinking water can reduce waterborne diseases, such as diarrhea, enteric fever, hepatitis, and so on.

>> **Improved nutrition:** Healthy food builds up a person's immunity and protects them from illnesses. Malnutrition and infectious diseases are a vicious cycle, meaning malnutrition brings more infections and infections cause more malnutrition. This cycle is more obvious among children who easily get sick if they're malnourished and their nutritional status goes down when the child is affected by several infections. Improving nutritional status can reduce many infections.

>> **Hand washing:** The simple practice of hand washing with soap can protect a person from spreading diseases or getting infections. Many infectious diseases such as Covid-19, flu, diarrheal diseases, and others can be prevented by proper hand washing.

TIP

Because of the importance of hand washing in disease prevention, the Centers for Disease Control and Prevention (CDC) maintain a website on "When and How to Wash Your Hands" in several languages at www.cdc.gov/handwashing/when-how-handwashing.html.

HAND WASHING 101

If you plan to work in public health, teaching people easy ways they can protect themselves from spreading diseases or getting infected can be a daily part of your job. Here are some tips for people to know when to wash their hands:

- Before, during, and after preparing food
- Before and after eating food
- Before and after caring for someone at home who is sick with vomiting or diarrhea
- Before and after treating a cut or wound
- After using the toilet
- After changing diapers or cleaning up a child who has used the toilet
- After blowing your nose, coughing, or sneezing
- After touching an animal, animal feed, or animal waste
- After handling pet food or pet treats
- After touching garbage

Here are the steps to hand washing:

1. **Wet hands with clean, running water.**

2. **Apply soap and rub hands, between the fingers, and under the nails.**

3. **Scrub for at least 20 seconds.**

4. **Rinse well under clean, running water.**

5. **Dry using a clean towel or air dry them.**

Studying Some Chronic Health Conditions

As a student of epidemiology, you're aware of the impact chronic diseases have on the worldwide populations. Here I examine a few chronic diseases that are prevalent in the United States and other countries. I also shed some light on the prevention of these diseases.

Hypertension

Hypertension, also referred to as high blood pressure, is a condition that's caused by many diseases. Sometimes, the cause of hypertension is unknown. At the same time hypertension may cause some other diseases as well.

The normal blood pressure (BP) of an adult is less than 120/80 mm of Hg (*Hg* means the mercury pressure). Here's what these two numbers mean:

>> **Systolic blood pressure:** This is top of the two numbers.

>> **Diastolic blood pressure:** This is the bottom number.

The following sections delve deeper into what you need to know about hypertension as an epidemiology student.

Naming the four categories of hypertension

The American College of Cardiology and the American Heart Association divide blood pressure into these four general categories:

>> **Normal BP:** BP is less than 120/80 mm of Hg.

>> **Elevated BP:** The systolic ranges from 120 to 129 mm Hg and the diastolic is above 80 mm Hg.

>> **Stage 1 hypertension:** The systolic BP ranges from 130 to 139 mm Hg or the diastolic BP is between 80 to 89 mm Hg.

>> **Stage 2 hypertension:** The systolic BP is 140 mm Hg or higher or the diastolic BP is 90 mm Hg or higher.

REMEMBER

Prior to labeling a person with hypertension, you should use an average of two or more readings obtained on two or more occasions.

Keep an eye open for these disguises:

>> **White coat hypertension:** In this type of hypertension, the BP is high during a doctor office visit, but it's normal at home.

>> **Masked hypertension:** It's just the opposite of white coat hypertension. In this case, a person's BP is high at home but is normal during a doctor's office visit.

Identifying risk factors of having hypertension

Excessive pressure damages blood vessels as well as many body organs. Some of these damages are noticed in the form of heart disease, stroke, heart failure and other symptoms such as heart pain (called angina) or a heart attack:

>> Research suggests that a 20 mm Hg higher systolic BP and 10 mm Hg higher diastolic BP are each associated with a doubling in the risk of death from stroke, heart disease, or other vascular diseases.

>> In people 30 years and older, higher systolic BP and diastolic BP are associated with an increased risk for heart disease, heart pain, myocardial infarction (heart muscle damage leading to heart attack), heart failure, and stroke.

Considering the causes of hypertension

Sometimes a doctor can detect the causes of a person's high BP. But often the cause is unknown. Based on whether the cause is known or not, high BP is divided into two groups:

>> **Essential hypertension:** Also called *primary hypertension,* the cause of high BP is unknown. Researchers think that genetics and an unhealthy lifestyle are responsible for it. Risk factors include smoking, drinking too much alcohol, stress, being overweight, eating too much salt, and not exercising enough.

>> **Secondary hypertension:** The cause of this type of hypertension is known. Most often, abnormalities of the kidney, such as narrowing of the kidney blood vessels, kidney stones, swelling of the kidney (*hydronephrosis*) cause it.

Other causes include obstructive sleep apnea (OSA), hormone abnormalities (thyroid and adrenal hormones), and side effects of medicines (diet medicines, birth control pills, and antidepressants).

Managing hypertension

Elevated blood pressure tends to get worse over time unless it's properly managed. That's why it's important for a person to regularly check and control their blood pressure. Elevated BP doesn't have symptoms; therefore, the only way to detect is to check BP regularly. An early morning checkup can give a more accurate reading of BP. A person can check it at home with a home blood pressure monitoring device. Lifestyle, such as eating a healthy diet and exercising regularly, can keep BP under control.

REMEMBER

People with high BP should limit their intake of salt. In general, Americans (also Asians) eat more salts. The 2020–2025 Dietary Guidelines for Americans suggest that people of all ages should limit salt intake to the Chronic Disease Risk Reduction (CDRR) levels as follows: 1,200 mg/day for ages 1 through 3; 1,500 mg/day for ages 4 through 8; 1,800 mg/day for ages 9 through 13; and 2,300 mg/day (less than one teaspoon) for all other age groups. Anyone with high BP, diabetes, and chronic kidney disease should limit daily salt intake to 1,500 mg/day.

Cholesterol and cardiovascular diseases

Increased levels of cholesterol remain one of the main culprits of cardiovascular diseases (CVDs). Cholesterol comes from food and the body and in two forms:

>> **Low density lipoprotein (LDL):** Generally called bad cholesterol. Too much LDL can clog arteries, which leads to CVDs.

>> **High density lipoprotein (HDL):** Generally called good cholesterol. More HDL lowers the risk for CVDs.

These sections explain what you need to know about cholesterol and CVDs.

Assessing risks — American Heart Association Guideline for LSS

When working in public health, you can direct populations to conduct a self-assessment of where they stand in the Life's Simple Seven (LSS) levels. Try to maintain an ideal level of LSS, as Table 8-2 demonstrates.

TABLE 8-2: **American Heart Association Guidelines for Life's Simple Seven (LSS)**

Factors	Ideal level	Intermediate level	Poor level
Body mass index (BMI)	Less than 25	25 to 29.9	More than and equal to 30
Physical activity	Moderate activity: 150 min or more per week; or vigorous activity: 75 min or more per week	Moderate activity: less than 150 min per week; or vigorous activity: less than 75 min per week	No physical activities
Smoking	Never smoker	Quit smoking within past 1 year	Current smoker
Blood pressure	Systolic >120, diastolic 80	Systolic between 120 – 140; diastolic between 89 – 90	Systolic 140 or more; diastolic 90 or more
Fasting sugar	Less than 100 mg/dL	100 or more mg/dL	126 or more mg/dL
Hemoglobin A1C	Less than 5.7	5.7 to less than 6.5	More than 6.5
Total cholesterol	Less than 200 mg/dL	200 to less than 240 mg/dL	240 and more mg/dL

In addition to the problem of high cholesterol, several other risk factors such as high BP, physical inactivity, obesity or being overweight, too much alcohol intake, unhealthy diet, diabetes, and genetics are independent risk factors for CVDs.

Controlling CVDs

Several factors such as early and improved treatments, awareness of the risk factors, and healthy lifestyle choices can curtail the incidence and complications of CVDs. In fact, the incidence of CVDs has slowed down in the United States; however, the CVD rates are still disproportionately high among Blacks compared to Whites. Researchers have uncovered genetic variants that make African Americans more susceptible to high blood pressure and increased CVDs.

After adjusting for socio-demographics and unhealthy dietary pattern characteristics, people in the U.S. southern states had a 56 percent greater hazard of CVDs. These diets are characterized by high salt, added fats, fried food, eggs, organ and processed meats, and sugar-sweetened beverages. People should be warned about their salt intake and unhealthy diets to control high BP and CVDs.

REMEMBER

Advise people to follow the LSS steps to improve heart health:

>> Reduce obesity.

>> Reduce cholesterol.

>> Reduce blood pressure.

>> Reduce blood sugar.

>> Stop smoking.

>> Exercise.

>> Eat a healthy diet.

Diabetes

Diabetes and heart disease work hand-in-hand. According to a CDC report, racial and ethnic minority groups are disproportionately affected by diabetes compared to non-Hispanic whites. Ethnic minorities suffer a greater burden of the disease, exhibit poorer self-management abilities, and experience worse complications and death due to diabetes compared to non-Hispanic whites.

Understanding how diabetes can lead to hypertension

Over time, high blood sugar can damage blood vessels and the nerves that control the heart. People with diabetes are also more likely to have other conditions such as hypertension. Hypertension increases the force of blood through the arteries and can damage artery walls. The combination of diabetes and hypertension increases the risk of heart disease. Furthermore, people with diabetes tend to develop heart disease at a younger age than people without diabetes. Adults with diabetes are nearly twice as likely to have heart disease or stroke as adults without diabetes.

Managing diabetes

When you're working in the public health field, tell your clients about the ABCs to manage their diabetes, which stands for the following:

>> **A for A1C:** A1C levels in the blood give an average blood sugar in the past three months. The ideal A1C level should be below 5.7 percent. The level increases with the increase of blood sugar and also with the increase of age. High levels of blood sugar can hurt the heart, blood vessels, kidney, feet, and eyes.

- **B for blood pressure:** High blood pressure forces a person's heart to work hard. Controlling blood pressure keeps the heart healthy.

- **C for cholesterol:** Cholesterol is a silent killer of the heart. It gradually increases plaque formation of the heart vessels, making blockage and poor blood supply to the heart. Lack of blood supply can damage the heart muscles, leading to heart attack.

- **S for stop smoking:** Smoking and diabetes narrow the heart blood vessels. Stop smoking to reduce blood pressure. E-cigarettes aren't a safer option.

Obesity

Being overweight or being obese can make it harder to manage diabetes and increase the risk for many health problems, including heart disease and high blood pressure. If a person is overweight, a healthy eating plan with fewer calories and more physical activity often will lower blood sugar levels and reduce the need for diabetes medicines.

Excess belly fat, even if the person isn't overweight, can increase their risk of developing heart disease.

TIP

A person has excess belly fat if their waist measures:

- **For men:** more than 40 inches

- **For women:** more than 35 inches

MISSISSIPPI — THE FATTEST STATE

Obesity in the United States is reaching epidemic proportions with a steady rise in obesity prevalence over the last three decades. Obesity prevalence was 15.6 percent in 1995, 19.8 percent in 2000, and 23.7 percent in 2005. Just in one decade, the total number of obese people rose from 317 million in 2012 to more than 338 million in 2022 when the national average figure for obesity was 32 percent.

In 2012, only 16 states had obesity percentages of 30 percent or more. In 2022, 39 states have reached that level. In 2008, the prevalence rates of obesity increased to 25 to 29 percent from only 14 percent or less in 1985; six states — Alabama, Mississippi, Oklahoma, South Carolina, Tennessee, and West Virginia — had prevalence rates

30 percent or more in 2008, whereas, in 2022, 35 states have obesity prevalence rates 30 percent or higher. Mississippi has the highest prevalence of obesity, amounting to 40.8 percent, which translates to more than 2.9 million Mississippians being obese or morbidly obese.

Morbidly obese is a term used to define clinically severe obesity when the BMI is 40 or higher. Four other states follow Mississippi based on the obesity rates — West Virginia (39.7 percent), Arkansas (37.4 percent), Oklahoma (36.8 percent), and Tennessee (36.5 percent). Colorado was the healthiest state in the nation with an obesity rate of 23.8 percent in 2022.

Obesity is now recognized as a separate disease entity. Obesity invites many other diseases including heart disease, type 2 diabetes, cancer, stroke, and osteoporosis. A person can curtail most of these chronic diseases by reducing their body fat and obesity, watching their food intake and energy expenditure, and making a balance between how many calories they're consuming and how much they're burning on a daily basis.

Understanding How Epidemiologic Transition Affects Healthcare

The results of epidemiologic transition are a reduction in the death rate of children before the age 5, a reduction in the overall death rate, and an improvement in people's life expectancy. All combined, they help in increasing the number of elderly populations, which is termed *graying of America*. The aging population in the United States will be shaping the future of the medical industry. These sections describe the effects of epidemiologic transition on overall healthcare.

Increasing healthcare cost

The field of medicine that provides care for seniors is known as *geriatrics*. According to the American Medical Association, the population of senior citizens (those older than 65) will increase by 73 percent between 2010 and 2030; in other words, one in five Americans will be a senior citizen. Older patients are a major portion of those who will be seeking medical care in the coming days and years. The healthcare industry will be dealing with more chronic and debilitating diseases than ever before.

The elderly health problems, such as risk of falls and injuries, senile dementia, hearing defects, eye defects, pain, suicide, and mental health problems are likely to increase in number as well. As a result, as more and more seniors need more healthcare, the field of geriatrics will need more attention. In order to provide the best care for the elderly who are faced with chronic diseases and disabilities, healthcare cost will undoubtedly rise.

Compromising quality of life

As people are living longer, an increased attention for social support, greater independency, and a better quality of life are needed for a growing number of senior citizens. Poorer physical and mental functioning is the most common reason for having senior citizens rely on others. This is called the *dependency ratio*. One of the goals of the healthcare system should be improving independence and at the same time providing an efficient support system in the society where senior citizens live.

Quality of life of the elderly — similarly to that of younger people — as defined by the World Health Organization (WHO) doesn't depend only on physical health but also on mental, social, cultural, and spiritual wellbeing. Because standard of living and quality of life are broad, there's no universal agreed-upon technique for measuring them. However, at a minimum, physical and mental health illnesses, which are measurable, should be given the most attention.

REMEMBER

Healthcare plans for senior citizens should provide the best possible curative as well as preventive services. To improve the quality of life, seniors can do the following:

>> **Make strong social bonds.** Tell people you know that you care about them.

>> **Do something that makes them happy.** Practice regular acts of kindness.

>> **Practice independence whenever possible.** For example, try to take daily medicines on time.

>> **Eat healthy and stay active.** Avoid fried food and fast food; make a daily practice of walking even for ten minutes.

>> **Stay in mental motion.** Reading makes your brain active.

>> **Practice good personal hygiene.** Examples include washing hands with soap after going to the toilet, brushing teeth twice a day, covering the mouth and nose with a tissue when sneezing or coughing.

What's the best medicine for seniors? Give love — if it doesn't work, increase the dose!

Chapter **9**

Linking Demography and Disease

D emographic characteristics — such as age and sex, racial differences, and many others — greatly influence a disease occurrence. Migration is another factor that's responsible for the reemergence of many infectious diseases.

As an epidemiology student, you need to be familiar with demographic changes and their relationship with morbidity and mortality. This chapter provides in-depth information on how changes in the disease pattern and demographics are connected. Furthermore, this chapter provides you information on how to calculate a future population of a country given certain basic demographic factors such as birth, death, migration, and growth rates.

Defining Demography — Why It's Important

Demography is the study of human populations. *Demos-* means population and *-graphy* means measurement. Demography encompasses the study of the structure, composition, and distribution of a population, and the spatial and temporal changes in the population in terms of birth, death, migration, and aging.

REMEMBER

Several factors known as *demographic variables*, such as age, sex, race/ethnicity, religion, occupation, income, home ownership, and so on, are important to demonstrate their influence on disease characteristics such as new occurrences (incidence) and deaths (mortality) in the population. For example, John Graunt was among the earliest scientists who described how age influences mortality.

Here are some other basic demographic variables:

» **Fertility:** Additional people enter the population naturally due to birth.

» **Mortality:** People leave the population naturally because of death.

» **Migration:** People enter (immigration) or leave (emigration) by moving.

» **Natural increase:** The difference between birth and death.

REMEMBER

Demographic trends describe the historical changes in demographics in a population over time. *Demographic transition* refers to the transition from high birth and death rates to low birth and death rates. Figure 9-1 demonstrates the four stages:

» **Stage 1:** Birth rates and death rates are high and roughly in balance. Population growth is very slow at this stage. This stage happened in pre-industrial society.

» **Stage 2:** In this stage, death rates drop. The reasons for the reduction in deaths is because of vaccination coverage against many infectious diseases, improved nutrition, and proper sanitation. The impact of lower death rates in children younger than 5 resulted in an increase in life expectancy. Many developing countries are seeing this stage of demographic transition now.

» **Stage 3:** At this stage, birth rates start falling. The reasons behind this decrease include increased access to contraception, breastfeeding, urbanization, more females getting formal education, increased female employment, and other social changes. During this stage, the death rates fall slowly and the overall increase in population growth also slows down. This stage of transition is occurring in countries, such as the United Arab Emirates and Jamaica.

» **Stage 4:** Both birth rates and death rates are low. Birth rates may drop below the replacement level. This stage of transition is happening in developed countries.

REMEMBER

Replacement level fertility is the level necessary to replace each person in the parents' generation. *Zero population growth* means there's no change in population size over time. In the long run, replacement level fertility will lead to zero population growth. Some countries, such as Germany, Italy, and Japan, have achieved the final stage of demographic transition where the population is actually shrinking.

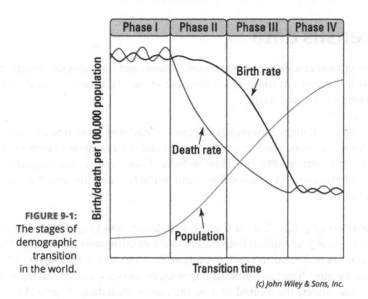

| Phase I | Phase II | Phase III | Phase IV |

Birth/death per 100,000 population

Birth rate

Death rate

Population

Transition time

(c) John Wiley & Sons, Inc.

FIGURE 9-1:
The stages of
demographic
transition
in the world.

Some countries, such as China, Thailand, and Brazil have passed through the demographic transition model very quickly and reached the final stage of demographic transition due to rapid social changes and economic growth. On the contrary, some societies in Africa still remain at Stage 2 of demographic transition because of disproportionately high death rates from diseases such as malaria, neonatal conditions, lower respiratory infections, diarrheal diseases, and HIV/AIDS, and poor economic development.

Using Demographic Data to Identify Population at Risk

Demographic data is crucial in health because healthcare policymakers and healthcare workers need to know how many people are sick. If you understand pertinent demographics for a specific region, you can study the disease trends, make future projections, and determine the proper strategies in order to help the target population. These sections explain the use of census data and other sources of demographic data.

Using census data

Data from the census can help you understand where and how specific groups of people live. You can find out more about their backgrounds, their economic situation, their family lives, and more.

For example, the U.S. Census Bureau has released an updated version of the population clock. This enhanced clock provides a quick and interactive overview of the population in the United States. This website (`www.census.gov/popclock/?intcmp=sldr1`) gives you an updated live count of the U.S. and the world population at every moment.

Near the time of writing this chapter the U.S. population was 333,338,656 and the world population was 7.94 billion; both numbers are continuously increasing. The world population is projected to reach 8.5 billion by 2030 and 9.7 billion by 2050 and 11.2 billion by 2100. The top ten most populous countries on July 1, 2022, were as follows: China, India, the United States, Indonesia, Pakistan, Nigeria, Brazil, Bangladesh, Russia, and Mexico. To discover more about world population projections, go to `www.worldometers.info/world-population/world-population-projections/`.

Census data doesn't only help in planning and understanding the health of a population, but also in the development of almost all areas of business. By using census data, you can study the location of businesses and people's buying trends, make future projections, and determine the proper marketing strategies to reach consumers. The U.S. Census Bureau's new mobile application America's Economy allows economists, planners, and policy makers to have greater access to key indicators about the health of the U.S. economy via their mobile devices.

The Census Bureau also produces timely local data that is critical to the emergency planning of a disease, disease preparedness, and recovery efforts. For example, the Emergency Management page of the U.S. Census Bureau website now provides access to information about hurricane forecast too at `www.census.gov/topics/preparedness.html`.

Focusing on population density

Population density is a measurement of population per unit area. To calculate population density of a country, you divide the number of people in the country by the total area in square kilometers or in miles. Population density data can be used to quantify demographic information and to assess relationships with ecosystems, human health, and infrastructure.

AMERICAN HOUSING SURVEY — A SOURCE FOR HOUSING INFORMATION

The American Housing Survey (AHS) is the largest, regular national housing sample survey in the United States. The U.S. Census Bureau conducts the AHS to obtain up-to-date housing statistics for the Department of Housing and Urban Development (HUD). The housing conditions of the population is directly related to people's lifestyle and occurrence of diseases.

The AHS contains a wealth of information that professionals in nearly every field can use for planning, decision making, market research, or various kinds of program development. It provides data on apartments, single-family homes, mobile homes, vacant homes, family composition, income, housing and neighborhood quality, housing costs, equipment, fuels, size of housing unit, and recent movers.

For example, here are the ten states with the highest population density in the United States at the time of writing this book:

>> New Jersey: 1,277 people per square mile

>> Rhode Island: 1,070 people per square mile

>> Massachusetts: 914 people per square mile

>> Connecticut: 746 people per square mile

>> Maryland: 645 people per square mile

>> Delaware: 517 people per square mile

>> New York: 432 people per square mile

>> Florida: 412 people per square mile

>> Pennsylvania: 292 people per square mile

>> Ohio: 290 people per square mile

Population density at a global level is also important. Why do you need to know population density in epidemiology? You can allocate your available resources efficiently, and you may get a better idea why a communicable disease is so rampant in a certain place compared to others.

You may have noticed that among the top ten states, the population density is highest in New Jersey. Similarly, you can get an idea about the population density of another country. As an epidemiologist your work scope isn't just limited to one country; you may want to work for other countries too. For example, take a job as an epidemic intelligence officer at the CDC. You may be placed to work in Rwanda, a country in East Africa to combat a malaria outbreak in that country.

Finding demographic data

Here, I discuss the source of the event such as birth, death, marriage, divorce, and so on, as well as population data. You use the event as the numerator and the population as the denominator for calculating a rate.

>> **Vital statistics:** Events documented by health departments — birth, death, marriage, and divorce. These are the numerator data for calculating rates. For example, birth rate = total birth / population. Here, *total birth* is the numerator and *population* is the denominator (or the divider of the formula).

>> **Census:** Generated by the federal government, this is the source of *population* or the denominator data for calculating rates.

>> **Population surveys:** Several organizations do population surveys for specific studies. It's also used for the source of population data or the denominator.

MORE INFORMATION ABOUT DEMOGRAPHIC DATA

Always use the U.S. Census Bureau as the primary data source for demographic information. The following are resources for additional demographic data (some of them charge a fee for information and some are free):

- *American Demographics*: This magazine reports on the trends of consumer marketing. It analyzes and publishes the impact of demographic and economic changes on consumer behavior by tracking households over time. It also publishes reports on the demographics of healthcare by showing trends of diseases by area.

- *American Sociological Association*: This is a nonprofit membership association that gives you free data briefs, articles, and research findings in the field of sociology.

- *Bureau of Census:* The U.S. Constitution mandates the census be conducted every ten years. The Census Bureau is responsible for the U.S. census and more than 200 annual surveys.

- *Central Intelligence Agency: World Factbook* (www.cia.gov/the-world-factbook/): It provides current demographic information by country. After you select a country, you get information on the country's geography, people and society, government, economy, energy, communication, transportation, military, and transnational issues.

- *Demographic Research*: This peer-reviewed journal provides international demographic data.

- *Population Reference Bureau* (www.prb.org): It informs about world population, health, and the environment and empowers users to utilize that information to advance the well-being of current and future generations.

- *UNESCO Institute for Statistics*: It provides global statistics on education, culture, sciences, and technology.

- *United States Bureau of Labor Statistics* (http://stats.bls.gov): It's the official site for labor economic statistics. It provides data on employment and unemployment, payroll, consumer price index, producer price index, employment cost index, and so on.

- *United States Demographic Research*: It provides demographic data for the United States and its geographic subdivisions. In addition to total population, it supplies information on age, race, sex, and so on.

- *Vital Statistics of the United States* (www.cdc.gov/nchs/products/vsus.htm): It contains data on births, deaths, and life expectancy as well as health reports.

- *World Bank* (www.worldbank.org): It provides demographic information on a wide variety of topics, browsed by country.

Tackling Population Pyramids: Not the Ones in Egypt

A population pyramid looks like a pyramid in Egypt because of its shape, with a broad base and a narrow tip. In fact, this was the typical shape of a graphical presentation of population in earlier days. The total population of a country is divided by age group and gender.

Males are displayed at the left and females are at the right side of the pyramid. Age groups are numbered from younger ages at the base, gradually increasing in age to the top. The broad base of the pyramid represents more people in younger age groups. Over time, the number of younger people is shrinking and the middle age group is expanding, making the pyramid fattier in the middle.

Here I examine changes of population pyramids of several countries and the distribution of the population by age group, including the elderly population of a country.

Shaping population pyramids

A *population pyramid* is a pyramid-shaped diagram illustrating the distribution of population by age group and sex, the youngest age groups being represented by a rectangle at the base, and the oldest by a rectangle at the apex of the pyramid. Diseases affect different age groups differently. It's important that you learn the population size of different age groups (and genders) to calculate the rate of a disease by age group and compare that with another age group. By this simple measurement, an epidemiologist can identify a risk factor and take appropriate actions.

The population pyramid of a developed country and that of a developing country contrasts sharply (see Figure 9-2). For example, the population pyramid of the United States has the largest number of people in the middle age-group, whereas the population pyramid of India has a broader base having the most people living in the younger age-group.

Calculating the dependency ratio

Because of increasing life expectancy, the age-structure is changing over time in all countries. However, as you may have noticed in Figure 9-2, the growth in the number of elderly population is much higher in developed countries (such as the United States) compared to a developing country (such as India). As the population gets older, the nation encounters more chronic health conditions and increasing treatment costs than earlier centuries due to the aging population.

As developing countries like the United States experience an increase in the number of people who are living longer, they have an increase in the proportion of elderly people. In other words, the *dependency ratio* is increasing.

Dependency ratio

$$= \frac{\text{No. people typically not in the labor force (ages 0 to 14 and 65+)}}{\text{No. people who are typically in the labor force (ages 15 to 64)}}$$

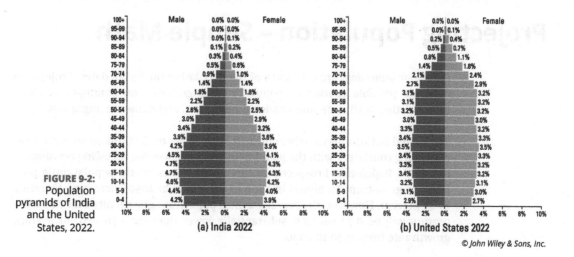

FIGURE 9-2: Population pyramids of India and the United States, 2022.

(a) India 2022   (b) United States 2022

© John Wiley & Sons, Inc.

Likewise, the populations of many other developed nations are experiencing a growing number of senior citizens and dealing with related old-age health conditions.

The following list identifies the top ten countries with the most senior citizens in the world (the proportion of the total population 65 and older):

» Japan: 28.2 percent

» Italy: 22.8 percent

» Greece: 21.8 percent

» Portugal: 21.8 percent

» France: 20.3 percent

» Sweden: 19.9 percent

» Hungary: 19.3 percent

» Spain: 19.1 percent

» Netherlands: 18.9 percent

» United Kingdom: 18.3 percent

In terms of the total number of people older than 65, the world's three largest countries unsurprisingly have the most: China ranks No. 1 with 166.37 million, followed by India with 84.9 million, and the United States with 52.76 million older people. Of the total people in the United States, 16.5 percent are older than 65.

Projecting Population – Simple Math

Population projections are estimates of the population for future dates. Projections illustrate possible courses of population change based on assumptions about future births, deaths, net international migration, and domestic migration.

The United Nations previously published long-range projections on six occasions, each being consistent with the population projections of the following revisions of the World Population Prospects. In these projections, world population is projected to grow from 6.1 billion in 2000 to 8.9 billion in 2050, increasing therefore by 47 percent. However, the average annual population growth rate over this half-century will be 0.77 percent, substantially lower than the 1.76 percent average growth rate from 1950 to 2000.

Most of the indicators of health measure (such as incidence and death rates) are calculated in terms of population and time. As an epidemiologist you must know the population size. In the following section, I provide a step-by-step guide on how to calculate the future population of a country based on the baseline population and the population growth rate. Remember, this is just an estimation because the growth rate may vary.

Calculating population

Use the following formula for calculating population of a country:

$$p_2 = p_1(1+r)^n$$

where

>> P_2 = Projected population

>> P_1 = Current population

>> r = Rate of population growth

>> n = Number of years to achieve from the present population to the projected population

In the following calculations, consider these two important factors:

>> **The rate of population growth:** The rate of population growth depends on total fertility (number of childbirths per woman in her lifetime) and the figure of total fertility varies.

>> **The current population:** The total population of a place at the time of your calculations.

Therefore, the figures of population projection work only if certain assumptions are true. For example, over the long run, total fertility is projected to settle at 1.85 children per woman in each country — in between the current rate for Northern America (which is just below the replacement level) and the rate for Europe (which is currently well below).

Here are a few other key terms for further information:

>> **Replacement-level fertility:** This term refers to the level of fertility at which a population replaces itself from one generation to the next. The number used to explain this term is 2.1 children per women. If the rate of fertility (per woman) falls below 2.1, it's called *sub-replacement level fertility*. In that case, each new generation will be less populous than the previous one in a given area. According to the most recent U.N. estimates, almost one half of the world's population lives in countries with below replacement level fertility, whereas several countries still have high total fertility rates, such as Niger, Somalia, Congo, Chad, Nigeria, and Gambia.

>> **Migration:** Assumptions about the number of future migrations is difficult to make because it largely depends on public policy toward migrations and other factors (such as political turmoil, war, disasters). Therefore, an assumption is made based on past migration estimates.

Working out some exercises

Here are some examples you can work through to practice your calculations.

Exercise 1

The current population of Mississippi is estimated to be 2,961,279. Calculate the time (in years) needed to get the population size of 3.5 million. The current rate of population growth in Mississippi is 0.30 percent. Assume that the rate of population growth will remain unchanged. Scientists often make such an assumption to get a future number.

$r = 0.30$ percent $= 0.003$ (just divide 0.30 by 100)

$P_1 = 2,961,279$

$P_2 = 3,500,000$

$$p_2 = p_1(1+r)^n$$
$$3{,}500{,}000 = 2{,}961{,}279(1+0.003)^n$$

Now, change the sides of the equation.

$$2{,}961{,}279(1+0.003)^n = 3{,}500{,}000$$
$$(1+0.003)^n = 3{,}500{,}000 / 2{,}961{,}279$$
$$(1.003)^n = 1.1819$$

TIP

Now, use the *log* function on your calculator for both sides of the equation.

$$log(1.003)^n = log\,1.1819$$
$$n \times log\,1.003 = log\,1.1819$$
$$n = log\,1.1819 / log\,1.003$$
$$n = 0.0726 / 0.0013$$
$$n = 55.8 \; years$$

It will take about 56 years to get the population of 3.5 million in Mississippi, provided the rate of population growth per year remains the same.

WARNING

Always keep in your mind that although the way the population grows may not be the same from year to year, still for the purpose of projection, you have to assume many factors such as population growth, fertility, migration, and others (discussed in the previous section) remain constant.

Exercise 2

Suppose the hypothetical figure of population growth rate of a future world, such as Mars, is extremely low (about 0.1 percent). How many years will it take to double the population?

$$r = 0.1 \text{ percent}$$

$$r = 0.001$$

Because the population doubles, $P_2 = 2P_1$

Insert the data in the following formula:

$$P_2 = P_1(1+r)^n$$
$$2P_1 = P_1(1+0.001)^n$$
$$2 = (1.001)^n$$

Use the *log* function for both sides of the equation to get:

$$log(2) = log(1.001)^n$$
$$log(1.001)^n = log(2)$$
$$n \times log(1.001) = log(2)$$
$$n = log(2) / log(1.001)$$
$$Log\ 2 = 0.3010$$
$$Log\ (1.001) = 0.00043$$
$$n = 0.3010 / 0.00043 = 700$$

It will take about 700 years to double the population size, assuming that the population growth rate is 0.1 percent on Mars.

Projecting more populations

Here are a few more examples for you to practice.

Canada

The population of Canada is 38,415,364 as of July 2022. The rate of population growth of the country is 0.78 percent per year. What would the population size of Canada be after ten years?

$$r = 0.78 \text{ percent}$$
$$r = 0.0078$$
$$n = 10$$
$$P_2 = 38,415,364\ (1 + 0.0078)^{10}$$
$$P_2 = 38,415,364\ (1.0078)^{10}$$
$$P_2 = 41,519,153$$

After ten years, the population of Canada would be approximately 41,519,153.

India

According to the United Nations estimate, India's current population is 1,406,631,776 and the population growth rate is about 0.97 percent. Find out how long it will take to increase the population to 2 billion.

$$r = 0.97 \text{ percent}$$
$$r = 0.0097$$
$$P_1 = 1,406,631,776$$
$$P_2 = 2,000,000,000$$

$$p_2 = p_1(1+r)^n$$

$$2,000,000,000 = 1,406,631,776(1+0.0097)^n$$

$$1,406,631,776(1+0.0097)^n = 2,000,000,000$$

$$(1+0.0097)^n = 2,000,000,000 / 1,406,631,776$$

$$(1.0097)^n = 1.4218$$

Now, use the *log* function for both sides of the equation.

$$\log(1.0097)^n = \log(1.4218)$$

$$n \times \log(1.0097) = \log(1.4218)$$

$$n = \log(1.4218) / \log(1.0097)$$

$$n = 0.1528 / 0.00419$$

$$n = 36.5 \text{ years}$$

It will take approximately 36.5 years to reach a population of 2 billion in India.

The United States

The 2022 population of the United States is 331,002,651, and the population growth rate of the country is 0.35 percent. Having this rate of growth, how long will it take to increase the population to 400 million?

$$r = 0.35 \text{ percent}$$

$$r = 0.0035$$

$$P_1 = 331,002,651$$

$$P_2 = 400,000,000$$

$$p_2 = p_1(1+r)^n$$

$$400,000,000 = 331,002,651(1+0.0035)^n$$

$$331,002,651(1+0.0035)^n = 400,000,000$$

$$(1+0.0035)^n = 400,000,000 / 331,002,651$$

$$(1.0035)^n = 1.208$$

Now, use *log* function for both sides of the equation.

$$\log(1.0035)^n = \log(1.208)$$

$$n \times \log(1.0035) = \log(1.208)$$

$$n = \log(1.208) / \log(1.0035)$$

$$n = 0.0821 / 0.00152$$

$$n = 54 \text{ years}$$

It will take approximately 54 years to reach a population of 400 million in the United States, provided the rate of population growth remains the same.

Chapter **10**

Digging into Math: Calculating Rates and Risks

I n epidemiology, you compute morbidity and mortality data of a disease to assess how big the problem is in your community, including how many people are affected, what's the death rate, what percentage of the affected people are getting the treatment, what's the ratio between those who received the treatment versus those who didn't respond to the treatment, and so on. This chapter introduces many statistical terms, their uses, and their calculations.

Addressing Some Basics When Calculating Descriptive Epidemiology

Before you start working on statistical functions, it's important to get familiar with statistical terms. This section explains some basics you need to know when calculating the descriptive measurements of people's health status.

Recognizing the key elements of a formula

When doing this calculation, here are four basic elements of the formula that are important:

>> **Numerator:** It's the number of cases or deaths that is used at the top of a formula; for example, in $\frac{a}{b}$ the variable a is the numerator.

>> **Denominator:** It's the total number of people who are at risk. This number is the divider, which is the bottom of the equation — in $\frac{a}{b}$ the variable b is the denominator.

>> **Measurement period:** Usually the data is expressed per year.

>> **Unit:** This is a constant. If you multiply the number by 100, the rate is expressed as a percentage. Usually when the rate is very small (such as a fraction), it's multiplied by 10,000 or 100,000.

Focusing on rate, ratio, and proportion

Here are three more terms you need to know — rate, ratio, and proportion.

Rate — The frequency a disease or event occurs

Rate is used to calculate the frequency that a disease or event occurs. Here is the formula:

$$\text{Rate} = \frac{a}{a+b} \times k$$

In a rate, the values of the numerator are included in the denominator. Here, k is a constant; it can be 100, 1000, 10,000, or 100,000.

Ratio — The relation between two amounts

A *ratio* is the quantitative relation between two amounts. In a ratio, one quantity is divided by another quantity. The values of the numerator and the denominator are distinct — the numerator isn't included in the denominator. For example, if you have 10 males and 15 females in a study, then the ratio of males to females is 10 to 15.

Here are a few examples:

>> Male / Female

>> Present in the class / Absent in the class

>> Immunized people / Nonimmunized people

>> Those who like math / Those who don't like math

The formula for ratio is as follows:

$$\text{Ratio} = \frac{a}{b} \times k$$

Here, k is usually 100.

Suppose you're recruiting 1 boy for 3 girls in your study; the ratio of boys and girls is expressed as 1:3.

Proportion — A comparison of a part in a whole

A *proportion* is the comparison of a part in the whole. In epidemiology, proportion is a special type of ratio, where the numerator is included in the denominator. The proportion is usually expressed as a percentage:

$$\text{Proportion} = \frac{x}{\text{Total}} \times k(100)$$

Here $k = 100$.

For example, in my epidemiology class, I have a total of 50 students. Of them, 20 are men and 30 are women. In terms of proportion, $\frac{20}{50} \times 100 = 40$ percent are men; and $\frac{30}{50} \times 100 = 60$ percent are women in my class. Alternatively, you can use a ratio. In that case, the ratio of men to women is 20:30 or 2:3.

Calculating Crude Morbidity and Crude Mortality Rates

A crude morbidity (or birth) rate and crude mortality (or death) rate are good indicators of the general health status of a population. However, these rates may not be appropriate for comparing different populations because there could be large differences in age-distributions. Other age-specific rates such as infant mortality rate, neonatal mortality rate, and post-neonatal mortality are better indicators of health for age-specific data.

Several rates are conventionally used to know the health status of a nation, including infant mortality rate, maternal mortality rate, life expectancy, and others. These sections describe these rates and explain how to calculate them.

Focusing on the terms and formulas

Here are the important terms you need to know and the formulas to calculate each.

Mid-year population

The *mid-year population* is the term used for the population that is counted in the middle of a calendar year, which means the population on June 30. It provides a more comprehensive statistical picture than the total population. It's better to use the mid-year population instead of the total population as the denominator in the following formulas.

TECHNICAL STUFF

The term in the denominator is labeled "mid-year population" or "total population." But technically, the term is known as "person-years at risk." *Person-year* is a measurement that considers both the number of people in the study and the amount of time each person spends in the study. For example, a study that follows 1,000 people for one year would contain 1,000 person-years provided all the people remain in the study for one year.

Crude birth rate (CBR)

Crude birth rate (CBR) is the proportion of live births out of total population or mid-year population. Use this formula:

$$\text{Crude birth rate} = \frac{\text{Number of live births}}{\text{Mid - year population}} \times 1,000$$

Crude death rate (CDR)

Crude death rate (CDR) is the proportion of total deaths out of total population or the mid-year population:

$$\text{Crude death rate} = \frac{\text{Number of deaths}}{\text{Mid - year population}} \times 1,000$$

Doing the math

Use the data presented in Table 10-1 and do the math.

TABLE 10-1 **Data for Calculating Crude Birth Rate and Crude Death Rate**

Event	Whites	Blacks	Total Population (Whites and Blacks)
Mid-year population	326,500	348,350	674,850
Live birth	4,800	6,750	11,550
Total death	3,150	4,280	7,430

Calculate the CBR for Whites and the CBR for Blacks and express the rates per 1,000 population.

To solve the CBR in Whites, fill the data in the formula:

$$\frac{4800}{326,500} \times 1,000 = 14.7 \text{ per 1,000 population}$$

To solve the CBR for Blacks, fill the data in the formula:

$$\frac{6750}{348,350} \times 1,000 = 19.4 \text{ per 1,000 population}$$

The difference in CBR rates between Blacks and Whites is $19.4 - 14.7 = 4.7$. That means the CBR for Blacks is 4.7 points higher than Whites.

Now using Table 10-1, calculate the CDR for Whites and the CDR for Blacks and express the rates per 1,000 population.

To solve the CDR in Whites, fill the data in the formula:

$$\frac{3150}{326,500} \times 1,000 = 9.6 \text{ per 1,000 population}$$

To solve the CRD for Blacks, fill the data in the formula:

$$\frac{4280}{348,350} \times 1,000 = 12.3 \text{ per 1,000 population}$$

The difference in CDR rates between Blacks and Whites is $12.3 - 9.6 = 2.7$. That means the CDR in Blacks is 2.7 points higher than Whites.

Figuring Out Commonly Used Rates

This section gives you an overview of several parameters that are most commonly used to define a nation's heath. Some of them are age-specific rates, sex-specific rates, and disease or cause-specific rates.

Infant mortality rate (IMR)

Infant mortality rate (IMR), which is a major health status indicator of populations, is the number of infant deaths for every 1,000 live births. IMR reflects the health status of the child throughout the pregnancy and birth process.

Factors responsible for IMR include the following:

>> Prenatal and postnatal nutritional care

>> Birth weight

>> Immediate medical care sought upon becoming pregnant and throughout the pregnancy

>> Abstinence from any drugs, chemicals, alcohol, and smoking

>> Proper immunization

>> Basic public health measures, including sanitation, personal hygiene, and infection control

>> Safe delivery

Here is the formula used to calculate IMR:

$$\frac{\text{Number of deaths under 1 year during a year}}{\text{Total live births during the year}} \times 1,000$$

Use the data in Table 10-2 to find the IMR.

Calculate IMR for Whites, Blacks, and the total population. Express the rates per 1,000 population.

To solve the IMR for Whites, fill the data in the formula:

Infant deaths (use item no. 4, Table 10-2) = 43

Total live births (use item no. 1, Table 10-2) = 4,800

$$IMR = \frac{43}{4,800} \times 1,000 = 8.96 \text{ per 1,000 population}$$

TABLE 10-2   Data for Calculating Age-Specific Death Rates

Event	Whites	Blacks	Total Population (Whites and Blacks)
1. Total Live births	4,800	6,750	11,550
2. Total births (stillbirth plus live birth)	4,840	6,798	11,638
3. Total deaths	3,150	4,280	7,430
4. Infant deaths	43	67	110
5. Fetal deaths plus Infant deaths under 7 days (perinatal death)	50	73	123
6. Neonatal deaths	8	60	68
7. Post neonatal deaths	11	42	53
8. Maternal deaths	3	7	10

To solve the IMR for Blacks, fill the data in the formula:

Infant deaths (use item no. 4, Table 10-2) = 67

Total live births (use item no. 1, Table 10-2) = 6,750

$$\text{IMR} = \frac{67}{6,750} \times 1,000 = 9.93 \text{ per 1,000 population}$$

To solve the IMR for the total population, fill the data in the formula:

Infant deaths (use item no. 4, Table 10-2) = 110

Total live births (use item no. 1, Table 10-2) = 11,550

$$\text{IMR} = \frac{110}{11,550} \times 1,000 = 9.52 \text{ per 1,000 population}$$

Maternal mortality rate (MMR)

The *maternal mortality rate (MMR)* refers to the number of deaths of women during pregnancy, at delivery, or soon after delivery due to causes related to pregnancy or *puerperium* (the phase of childbearing).

Here are factors responsible for a higher MMR:

>> Poverty

>> Lack of public health measures

>> Maternal age

>> Lack of prenatal care

>> Poor nutrition

>> Drug, smoking, and alcohol abuse

>> Complications of pregnancy and the birth process, such as hemorrhage, toxemia, and infection

Use this formula:

MMR

$$= \frac{\text{Number of maternal deaths from puerperal causes in a given years}}{\text{Total number of live births in the same year}} \times 100,000$$

Notice that the k here is 100,000 because the rate is very small.

Use the data in Table 10-2, calculate the MMR for Whites, Blacks, and the total population. Express the rates per 1,000 population.

To solve the MMR for Whites, fill the data in the formula:

Maternal deaths (use item no. 8, Table 10-2) = 3

Total live births (use item no. 1, Table 10-2) = 4,800

$$MMR = \frac{3}{4,800} \times 100,000 = 62.5 \text{ per } 100,000 \text{ population}$$

To solve the MMR for Blacks, fill the data in the formula:

Maternal deaths (use item no. 8, Table 10-2) = 7

Total live births (use item no. 1, Table 10-2) = 6,750

$$MMR = \frac{7}{6,750} \times 100,000 = 103.7 \text{ per } 100,000 \text{ population}$$

To solve the MMR for the total population, fill the data in the formula:

Maternal deaths (use item no. 8, Table 10-2) = 10

Total live births (use item no. 1, Table 10-2) = 11,550

$$MMR = \frac{10}{11,550} \times 100,000 = 86.6 \text{ per } 100,000 \text{ population}$$

Neonatal mortality rate (NNMR)

A *neonate* is a baby who is younger than 4 weeks old. The *neonatal mortality rate (NNMR)* refers to the number of deaths of infants younger than 28 days old (aged 0 to 27 days) per 1,000 live births.

Here are the factors responsible for the NNMR:

>> Poor prenatal care

>> Low birth weight

>> Infection

>> Lack of proper medical care

>> Injuries

>> Prematurity

>> Congenital defects

The formula for NNMR is as follows:

$$\frac{\text{Number of deaths under 28 days of age during a year}}{\text{Total number of live births during a year}} \times 1,000$$

Use the data in Table 10-2, calculate the NNMR for Whites, Blacks, and the total population. Express the rates per 1,000 population.

To solve the NNMR for Whites, fill the data in the formula:

Neonatal deaths (use item no. 6, Table 10-2) = 8

Total live births (use item no. 1, Table 10-2) = 4,800

$$\text{NNMR} = \frac{8}{4,800} \times 1,000 = 1.67 \text{ per 1,000 population}$$

To solve the NNMR for Blacks, fill the data in the formula:

Neonatal deaths (use item no. 6, Table 10-2) = 60

Total live births (use item no. 1, Table 10-2) = 6,750

$$\text{NNMR} = \frac{60}{6,750} \times 1,000 = 8.89 \text{ per 1,000 population}$$

To solve the MMR for the total population, fill in the data in the formula:

Neonatal deaths (use item no. 6, Table 10-2) = 68

Total live births (use item no. 1, Table 10-2) = 11,550

$$NNMR = \frac{68}{11,550} \times 1,000 = 5.89 \text{ per } 1,000 \text{ population}$$

Post-neonatal mortality rate (PNNMR)

The *post-neonatal mortality rate (PNNMR)* is the number of deaths among infants aged 28 to 364 days per 1,000 live births. In the United States, 2016 data shows the five leading causes of PNNMR as follows:

>> Congenital malformation

>> Sudden infant death syndrome (*SIDS*)

>> Unintentional injury

>> Diseases of the circulatory system

>> Homicide

The formula for PNNMR is as follows:

$$\frac{No.\,deaths\,between\,28\,days\,to\,1\,year\,of\,age\,during\,a\,year}{Total\,number\,of\,live\,births} \times 1,000$$

Use the data in Table 10-2, calculate the PNNMR for Whites, Blacks, and the total population. Express the rates per 1,000 population.

To solve the PNNMR for Whites, fill the data in the formula:

Post-neonatal deaths (use item no. 7, Table 10-2) = 11

Total live births (use item no. 1, Table 10-2) = 4,800

$$PNNMR = \frac{11}{4,800} \times 1,000 = 2.29 \text{ per } 1,000 \text{ population}$$

To solve the NNMR for Blacks, fill the data in the formula:

Post-neonatal deaths (use item no. 7, Table 10-2) = 42

Total live births (use item no. 1, Table 10-2) = 6,750

$$PNNMR = \frac{42}{6,750} \times 1,000 = 6.22 \text{ per } 1,000 \text{ population}$$

To solve the PNNMR for the total population, fill the data in the formula:

Post-neonatal deaths (use item no. 7, Table 10-2) = 53

Total live births (use item no. 1, Table 10-2) = 11,550

$$PNNMR = \frac{53}{11,550} \times 1,000 = 4.59 \text{ per 1,000 population}$$

Perinatal mortality rate

The perinatal mortality rate (PMR) means the number of fetal deaths (or still-births) of 28 or more weeks of gestation plus the number of newborns dying younger than 7 days after birth. In the United States, stillbirth occurs in 1 out of 160 pregnancies.

REMEMBER

You may have noticed that the denominator used for the formulas for infant mortality rate, maternal mortality rate, neonatal mortality rate, and post-neonatal mortality rate was the same – *total number of live births*. For perinatal mortality rate, the denominator is the *Total births (stillbirth plus live birth)*.

Here's the formula for PMR:

$$\frac{\text{Fetal deaths of 28 wk or more} + \text{infant deaths} < 7 \text{ days}}{\text{Total births (stillborn} + \text{live born)}} \times 1,000$$

Use the data in Table 10-2, calculate the PMR for Whites, Blacks, and the total population. Express the rates per 1,000 population.

To solve the PMR for Whites, fill the data in the formula:

Perinatal death (use item no. 5, Table 10-2) = 50

Total births (use item no. 2, Table 10-2) = 4,840

$$PMR = \frac{50}{4,840} \times 1,000 = 10.3 \text{ per 1,000 population}$$

To solve the PMR for Blacks, fill the data in the formula:

Perinatal death (use item no. 5, Table 10-2) = 73

Total births (use item no. 2, Table 10-2) = 6,798

$$PMR = \frac{73}{6,798} \times 1,000 = 10.7 \text{ per 1,000 population}$$

To solve the PMR for the total population, fill the data in the formula:

Perinatal death (use item no. 5, Table 10-2) = 123

Total births (use item no. 2, Table 10-2) = 11,638

$$PMR = \frac{123}{11,638} \times 1,000 = 10.6 \text{ per } 1,000 \text{ population}$$

Cause-specific mortality rate

Cause-specific mortality rate (CSMR) is the number of deaths from a specified cause per 100,000 population. As I mention in the section, "Focusing on the terms and formulas," earlier in this chapter, it's better to use the mid-year population as the denominator to calculate a rate.

If the numerator uses the sum of the number of deaths across multiple years, the denominator should use the sum of the population over the same years. Alternatively, you can use the average annual deaths of a disease in the numerator. In that case, you can use the population in a single year in the middle of the time period or the average annual populations to represent the person-years at risk for the denominator.

Cancer and heart disease deaths

Use the data in Table 10-3 to calculate the following:

TABLE 10-3   **Data for Calculating Cause-Specific Death Rates**

Event	Whites	Blacks	Total Population (Whites and Blacks Only)
Mid-year population	326,500	348,350	674,850
Cancer deaths	522	730	1,252
Heart disease deaths	614	862	1,476

Determine the cancer death rates for Whites, Blacks, and the total population. Express the rates per 100,000 population.

The formula is as follows:

$$\text{Cancer death rate} = \frac{\text{No. of deaths due to cancer}}{\text{Mid-year population}} \times 100,000$$

To calculate the cancer death rate for Whites, fill the data in the formula:

$$\text{Cancer death rate} = \frac{522}{326,500} \times 100,000 = 159.9 \text{ per } 100,000 \text{ population}$$

To calculate the cancer death rate for Blacks, fill the data in the formula:

$$\text{Cancer death rate} = \frac{730}{348,350} \times 100,000 = 209.6 \text{ per } 100,000 \text{ population}$$

To calculate the cancer death rate for the total population, fill the data in the formula:

$$\text{Cancer death rate} = \frac{1252}{674,850} \times 100,000 = 185.5 \text{ per } 100,000 \text{ population}$$

Refer to Table 10-3 and calculate the heart disease death rates for Whites, Blacks, and the total population. Express the rates per 100,000 population.

The formula is as follow:

$$\text{Heart disease death rate} = \frac{\text{No. of deaths due to heart disease}}{\text{Mid} - \text{year population}} \times 100,000$$

To calculate the heart disease death rate for Whites, fill the data in the formula:

$$\text{Heart disease death rate} = \frac{614}{326,500} \times 100,000$$

$$= 188.1 \text{ per } 100,000 \text{ population}$$

To calculate the heart disease death rate for Blacks, fill the data in the formula:

$$\text{Heart disease death rate} = \frac{862}{348,350} \times 100,000$$

$$= 247.5 \text{ per } 100,000 \text{ population}$$

To calculate the heart disease death rate for the total population, fill the data in the formula:

$$\text{Heart disease death rate} = \frac{1476}{674,850} \times 100,000$$

$$= 218.7 \text{ per } 100,000 \text{ population}$$

Homicide rates

You can also calculate homicide rates by state. Table 10-4 presents the total number of homicides in selected U.S. states in 2020. The calculated homicide rates are per 100,000 population.

The formula for calculating homicide rates is as follows:

$$\text{Homicide death rate} = \frac{\text{Number of homicide deaths}}{\text{Midyear population}} \times 100{,}000$$

TABLE 10-4   **Calculating Homicide Rates in Five States**

State	Number of homicides	2020 Population	Homicide rate per 100,000
California	2,203	39,538,223	$2{,}203 / 395{,}388{,}223 \times 100{,}000 = 5.57$
Texas	1,931	29,145,505	$1{,}931 / 29{,}145{,}505 \times 100{,}000 = 6.63$
Florida	1,290	331,449,281	$1{,}290 / 331{,}449{,}281 \times 100{,}000 = 0.39$
Illinois	1,151	12,812,508	$1{,}151 / 12{,}812{,}508 \times 100{,}000 = 8.98$
Pennsylvania	1009	13,002,700	$1{,}009 / 13{,}002{,}700 \times 100{,}000 = 7.76$

From the analyses of homicide rates, you may notice that the absolute number of an event doesn't make much sense. For example, the number of homicides is highest in California, but the homicide rate is highest in Illinois. Bottom line: Both the numerator and the denominator are important.

Colorectal cancer incidence

To determine the population at risk, you need to find out who is commonly affected by the disease. Take colorectal cancer where the majority of colorectal cancers occur in people older than 50. For colon cancer, the average age at the diagnosis for men is 68 and for women is 72. For rectal cancer, it's age 63 for both men and women. Can it occur in younger adults? In fact, about 20 percent of people diagnosed with colorectal cancer are between ages 20 and 54, according to the Colon Cancer Coalition.

Colorectal cancer is now the third leading cause of death in young adults. Having known the age-groups of the people who can be affected with colorectal cancer, you can now consider all adults ages 19 and older as the population at risk. Adults older than 18 years comprise 76.5 percent of the total population. They are the population at risk for colorectal cancer. You can use the following formula to calculate the "population at risk".

$$\text{Population at risk} = \text{Total population} \times \text{Percent at risk}$$

To calculate the population at risk of colorectal cancer, fill the data in the formula:

Total population (based on 2020 census) = 2,961,279

Population at risk = 76.5 percent = 0.765 (by dividing 76.5 percent by 100)

Population at risk of colorectal cancer = 2,961,279 × 0.765 = 2,269,968

New cases of colon cancer = 104,610

New cases of rectal cancer = 43,340

Total new cases of colorectal cancer = 104,610 + 43,340 = 147,950

To calculate the incidence of colorectal cancer, use the following formula:

$$\text{Incidence} = \frac{\text{New cases}}{\text{Population at risk}} \times 1,000$$

$$\text{Incidence of colorectal cancer} = \frac{147950}{2,269,968} \times 1,000$$

$$= 65.2 \text{ per 1,000 population}$$

Gender-specific rates

Denominators for certain diseases are calculated for a single gender and not for the whole population. For example, breast cancer rates are different among males and females. They're usually calculated for specific gender. Certain diseases occur only in either males or females because they're sex-organ specific (such as prostate cancer, ovarian cancer, cervical cancer, and uterine cancer).

Prostatic cancer rates

From 2004 through 2018, a total of 836,282 patients were recorded with prostate-specific antigen (PSA)-based prostate cancer (PCa) in 18 states in the United States.

Because prostate cancer is a male condition, the denominator is only the male population. Males were 49.5 percent of the total population of 331,449,281, so the calculation is as follows:

Number of males = 331,449,281 × 0.495 = 164,067,394

$$\text{PCa rate} = \frac{836,282}{164,067,394} \times 100,000 = 509.7 \text{ per 100,000 population}$$

Female breast cancer incidence and mortality

Compared to other states, the age-adjusted mortality rate for female breast cancer in Mississippi is the second highest in the nation. Here I calculate female breast cancer incidence and mortality in Mississippi.

Similar to other diseases, you need the number of new cases of female breast cancer for the incidence calculation and the number of deaths due to breast cancer for the mortality rate of female breast cancer.

According to the Mississippi State Plan for Comprehensive Cancer Control 2018–2022, an average of 2,021 new cases are diagnosed with female breast cancer, and 429 women died from breast cancer each year from 2011–2015. According to the 2020 U.S. standard population, the female population is 51.3 percent of the total of 2,961,279 population in Mississippi.

Therefore, female population in Mississippi is $2,961,279 \times 0.513 = 1,519,136$

To calculate the incidence of female breast cancer in Mississippi, do the following:

$$\text{Incidence of female breast cancer} = \frac{2021}{1,519,136} \times 100,000 = 133.04 \text{ per } 100,000$$

To calculate the mortality rate of female breast cancer in Mississippi, do the following:

$$\text{Mortality of female breast cancer} = \frac{429}{1,519,136} \times 100,000 = 28.2 \text{ per } 100,000$$

Cervical cancer incidence and mortality rates

In Mississippi, an average of 149 new cases are diagnosed with cervical cancer, and 58 women die of cervical cancer each year. The age-adjusted mortality rate from cervical cancer in Mississippi is highest in the nation.

Using the female population of 1,519,136 in Mississippi in 2020, the calculated rates are as follows:

To calculate the cervical cancer incidence in Mississippi, do the following:

$$\text{Cervical cancer incidence} = \frac{149}{1,519,136} \times 100,000 = 9.8 \text{ per } 100,000$$

To calculate the cervical cancer mortality in Mississippi, do the following:

$$\text{Cervical cancer mortality} = \frac{58}{1,519,136} \times 100,000 = 3.8 \text{ per } 100,000$$

Age-specific rates

Many diseases are more common in certain age-groups. A generalization of the rates for the entire population doesn't make sense if the disease is commonly found in either children or the elderly people.

Hospitalization rate due to rotavirus diarrhea in children

Rotavirus diarrhea predominantly affects children under 5. Each year an estimated 54,000 to 55,000 infants and young children are hospitalized for rotavirus diarrhea in the United States,

To find the denominator, do the following: If you use the entire population, the burden of the disease *rotavirus* will be diluted. According to the 2020 census, 6 percent of the population is aged under 5 years.

Total 2020 population $= 2,961,279$

Population under $5 = 2,961,279 \times 0.06 = 177,677$

The average number of children hospitalized with rotavirus diarrhea = 54,500. Find the rate of hospitalization with rotavirus diarrhea per year, as expressed as a percent.

$$\text{Hospitalization rate due to rotavirus} = \frac{54500}{177,677} \times 100 = 30.7 \text{ percent}$$

Alzheimer's disease among seniors

Alzheimer's disease is one of the causes of dementia or memory loss in the elderly population. The risk of Alzheimer's disease and other types of dementia increase with age, affecting an estimated 1 in 14 people older than 65 and 1 in every 6 people older than 80. In 2020, an estimated 5.8 million Americans aged 65 years or older had Alzheimer's disease. The total estimated number of seniors is 54.1 million.

To calculate the rate of Alzheimer's disease among seniors, do the following:

$$\text{Alzheimer's rate among seniors} = \frac{5.8 \text{ million}}{54.1 \text{ million}} \times 100 = 10.7 \text{ percent}$$

Proportionate mortality rate

To prioritize the impact of a disease mortality, epidemiologists often calculate the contribution of a particular disease mortality to all causes of mortality. In other words, what proportion of death from disease X contributes to all causes of death?

Table 10-5 shows the number of deaths of the top ten causes of death in 2003, and their relative contribution to the total number of all causes of deaths. For example, deaths due to heart disease accounted for 684,462 deaths, and the number of deaths from all causes were 2,442,930. The proportion of deaths due to heart disease was 28 percent of all deaths. You calculate it by dividing the number of heart disease deaths by the number of deaths from all causes and multiplied by 100.

TABLE 10-5

Proportionate Mortality (Percentage) of Top Ten Causes of Deaths, United States, 2003

Cause	Number of deaths	Percentage
All causes	2,443,930	100
Heart disease	684,462	28.0
Cancer	554,643	22.7
Stroke	157,803	6.5
Chronic lower respiratory disease	126,128	5.2
Unintentional injuries	105,695	4.3
Diabetes	73,965	3.0
Influenza and pneumonia	64,847	2.6
Alzheimer's disease	63,343	2.6
Kidney disease	33,615	1.4
Septicemia	34,243	1.4

Here is the formula:

$$\text{Proportionate mortality} = \frac{\text{Deaths due to specific disease}}{\text{Total deaths from all causes}} \times 100$$

Using data presented in Table 10-5, calculate proportionate mortality rates for:

» **Cancer:**

$$\frac{554643}{2,443,930} \times 100 = 22.7$$

>> **Stroke:**

$$\frac{157,803}{2,443,930} \times 100 = 6.5$$

>> **Chronic lower respiratory disease:**

$$\frac{126,128}{2,443,930} \times 100 = 5.2$$

>> **Unintentional injury:**

$$\frac{105,695}{2,443,930} \times 100 = 4.3$$

Case fatality rate

In epidemiology, case fatality rate is also known as case fatality ratio (CFR). It's the proportion of the people who die among those who have the disease.

CFR depends on the virulence of the disease, infective dose, host defense, and effectiveness of the treatment. CFR is widely used in epidemic situations and also in nonepidemic periods of a disease. Due to effective treatments, CFR has come down to less than one in the case of cholera epidemics. Table 10-6 lists the data for cases and deaths due to Covid-19 that has been analyzed to calculate CFR of the disease in several major countries which are mostly affected by Covid-19 today.

The formula is as follows:

$$CFR = \frac{\text{Deaths due to a disease}}{\text{Cases due to the same disease}} \times 100$$

TABLE 10-6 **Covid-19 Cases, Deaths, and Case-Fatality Rates, January 23, 2023**

Location	Cases	Deaths	CFR
World	673,382,584	6,746,906	1.00
United States	103,856,217	1,128,807	1.09
India	44,682,015	530,735	1.19
France	39,484,549	163,752	0.41
Germany	37,668,384	164,703	0.44
Brazil	36,734,089	696,323	1.90

Among the countries in Table 10-6, the CFR is highest in Brazil, followed by India, and the United States. A higher CFR may indicate a number of possibilities:

>> That the virus was probably more virulent (causing more complications and deaths)

>> That the people might have had more comorbidities

>> That the disease could have affected more elderly people who are more vulnerable

>> The management of the disease could be less effective

Measuring Incidence and Prevalence

Incidence is the new occurrence of disease or an event. *Prevalence* is the existing cases or a total of old and new cases in a population at a specified time. These measurements depend on the type of the study you're conducting. For example, in a cross-sectional study, you can measure prevalence but not incidence, whereas in a cohort study (or a longitudinal follow-up study), you can measure incidence, relative risk, and attributable risk. (Chapter 17 discusses these measurements in greater detail.)

Among 41,800 women, 620 are of premenopausal age, 1,450 have had their breasts surgically removed, and 2,225 women had a previous diagnosis of breast cancer. After five years of follow-up, 1,025 women were newly diagnosed with breast cancer. Calculate the prevalence and incidence rates of breast cancer among post-menopausal women at the end of five years. Express the rates per 1,000.

$$\text{Prevalence} = \text{old} + \text{new cases} = 2,225 + 1,025 = 3,250$$

$$\text{Denominator} = \text{Population at risk}$$

To calculate prevalence, the following women aren't at risk:

Those who had their breasts removed = 1,450

Premenopausal women = 620

Figure out who's at risk:

$$\text{Population at risk} = 41,800 - 1,450 - 620 = 39,730$$

$$\text{Prevalence rate} = \frac{3,250}{39,730} \times 1,000 = 81.8 \text{ per 1,000 population}$$

For incidence, you need to know new cases. Read the following statement mentioned in the problem, where it says: "After five years of follow-up, 1,025 women were newly diagnosed with breast cancer." Therefore, the new cases used for the calculations of incidence = 1.025.

Now check who're at risk. The following women aren't at risk for incidence:

Those who had their breasts removed = 1,450

Premenopausal women = 620

Those who already have had breast cancer (old cases) = 2,225

Population at risk = $41,800 - 1,450 - 620 - 2,225 = 37,505$

Incidence rate = $\frac{1025}{37,505} \times 1,000 = 27.3$ per 1,000 population

Standardizing Rates

Standardization is necessary when you want to compare the disease status (such as incidence or mortality) of two populations, which aren't comparable with respect to other exposure variables of interest, such as variability in age-group rates. You can reduce or eliminate the effect of age-specific rates (or other variability) and standardize the observed rates in your study population by using a method called *standardization*.

By standardization, you can remove the effect of a potential confounder (or a noise variable) between the association of an exposure and a disease. These sections discuss the two types of standardization: direct and indirect. The direct method is preferable over the indirect method.

Using the direct method

Suppose you have a mortality rate (or incidence rate) for the data in your study population. You want to standardize the observed mortality rate in your study population.

For the direct method of standardization, you want to calculate the overall mortality rate (or incidence rate) that you would have expected to find if your study population had the same age-specific rates as the standard population.

To select a standard population, use one of the following methods:

>> Use the least exposed population.

>> Use a sum of two populations.

>> Use the standard population that has been used by others (such as an international organization)

Here I show you a step-by-step method of using the direct method. Table 10-7 shows the data of your study population.

TABLE 10-7

Distribution of Deaths by Age-Group and Person-Year in the Study Population

Age Group	Person-Year	Death
0–15	52	13
16–45	76	7
46–85	112	7
Total	240	27

Select the standard population. Table 10-8 shows the data of your standard population.

TABLE 10-8

Distribution of Deaths by Age-Group and Person-Year in the Standard Population

Age Group	Person-Year	Death
0–15	130	3
16–45	100	9
46–85	33	2
Total	263	44

Here are the steps to follow:

1. **Calculate the observed death rate for the study population.**

   Here's the formula for observed population (O):

   $$O = \frac{\text{Total deaths in the study population}}{\text{Total person} - \text{year}}$$

   Use Table 10-7 (for study population) to fill in this equation:

   $$O = \frac{22}{240} = 0.1125$$

2. **Calculate age-specific weights for the standard population.**

   Here is the equation for calculating weight:

   $$\text{Weight} = \frac{\text{Age} - \text{specific person} - \text{year in the standard population}}{\text{Total person} - \text{year}}$$

   Use Table 10-8 (for standard population) to fill in this equation:

   $$\text{Weight for age} - \text{group} (0 - 15) = \frac{130}{263} = 0.49$$

   $$\text{Weight for age} - \text{group} (16 - 45) = \frac{100}{263} = 0.3$$

   $$\text{Weight for age} - \text{group} (46 - 85) = \frac{33}{263} = 0.13$$

3. **Calculate age-specific death rates for the study population.**

   Here is the formula:

   $$\text{Age} - \text{specific death rate} = \frac{\text{Age} - \text{specific death in study population}}{\text{Age} - \text{specific person} - \text{year}}$$

   Use Table 10-7 (for study population) to fill in the equation:

   $$\text{Death rate for age} - \text{group}(0 - 15) = \frac{13}{52} = 0.25$$

   $$\text{Death rate for age} - \text{group} (16 - 45) = \frac{7}{76} = 0.0921$$

   $$\text{Death rate for age} - \text{group} (46 - 85) = \frac{7}{112} = 0.0625$$

4. Calculate expected death rate for the study population.

Here is the formula for expected death rate (E):

$$E = \sum (\text{Age} - \text{specific death rate in study population})$$
$$(\text{Age} - \text{specific weight in standard population})$$

$$E = (0.25)(0.49) + (0.0921)(0.38) + (0.0625)(0.13) = 0.1656$$

5. Calculate the standardized mortality ratio (SMR) of the observed death rate and the expected death rate.

Here is the formula:

$$SMR = \frac{O}{E} \times 100 = \frac{0.1125}{0.1656} \times 100 = 67.9\%$$

The expected death rate would be 67.9 percent higher than the observed death rate in the study population if the study population had the same age-specific rates as the standard population.

Utilizing the indirect method

The indirect method is the easier way to calculate standardization. In this method, you also calculate the observed mortality rate (or another parameter, such as incidence rate) in your study population, and then compare that with the rate in the standard population.

Here is an exercise: In Mississippi, you *observed* 782 deaths from pneumonia and flu in a year. Is this number in excess of the number you had *expected*?

To calculate, select a standard population.

Find the death rate from pneumonia in the standard population. Suppose it's 1 in 10,000 or 0.0001.

According to the 2020 census, Mississippi's population is 2,961,279. If Mississippians die from this disease at the same rate as do people in the comparison (or standard) state, you'd expect:

Total deaths = Death rate × Population

Total death = 0.0001 × 2,961,279 = 296

$$SMR = \frac{O}{E} \times 100 = \frac{782}{296} \times 100 = 264\%$$

If you take the rate of the standard population, the death rate is expected to be 264 percent lower than the observed rate in the study population.

3
Prevention Is Better Than a Cure

Chapter **11**

Focusing on the Levels of Prevention

hree levels of prevention have been established in public health. They are primary prevention, secondary prevention, and tertiary prevention. This chapter examines the methods and means of carrying out these three levels of prevention.

Identifying Primary Prevention

Primary prevention concentrates on averting the occurrence of a disease in a person who is apparently healthy and doesn't have the disease in question. The following sections discuss how you get primary prevention from vaccines, health education, personal hygiene, and proper nutrition.

Combating diseases by vaccines

You can prevent a number of diseases, known as *vaccine-preventable diseases*, by using vaccines. These diseases are as follows:

» **Covid-19:** Although most people who get this viral infection show mild to moderate symptoms, some can develop severe life-threatening illnesses.

Covid-19 vaccines remain the single most important tool to protect people against serious illness, hospitalization, and death. More studies are ongoing to investigate the efficacy of the vaccines against newer variants of the virus.

>> **Measles:** In some cases, this highly infectious viral disease can cause major complications including pneumonia, brain swelling, and death. One dose of MMR vaccine is 93 percent effective against measles, 78 percent effective against mumps, and 97 percent effective against rubella. Two doses of MMR vaccine are 97 percent effective against measles and 88 percent effective against mumps.

>> **Whooping cough:** Serious complications of this bacterial infection are pneumonia, seizures, and slowed or stopped breathing. Four doses of DTP vaccine — diphtheria, pertussis (also called whooping cough), and tetanus vaccine — can protect against these three diseases.

>> **Influenza (flu):** Up to 61,000 Americans die from this disease, commonly known as flu, each year. The flu can create severe complications for people with asthma or diabetes. In the United States flu is a seasonal disease, from October to May. Most cases happen from late December to early March. Getting a flu vaccine early in flu season — by the end of October — is ideal. A flu vaccine can't protect a person 100 percent from getting the illness, but it prevents major complications.

>> **Polio:** Two doses of inactivated polio vaccine (IPV) are 90 percent effective or more against paralytic polio; three doses are 99 percent to 100 percent effective. Although polio is almost eradicated from the world, a recent report of two cases of wild poliovirus type 1 (WPV1) from Khyber Pakhtunkhwa, one of the four provinces of Pakistan, is a public health concern. The Global Polio Eradication Initiative (GPEI), spearheaded by national governments, the World Health Organization (WHO), the Centers for Disease Control and Prevention (CDC), Rotary International, UNICEF, and other partners have been successful to reduce the disease to 99.9 percent. GPEI has set a new target of polio eradication by 2030.

>> **Pneumococcal disease:** This bacterial infection can cause pneumonia, and infections of ear, blood, and the brain (meningitis). Pneumococcal vaccine protects you from infections caused by *Streptococcus pneumoniae* bacteria. The primary series consists of three doses routinely given at 2, 4, and 6 months of age. If a person gets pneumococcal vaccines for the first time at 65 or older, they'll need two shots, one year apart.

>> **Tetanus:** *Clostridium tetani* bacteria causes this bacterial disease. The bacteria can enter the body from a cut or a wound. The CDC recommends tetanus vaccination for all babies, children, preteens, teens, and adults. Adults need booster shots every ten years to get protected.

>> **Meningococcal disease:** This bacterial infection can cause serious illnesses such as septicemia (blood infection) and meningitis (infection of the brain). All children ages 11 through 12 should receive meningococcal vaccine, followed by a booster dose at age 16.

>> **Hepatitis B:** The hepatitis B virus causes this chronic liver disease. A person gets the virus through sex or needle sharing, and a pregnant mother can pass it to the baby. This virus is 100 times more infectious than HIV (the human immunodeficiency virus), which causes AIDS. Infants should get their first dose of hepatitis B vaccine at birth and will usually complete the series at 6 to 18 months of age. An adult needs three doses of the vaccine.

>> *Haemophilus influenzae* **type B (Hib):** This bacterial infection affects lungs (pneumonia), blood (sepsis), brain (meningitis), bone, or joints. The CDC recommends Hib vaccination for all children younger than 5 years old in the United States.

Giving health education

Health education offers a big role in improving people's health. Health education is both a process and a product:

>> **Education:** The process of education encompasses education at home, at school, at daycare, through the community, and from the parents, friends, and others. In other words, not all education comes from a formal institution. If your child spends only 4 to 5 hours in school, imagine how much education they're getting from their teachers. Most of the learning is through interactions with others. The same is true for getting information about your health.

>> **Product:** Health education products vary — information in the form of leaflets or brochures for smoking cessation given through an outreach program in the community, an exercise education session for young adolescents to prevent overweight and obesity, an educational intervention aiming to prevent cavities in small children, and so on. Therefore, health education includes information on supplies of vaccines, proper nutrition, lifestyle changes, safety at work, safe water and sanitation, food safety, environmental pollution, and many others.

Taking prenatal care

Prenatal care is when someone pregnant get checkups and services from a health-care professional — doctor, nurse, or midwife — throughout the pregnancy. Prenatal care aims to reduce or prevent pregnancy-related health problems of the mother and the baby. A good prenatal care focuses on

>> Reducing the risk of pregnancy complications

>> Reducing the fetus's and the baby's risk for complications

>> Providing necessary medications and supplements

Here's what happens and why prenatal care is important:

1. **At the first prenatal visit, the healthcare provider takes a comprehensive history.**

A proper history is the key to ensuring proper care. The healthcare provider asks several questions about any present and past illnesses, any previous surgeries, history of previous pregnancies, current medications, and a family history.

2. **During this visit the provider performs a thorough physical exam.**

They take blood and urine for lab tests and check weight, height, and blood pressure. They might also do a breast exam, pelvic exam to check the uterus, and a cervical exam, including a Pap test.

3. **After the first visit, the healthcare provider schedules follow-up visits in a regular interval depending on the patient's condition.**

4. **In follow-up visits, the healthcare provider performs a physical exam, takes some routine blood and urine tests, and checks the fetus's conditions, such as its heartbeat and growth.**

Using an ultrasonography, the healthcare provider can detect any abnormalities of the baby and identify the fetus's gender.

During a pregnancy ultrasound, a healthcare provider uses a small handheld machine called a transducer to produce high-frequency sound waves through the patient's uterus. These sound waves send a signal back to a machine where they're converted to images on a monitor.

REMEMBER

An ultrasonography is important in detecting any pregnancy complications. An ultrasonography during a prenatal visit does the following:

>> Confirms the pregnancy and its location (within or outside the uterus)

>> Determines the fetus's gestational age

>> Confirms the number of fetuses

>> Evaluates the fetus's growth

>> Identifies any birth defects

>> Studies the position of the placenta and amniotic fluid

>> Identifies any complications

>> Helps in performing other tests

Prenatal care is especially crucial for women with high-risk pregnancies. Here are women who are likely to be at high-risk:

>> Teens and women older than 35

>> Women who have had problems in previous pregnancies

>> Women pregnant with multiples (twins, triplets, or more)

>> Women who are overweight or obese

>> Women who are undernourished

>> Women who have current or past health problems, such as high blood pressure, diabetes, asthma, HIV infection, autoimmune disease, cancer, and others

Assuring proper nutrition

Proper food and nutrition keeps a person healthy. A balanced diet provides *immunity*, meaning the power to protect oneself from illnesses, whereas an unbalanced diet can weaken a person's immune system and invite illnesses. In this section, I discuss the importance of different kinds of food that people need for growth and for sufficient energy to fight illnesses.

With a balanced diet a person needs all kinds of important food and the right amount of each of them. The right kind of balanced diet depends on a person's age. For instance, a young growing child needs protein-rich foods important for growth and muscle development.

As an epidemiologist, you may take care of the health of senior citizens. You may advise seniors about the following foods:

REMEMBER

>> **Raw eggs:** Limiting raw eggs is important for seniors to lower the risk of foodborne illnesses. Some products to avoid are homemade mayonnaise, eggnog, and hollandaise sauce.

>> **Uncooked meat and seafood:** Uncooked meat also poses a risk of foodborne illness especially on a compromised immune system. If you love red meat, avoid rare steak. Furthermore, seniors should avoid raw oysters, crab, scallops, eel, octopus, or any other fish that is eaten raw.

>> **Deli meats:** Seniors are encouraged to eat protein; however, deli meats may be loaded with salt and harmful additives. The American Institute of Cancer Research has suggested that processed meats, such as cured bacon, sausage, and ham increase the risk of colorectal cancer. Seniors can reduce their consumption of deli meats; tuna, salmon, or egg salad are healthier choices.

>> **Unpasteurized dairy and juices:** Calcium-rich milk and dairy products are great for bone health. However, seniors should avoid unpasteurized milk, unpasteurized juice, and soft cheeses due to a higher risk of foodborne infections.

- **Soda:** Soda is full of carbohydrates or sugar; products high in sugar can accelerate demineralization of teeth and bone. Drinking water sweetened with some orange or lemon juice can give added natural flavors.

- **Alcohol:** Mixing alcohol with certain medications may lessen their effectiveness or cause serious side effects. Alcohol may also lower blood pressure, which is a serious concern for many seniors. For some people, excessive drinking may cause disturbed sleep. Moderation in alcohol consumption is the key.

- **Salt:** Keeping salt intake as low as possible. According to the CDC, all persons older than 50 should consume no more than 1.5g of sodium per day, which is slightly more than a half teaspoonful of salt.

A balanced diet for a healthy adult should contain six food groups in the proper amount in a person's diet. The following lists these food groups:

- **Carbohydrates:** Carbohydrates are an excellent source of energy and a key component of a balanced diet. One gram of a carbohydrate provides 4 calories, and carbohydrates should comprise roughly 60 percent of a person's diet or approximately 310 grams. Food sources of carbohydrates are rice, pasta, potatoes, and wheat.

- **Protein:** One gram of protein provides 4 calories with the maximum daily amount of protein being 50 grams for an adult. Protein primarily helps with the development of muscles and skin. Lean meats are an excellent source of protein. Here are 15 other foods that are great sources of protein:

  - **Tofu, tempeh, edamame:** These soy products are rich in protein, iron, and calcium.

  - **Lentils:** They're good sources of protein, fiber, calcium, and potassium. Cooked lentil contains 8.8g of protein per $\frac{1}{2}$ cup.

  - **Chickpeas:** Also called garbanzo beans, they can be added to stews and curries. They contain 7.25g of protein per $\frac{1}{2}$ cup.

  - **Peanuts:** They're a protein-rich, heart-healthy food. They contain about 20.5g of protein per $\frac{1}{2}$ cup serving.

  - **Almonds:** They offer 16.5g of protein per $\frac{1}{2}$ cup.

  - **Spirulina:** Spirulina is a dietary supplement that provides mostly protein. It can be added to water, smoothies, or fruit juices.

  - **Quinoa:** This grain can fill in for pasta in soups and stews.

  - **Mycoprotein:** This fungus-based protein provides 13g of protein per $\frac{1}{2}$ cup serving.

- **Chia seeds:** A complete source of protein, they contain 2g of protein per tablespoon.

- **Hemp seeds:** They provide 5g of protein per tablespoon.

- **Potatoes:** A large baked potato provides 8g of protein per serving.

- **Protein-rich vegetables:** Examples include broccoli, kale, and mushrooms.

- **Seitan:** Made from mixing wheat gluten and several spices; it provides high protein for vegetarians.

- **Ezekiel bread:** Made from whole sprouted barley, wheat, lentils, soybeans, and spelt; it's a good source of protein and carb.

» **Fat:** One gram of fat contains 9 calories. Healthy fats are unsaturated fats, which are in dairy products, lean meats, and fish. A person can eat up to 70 grams of fat per day.

» **Minerals:** Minerals promote organ growth. For example, calcium helps in bone and teeth development, and iron provides energy and facilitates blood formation.

» **Vitamins:** There are two groups of vitamins:

- **Water-soluble vitamins:** Examples are vitamins B and C. A person gets water-soluble vitamins from vegetables and fruits.

- **Fat-soluble vitamins:** Examples include vitamins A, D, E, and K. The best dietary sources of fat-soluble vitamins are fish fat and fish oil. Exposure to ultraviolet light can also provide vitamin D. Animal meat, fish liver, beef liver, eggs, dark green vegetables, sweet potatoes, carrots, cabbage, and asparagus are other sources of fat-soluble vitamins.

» **Water:** About 66 percent of food contains water. In addition to the water used for making food, an adult should drink 2.7 liters to 3.7 liters (or about 90 to 125 ounces) of water per day.

Providing safe water, sanitation, and hygiene (WASH)

Access to safe and clean water, adequate sanitation, and practice of hygiene are three prerequisites to ensure health and prevent many water-related diseases. However, many developing countries are facing challenges to ensure these basic needs for their populations. In this section, I explain how the global WASH program, which focuses on providing safe and clean water, sanitation, and hygiene, can help prevent diseases and improve health. Consider some of these staggering statistics:

>> One in three people globally don't have access to safe drinking water.

>> Nearly half the world's population, 3.6 billion people, don't have access to safely managed sanitation in their homes.

>> Lack of access to hand-washing facilities is responsible for 700,000 deaths each year.

>> In rural areas, only 1 in 3 people have access to basic hygiene services, such as soap and water at home.

Universal access to WASH programs can reduce the global disease burden by 10 percent. Between 2000 and 2016, improved sanitation saved 15 percent of deaths from diarrheal diseases alone in several countries in Southeast Asia, East Asia, and Oceania. According to a WHO report, every dollar invested in water safety and sanitation returns $4.30 and an estimated gain of 1.5 percent of global gross domestic product (GDP). These benefits are estimated based on the reduced healthcare costs, reduced pollution, increased workplace productivity, increased school attendance, and improved privacy and safety of the people.

Recognizing Secondary Prevention

Sometimes you may not prevent a disease from happening; however, by detecting a disease earlier, you may start the treatment early enough to reduce sufferings from the disease. *Secondary prevention* aims to identify diseases in the earliest stages before the onset of clinical sign and symptoms so that intervention measures will be more effective. For example, if a pregnant woman during her antenatal visits is screened for her hemoglobin status and found anemic, giving an iron treatment will keep her and the fetus healthy. Screening for iron status is a secondary prevention.

Here are some secondary prevention measures (Chapter 15 discusses screening programs in greater detail):

>> A breast self-exam and mammogram can detect breast cancer.

>> A stool of occult blood test can detect colon cancer.

>> A Pap smear test can detect cervical cancer.

>> A prostate-specific antigen (PSA) test can detect prostatic cancer.

>> A tuberculin skin test (also called a Manteaux test) and a chest X-ray can detect tuberculosis.

Examining Tertiary Prevention

Tertiary prevention seeks to reduce the impact of established disease by eliminating or reducing disability, minimizing suffering, and maximizing potential years of quality life. The disease already has occurred, it has been treated clinically, but the patient needs more care to limit the effects and damage caused by the disease and restore the patient to an optimal functioning state.

Here are the goals of tertiary prevention:

>> Helping those diseased, disabled, or injured individuals to avoid wasteful use of healthcare services

>> Avoiding dependency upon others, such as the family, healthcare professionals, and healthcare institutions

Components of tertiary prevention are as follows:

>> Rehabilitation

>> Patient education

>> Health counseling

>> Vocational training

These sections discuss two types of disabilities that can be prevented. Limiting disabilities fall under tertiary prevention.

Limiting any disability

One of the goals of tertiary prevention is to limit disabilities and promote a healthy life. The two types of disabilities are as follows:

>> **Visible:** Common examples of visible disabilities are amputations, paralysis, cerebral palsy, muscular dystrophy (a group of muscle diseases caused by alterations in the genes), multiple sclerosis (fatigue, vision problems, muscle spasm, stiffness, weakness, and muscle pain — due to multiple nerve damage), and autism (developmental disability).

>> **Invisible:** Invisible disabilities can include chronic diseases such as asthma, renal failure, depression, hearing loss, and sensory and processing difficulties.

TIP

As a public health professional, you can reduce the chance of disability or becoming disabled by providing the following health advice:

>> **Quit smoking.** Smoking invites a variety of life-threatening illnesses including cancer, heart disease, and asthma.

>> **Get a regular checkup.** Major complications of diseases can be prevented by early detection and a regular checkup.

>> **Get regular cancer screenings.** Because cancer is a major cause of disabilities, someone with possible risk factors should go for regular cancer screenings.

>> **Avoid excessive drinking.** Excessive drinking can further worsen complications such as liver damage or heart disease. The Substance Abuse and Mental Health Services Administration (www.samhsa.gov) can help answer any questions about alcohol habits.

>> **Get regular exercise.** Periodic physical activity and exercise can help restore functions in patients recovering after heart surgery or who have a chronic lung condition such as asthma or COPD.

>> **Stay active.** Recovering from major surgery or having chronic pain shouldn't stop someone from staying active. Spend time with others, take a walk with a friend, or just watch a movie together. Help people find purpose in living and leading a good life.

Providing rehabilitation

Rehabilitation is any attempt to restore an afflicted person to a reasonably healthy, useful, productive, and satisfying lifestyle. The purpose of rehabilitation is to promote the highest quality of life possible, given the extent of the damage and disabilities the person suffers from.

As a public health professional, you can consider some of the following methods of rehabilitation:

>> Helping the person change jobs suitable for their condition

>> Supplying resources to help them find vocational training

>> Offering education

>> Directing them to counseling

>> Providing recreational facilities for improving their quality of life

Chapter **12**

Preventing Disease with Vaccine

Vaccines prevent more than a dozen serious infectious diseases. In fact, vaccines have eradicated smallpox, and a global push for polio eradication is ongoing. However, a few new cases of wild polio make the global polio eradication program challenging. Humanity now faces a new challenge in controlling Covid-19.

Having a sound knowledge of vaccines and other preventive measures is important to tackling ongoing and emerging infectious diseases. This chapter primarily focuses on preventing diseases by vaccines. You can also find what vaccines are recommended for children at different ages. In addition, I also explain other ways immunity is obtained, such as the transfer from mothers to babies, the natural way, such as getting an infection, or by immunity transfer through using gamma globulins. I also discuss what vaccines and preventive measures you should take before traveling to an infectious disease–prone area.

Getting the Lowdown on Immunity

The human body is continuously being exposed to a number of infective agents such as bacteria, viruses, parasites, fungi, and molds, which can enter the body through air, water, food, soil, and physical contacts. But how come people aren't infected all the time? And why are some people infected and some aren't?

Here are several factors that are responsible for an infection to occur:

>> **Infective dose:** There must be enough of the infective agent to cause an infection.

>> **Infectivity or infectiousness:** *Infectivity,* also referred to as *infectiousness,* refers to how likely an agent that enters the body will cause an infection. For example, the measles virus is highly infectious.

>> **Virulence:** *Virulence* refers to how severe a disease is, which can include death. After an infection, a disease can progress to show many complications and death, or it may be cured quickly, sometimes even without any treatments. Such diseases that are cured with an intervention or treatment are called *self-limiting diseases,* whereas diseases that cause more complications and death are called more *virulent.*

>> **Host defense:** The human body offers a defensive mechanism against an infection, which is called *immunity.* Human organs such as bone marrow, spleen, thymus, tonsils, mucous membrane, and skin can protect many diseases or even kill infecting agents.

These sections discuss immunity in greater detail by looking closer at the immune system and identifying the different kinds of immunity.

Understanding the body's immune system

Here I discuss the organs and tissues in the human body that act in the defense against agents.

Bone marrow

Bone marrow, which is the soft tissue inside the bone, produces red blood cells, white blood cells, and platelets. White blood cells take part in the body's defense function. Lymphocytes, which are one type of white blood cells, play an important role in the body's immune system. The two types of lymphocytes that comprise the immune system are as follows:

> » **B cells:** B cells mature in the bone marrow.

> » **T cells:** T cells travel from the bone marrow to the thymus (see the later section) and mature there to become active for the defense function.

Spleen

This organ located on the left side of the abdomen filters all blood. The unwanted products such as old and damaged cells and germs get removed so clean blood is the end result that is circulated back in the body. Lymphocytes and macrophages, another type of white blood cell, kill the germs.

Thymus

The thymus is a small gland only found before puberty. After puberty it starts to slowly shrink and become replaced by fatty tissue. The thymus is located behind the flat chest bone called the sternum and between the lungs. The thymus secretes a hormone called thymosin. Thymosin stimulates the development of disease-fighting T cells.

Tonsils and lymph nodes

The tonsils are small glands located in different parts of the body and work like guards to protect germs from entering the body. For example, two relatively large-sized tonsils are located on each side of the throat and palate. They can stop germs from entering the body from the mouth and the nose.

There are also small lymph nodes under the armpit, in the chest and the abdomen, near the elbow, and groin. These lymph nodes contain immune cells that fight infection by attacking and destroying germs that are carried in lymphatic fluid.

Mucus membranes

Mucus membranes work like your winter clothes — they're protective physical and biochemical barriers. Mucus membranes cover the entire respiratory system, digestive system, and the urogenital tracts. They also cover the eye conjunctiva, the inner ear, and the ducts of all exocrine glands with powerful mechanical- and chemical-cleansing mechanisms. Exocrine glands are those that make sweat, tears, saliva, milk, and digestive juices in the stomach, pancreas, and intestines. The mucosal immune system prevents potentially dangerous germs from entering and growing inside the body.

Skin

The skin is the first layer of protection on your body. In addition to a physical barrier, the skin also acts as an active immune organ. Traversed by an extensive network of blood vessels and lymphatic vessels, the inner layer of skin called the *dermis* contains lymphocytes, leukocytes, mast cells, and tissue macrophages. The outer layer of skin called the *epidermis* is equipped with immune-competent cells, such as Langerhans cells, the macrophage-like cells, keratinocytes, epithelial cells, and melanocytes — all of which act like frontline defenses against environmental toxins and germs.

Comparing natural and acquired immunity

The human body has its own defensive mechanisms to fight off an infection. The entire system is a natural barrier against many infective agents. Here are examples of *natural immunity:*

>> The skin and the mucus lining from the mouth to the anus provides natural defense against any invading germ.

>> A person sneezes or coughs, which is often triggered when an irritant or foreign body tries to enter the nose or mouth.

>> When a person vomits, they expel many germs from the stomach and out the mouth. The natural system works as soon as they come into contact with a foreign substance or an infective agent.

A person can get immunity a second way — called *acquired immunity.* An acquired immunity usually takes several days to be fully developed and provide immunity in a naive host (who didn't have a disease or haven't received a vaccine). The acquired immune system with the help from the natural body system (such as immune organs and immune cells), makes special proteins, called *antibodies,* to protect the body from a specific invader. These antibodies are developed by cells called B lymphocytes after the body has been exposed to the invader. That's why it can take several days for antibodies to form. But after the first exposure, the immune system will recognize the invader and defend against it.

Comparing active and passive immunity

Immunity in the form of antibodies comes in four types:

>> Natural passive immunity

>> Artificial active immunity

>> Natural active immunity

>> Artificial passive immunity

The following sections delve deeper into these four kinds of immunity.

Natural passive immunity

A child can get natural passive immunity from their mother through the placenta while in the womb or from breastmilk after birth. Research indicates that a baby's passive immunity from the mother lasts for around six months of life.

One study examined passive immunity to measles in infants. The study found that the passive immunity gradually diminished and didn't last more than nine months.

Artificial active immunity

Because natural passive immunity only lasts around 6 to 9 months, a baby needs long-lasting immunity. This type, referred to as *artificial active immunity*, happens through an immunization. The immunizations train the child's immune system to make antibodies to protect them from harmful diseases for a longer period. The immunity provided by a vaccine varies with the type of disease.

Natural active immunity

Natural active immunity is the type of immunity that a person gets from an infection or a disease. After they recover from an infection with a virus or a bacterial pathogen, the immune system retains a memory of it. Immune cells and proteins that circulate in the body can recognize and kill the pathogen if they encounter it again, protecting against the disease and reducing its illness severity. This type of immunity varies with the type of disease and the severity of the disease that person had.

Artificial passive immunity

Another way a person can actively acquire immunity is called *artificial passive immunity.* In this manner, if a person doesn't naturally produce antibodies, they can receive an injection of antibodies, such as gamma globulin, shot directly into their bloodstream, giving them immediate immunity.

One major disadvantage of passive artificial immunity is that it provides immunity only for about 3 to 4 months. After the antibodies disappear, the person is just as susceptible as someone who had never been exposed. Only active immunity through an immunization is long lasting.

UNDERSTANDING HERD IMMUNITY

Herd immunity refers to the ability of a minority group of population or community living in a herd (or group) to protect themselves from an infectious disease because the majority (or a large proportion) of the population of the group have become immune or unable to contract the disease. Herd immunity occurs by passing immunity to nonimmune people from people who have been vaccinated, or by people who contracted the disease. For herd immunity to be effective, the number of immune persons — either by vaccination or by previous exposure to the disease, needs to be large enough to transfer immunity to other nonimmune persons living in the herd.

For example, if people living in an area where vaccine coverage is low and most children aren't vaccinated, it's likely that some infected people in a crowd may easily spread the infection to others. If one of these contacts has measles, the others in the population can easily get measles from the infected person. Herd immunity applies to any infectious diseases like diphtheria, measles, Covid-19, and others.

Furthermore, the percentage of the population that is required to be immune for herd immunity to be reached varies with the type of infectious disease. Basically, it depends on how easily the disease can spread from one person to another. For that reason, a large number of people need to be vaccinated for herd immunity to be successful.

Here are a few examples of the critical numbers of the vaccinated (or otherwise immune) population that is necessary to reach an effective level of herd immunity in order to prevent people (herd), who are unvaccinated or who have not contracted the disease from being infected:

- **Rubella:** Requires 85 to 95 percent of community residents to be vaccinated or immune to the disease by having the disease.

- **Diphtheria:** Requires only 70 percent immune people in the community to transfer herd immunity.

- **Measles:** Because measles is easily transferred from one person to another, a higher percentage of the community need to be immune to transfer immunity. The critical number for measles is 95 percent.

- **Polio:** The threshold is about 80 percent.

Herd immunity can be measured at the local, national, and global levels, and the level of protection may change over time. Suppose a large group of people in a local community didn't get vaccinated this year against a very contagious disease and the immunity of the people in the local community against the disease decreased, the disease may resurge the following year or sooner. This happened in Clark County, Washington in 2019, when a measles outbreak occurred in public schools because the vaccination rate in public schools fell to 77 percent.

However, setting a critical number for herd immunity in the case of Covid-19 is difficult because the disease agent is frequently changing and also becoming more virulent by mutation. For example, at the beginning of the Covid-19 pandemic scientists figured out that 60 to 70 percent of vaccinated people could probably protect the nonvaccinated population from contracting the disease. However because the virus that causes Covid-19 continues to evolve and change, this number of 60 to 70 percent wasn't working. Researchers don't yet know how long immunity to Covid-19 lasts after infection or vaccination. Hence, they advocate a *booster shot* (an additional vaccine dose). Because the increase in more infectious variants of the virus could potentially impact the effectiveness of available vaccines, researchers now estimate that the herd immunity threshold for Covid-19 is probably 85 percent, meaning at least 85 percent of the population should be vaccinated to get herd immunity to other nonvaccinated people.

Planning Shots for Children, from Birth through Adolescence

You may choose to work with childcare health and development after your epidemiology studies. If so, you already know that vaccinations can prevent many diseases before they affect a baby. With that knowledge, you should advise people that a parent needs to plan for the baby's good health. There's no alternative and no better method than giving timely vaccinations to protect the baby from common illnesses and help the child grow as a healthy adult.

The immunization programs of the Centers for Disease, Control, and Prevention (CDC), the Expanded Program of Immunization (EPI) of the World Health Organization (WHO), and the health programs of UNICEF and other healthcare organizations advocate and promote these vaccination guidelines to all people around the world.

TECHNICAL STUFF

The EPI was established in 1974 to develop and expand immunization programs throughout the world. Initially, six diseases — diphtheria, pertussis, tetanus, poliomyelitis, measles, and tuberculosis — were under the umbrella of the program. UNICEF works with partners to establish, maintain, and improve the cold chain for vaccines and other essential medical supplies, engage communities, procure and distribute vaccines, and help ensure affordable access for the vaccines for every family in more than 100 countries. Tremendous progress has been achieved over the past 40 years toward development of effective national immunization programs throughout the world.

REMEMBER

There are a number of vaccinations that infants and children should get:

>> Hepatitis B (Hep B)

>> Rotavirus (RV1 and RV5)

>> Diphtheria, tetanus and pertussis (DTaP)

>> *Haemophilus influenzae* Type B (Hib)

>> Pneumococcal vaccine (PCV13)

>> Injectable polio vaccine (IPV)

>> Influenza

>> Measles, mumps, and rubella (MMR)

>> Chickenpox (varicella)

>> Hepatitis A

>> Meningitis (meningococcal vaccine)

Table 12-1 provides specific guidelines for the vaccination of children starting at birth until the child is 15 months old.

TABLE 12-1   **Vaccination Schedule for Infants from Birth to 15 Months Old**

Vaccine	Birth	1 mos	2 mos	4 mos	6 mos	9 mos	12 mos	15 mos
Hepatitis B (Hep B)	1st	2nd					3rd	
RV1 (2 doses); RV5 (3 doses)			1st	2nd	3rd (RV5)			
DTaP			1st	2nd	3rd			4th
Hib			1st	2nd			3rd or 4th	
Pneumococcal (PCV13)			1st	2nd	3rd		4th	
IPV <18 years			1st	2nd	3rd			
Influenza					Annual 1 or 2 doses			
MMR							1st	
Varicella							1st	
Hepatitis A							1st	

To read this table, identify the vaccination in the left-hand column and then follow along that row to see when the series of vaccinations should be administered. Take hepatitis B in the first row. A baby should receive the first dose at birth, the second dose between 1 and 2 months old, and the third dose between 9 and 15 months old.

Table 12-2 lays out a vaccination schedule for children and teens starting at 18 months up to 18 years.

You can read Table 12-2 the same way as Table 12-1.

TABLE 12-2   ## Vaccination Schedule for Children and Teens

Vaccine	18 m	19-23 m	2-3 y	4-6 y	7-10 y	11-12 y	13-15 y	16 y	17-18 y
Hep B	3rd								
DTaP	4th			5th					
IPV	3rd			4th					
Influenza	Annual 1 or 2 doses				Annual 1 dose only				
MMR				2nd					
Varicella				2nd					
Hepatitis A	2 dose series								
Tdap ≥ 7 years									
HPV									
Meningococcal									

DO'S AND DON'TS FOR PREGNANT WOMEN AND VACCINES

Certain live vaccines, such as MMR and chickenpox (varicella), may not be safe during pregnancy and in mothers who are breastfeeding. Yellow fever vaccine also isn't advised in women while breastfeeding.

Although some people were concerned about the Covid-19 vaccine, data from American, European, and Canadian studies showed that receiving a vaccination with an mRNA Covid-19 vaccine during pregnancy wasn't associated with an increased risk of pregnancy complications, including preterm birth, stillbirth, bacterial infection of the placenta, and excessive maternal blood loss after birth.

(continued)

(continued)

A Chicago study also showed that women vaccinated against Covid-19 before or during the first trimester didn't have any added risk of pregnancy complications such as birth defects.

The CDC is also continuously monitoring any adverse effects of the Covid vaccines in pregnant and lactating mothers. A new CDC analysis of current data showed that among nearly 2,500 pregnant women who received an mRNA Covid-19 vaccine (Moderna and Pfizer vaccines) before 20 weeks of pregnancy, there was no increased risk of miscarriage.

When you're working with moms-to-be, share important information from the CDC about the safety for all vaccines. Check out www.cdc.gov/vaccines/pregnancy/vacc-safety.html. Here is a quick recap of what you can read at the site:

- Some vaccines made of a killed version of the germ that causes a disease are called *inactivated vaccines.* Pregnant and lactating mothers may safely receive inactivated vaccines. Here are some examples of inactivated vaccines:

  - **Hepatitis A:** This is a waterborne and foodborne disease.

  - **Flu:** A pregnant woman can receive the flu shot before *and* during pregnancy, depending on whether or not it's flu season during a pregnancy. The flu vaccine is also safe while breastfeeding.

  - **Polio:** This vaccine protects against paralytic polio.

  - **Rabies:** This disease is transmitted from animal bites.

  - **Tdap:** This vaccine helps protect against tetanus, diphtheria, and whooping cough during pregnancy.

- A second group of vaccines is prepared from live viruses, so pregnant mothers shouldn't take these vaccines during pregnancy. However, pregnant women should get them before or after pregnancy if they didn't receive the vaccine as a child. They include the following:

- **MMR:** To protect against measles, mumps, and rubella.

- **Chickenpox vaccine (varicella):** Nursing women who lack evidence of immunity should receive the varicella vaccine, administered during the postpartum visit (6 to 8 weeks after delivery). Women who get varicella vaccine may continue to breastfeed.

- **Yellow fever vaccine:** Until more information is available, breastfeeding women should avoid this vaccine.

Looking Closer at Cancer-Preventing Vaccines

Scientists are exploring ways to lower cancer risk at every stage of life, and they've recognized infections with certain type of viruses, bacteria, and parasites as risk factors for several types of cancers in humans. These infections are linked to about 15 percent to 20 percent of cancers.

Infections can raise your risk of cancer in different ways. For example:

>> Some viruses directly affect cellular growth and multiplication. These viruses work directly on the genes that control cell growth. The viruses can insert their own genes into the cell, causing the cell to grow out of control.

>> Some types of infections can cause long-term inflammation in a part of the body, which can lead to changes in the affected cells and in nearby immune cells, which can eventually lead to cancer.

>> Some infections can suppress the immune system, which normally helps protect the body from some cancers.

These sections describe several cancer-causing viruses, bacteria, and parasites and highlight a few vaccines that can be used to prevent cancers.

Identifying cancer-causing viruses

Scientists have linked several viruses with cancer in humans and have developed vaccines against some of these cancer-causing viruses. *Note:* These vaccines must be given before the person is exposed to the cancer-promoting virus. Chapter 15 discusses many of the screening tests available to identify many of these types of cancers.

Human papillomaviruses (HPVs)

More than 150 viruses are called *papillomaviruses* because some of them cause papilloma (also called *genital warts*). Sexually active people are more likely to be infected with HPVs at some point in their lives. About a dozen of these HPVs are known to cause cancers. If you're exposed to long-lasting infections of these high-risk types of HPV, you can develop cancer. However, not all HPV infections will cause cancers.

HPV can cause the following types of cancer:

>> **Cervical:** HPV is the main cause of cervical cancer. Because Pap smears are widely available for screening (see Chapter 15), cervical cancer has become less common in the United States. A Pap smear can detect precancerous cells on the surface of the cervix.

>> **Vaginal:** Vaginal cancer is a rare type of cancer. Older women can develop it after HPV infection.

>> **Vulval:** This type of cancer can occur at the outer surface of the female genitals.

>> **Anal:** Sexual activity increases the risk of anal cancer. It's common in both men and women. Men who have sex with men have a high risk of this cancer.

>> **Mouth and throat:** HPV is believed to cause 70 percent of cancers of mouth and throat (called oropharynx).

REMEMBER

Here is important information about HPV vaccines:

>> Both females and males can get HPV vaccines.

>> The best time for boys and girls to get the shot is between ages 9 and 12.

>> Children and young adults who haven't been vaccinated earlier, should get the vaccine between ages 13 and 26.

>> No one older than 26 should get the HPV vaccine.

Hepatitis B and hepatitis C viruses

Long-term infections with both hepatitis B and hepatitis C viruses can progress to chronic hepatitis and hepatocellular carcinoma (or liver cancer). Hepatitis C virus is also linked with another cancer called non-Hodgkin lymphoma.

The viruses spread through needle sharing for injectable drug users, blood transfusion, unprotected sex, and childbirth. In the United States, transmission of the viruses through blood donation is rare because a donor's blood is tested for several germs including the hepatitis viruses. Jaundice (or yellow coloration of skin, eyes, and urine) is a common symptom of hepatitis.

Vaccines are available for hepatitis A and hepatitis B, but not for hepatitis C.

The hepatitis A (HepA) vaccination is recommended as follows:

>> All children 12 to 23 months old, followed by a second dose after 6 months.

>> HepA can be given as early as 6 months of age if the baby travels to a place where hepatitis A is common. The baby will still need to follow the routine vaccination after their first birthday.

Meanwhile, the hepatitis B (HepB) vaccination is recommended as follows:

>> All infants, children, and adolescents younger than 19 years of age should be vaccinated.

>> Adults ages 19 through 50, and adults older than 60 with risk factors for hepatitis B infection should receive a vaccine.

>> Three doses of HepB should be taken — the second dose at a month after the first dose and the third dose at 6 months after the first dose.

Human immunodeficiency virus (HIV) and cancer risk

HIV infection is linked with a number of cancers:

>> **Kaposi sarcoma:** This type of cancer forms in the lining of blood vessels and lymph vessels.

>> **Non-Hodgkin's lymphoma:** This type of cancer begins in the lymphatic system, which is part of the body's germ-fighting immune system.

>> **Anal cancer:** Some cancers in the anal region (anal canal and anus) are malignant, others are benign (not malignant), and some are precancerous (may develop into cancer).

>> **Hodgkin's disease:** This type of cancer starts in the white blood cells called lymphocytes. Lymphocytes are part of the body's immune system.

>> **Lung cancer:** Lung cancer is the most frequent cause of cancer deaths in HIV-infected people.

>> **Mouth and throat cancers:** Data suggests that HIV-infected patients are at two to six times greater risk of cancers in the oropharynx (mouth and throat).

>> **Liver cancer:** Having coinfection with hepatitis B and hepatitis C, patients with HIV infection have a higher burden of hepatocellular carcinoma (liver cancer) and end stage liver disease compared to others who don't have HIV infection.

>> **Skin cancer:** HIV-infected patients have certain types of skin cancers more common than other skin cancers (more basal cell type than squamous cell type).

HIV VACCINE

No vaccine is available to prevent HIV infection. However, a person can lower the risk of cancers by taking HIV medicines regularly if they're HIV infected. They can also reduce the risk of getting HIV infection by several means:

>> Not having unprotected sex

>> Not sharing needles with someone who has HIV

>> Reducing the number of sex partners

>> Taking PrEP (pre-exposure prophylaxis)

Epstein-Barr virus (EBV)

Epstein-Barr virus (EBV), best known for its causing mononucleosis or the "kissing disease," is a type of herpes virus. In addition to kissing, the virus can be spread from one infected person to another through the air by coughing and sneezing and through sharing drinking and eating utensils.

EBV can increase the risk of some cancers, including:

>> **Nasopharyngeal cancer:** Cancer of the back of the nose

>> **Burkitt lymphoma:** A type of non-Hodgkin lymphoma or the cancer of the lymphatic system that is responsible for a person's immunity. In this cancer, the body makes abnormal B-lymphocytes.

>> **Hodgkin lymphoma:** Also called Hodgkin's disease (see the previous section).

>> **Stomach cancer:** Only 8 to 10 percent of stomach cancers (also called *gastric cancer*) are associated with EBV.

No vaccine is available to prevent EBV, and there currently is no cure for cancers caused by EBV.

Human herpes virus 8 (HHV-8)

HHV-8 is transmitted through sex, blood, and saliva. About 10 percent or less of the U.S. population is infected with this virus. People with a weakened immune system who have this virus may develop Kaposi sarcoma, which is more common among HIV-infected patients (refer to the section, "Human immunodeficiency virus (HIV) and cancer risk," earlier in this chapter.

Rarer types of viruses

Other rare types of cancer-causing viruses include:

» **Human T-lymphotrophic virus-1 (HTLV-1):** HTLV-1 is a retrovirus that causes a chronic lifelong infection in humans.

» **Merkel cell polyomavirus (MCPyV):** Infection with MCPyV is most frequently detected in skin.

» **Simian virus 40 (SV40):** It induces primarily brain and bone cancers.

Cancer-causing bacteria

The bacteria *Helicobacter pylori* (*H. pylori*) is commonly found in about two-thirds of the world population. It colonizes in the stomach and can cause stomach cancer and lymphomas. However, in one study, only 3 percent of *H. pylori*-infected patients developed gastric cancer. Several antimicrobial agents such as clarithromycin, metronidazole, and amoxicillin are effective against *H. pylori*. The standard treatment of *H. pylori* is called *triple therapy*, which includes proton pump inhibitors (PPI), clarithromycin, and amoxicillin or metronidazole.

Researchers have made some progress in the therapeutic use of bacteria in the cancer treatment, either alone or in combination with conventional therapies for cancer. They're continuing to find the use of genetically modified bacteria to treat cancer. For the first time they've used live bacteria for cancer treatment. Here are two examples:

» *Streptococcus pyogenes*, a bacteria that causes many serious diseases such as pneumonia, sepsis, and toxic shock syndrome, helped in the regression of cancer in a patient with cancer and *erysipelas* (a systematic infection caused by *Streptococcus*).

» *Clostridium* infection in patients with gas gangrene and cancer helped in tumor regression. A vaccine, known as *Bacillus Calmette-Guerin* (BCG), given for the prevention of tuberculosis in many countries (except the United States), has shown to reduce cancer frequency.

Cancer-causing parasites

A couple protozoan parasites are linked with cancer. They are as follows:

>> *Schistosoma haematobium:* Referred to as a *blood fluke*, it causes urinary bladder cancer. Praziquantel (an anti-parasitic medicine), given one to two days, can clear the infection.

>> *Plasmodium falciparum:* This parasite causes malaria. The parasite can act as a co-factor in the development of Burkitt lymphoma. Because of the potential risk of multidrug resistance of *P. falciparum*, the drug should be chosen cautiously. Generally, chloroquine or hydroxychloroquine are drugs of choice.

>> *Cryptosporidium:* This parasite commonly implicated for diarrhea in immuno-compromised patients such as in patients with AIDS can also cause diarrhea in children. The CDC published a report of 32 outbreaks of diarrhea in the United States in 2016, demonstrating that they were linked with *Cryptosporidium* infection from swimming pools and water playgrounds. Several epidemiologic and clinical studies suggest the link of the parasite with colon cancer and cancer of other digestive organs such as bile duct and pancreas. No vaccines are available for this parasite. Nitazoxanide is the only FDA-approved treatment for cryptosporidiosis in adults and children older than 12 months with a healthy immune system.

Identifying Common Vaccine-Preventable Diseases

This section describes vaccine effectiveness in a few vaccine-preventable diseases. I also provide some available information on the natural immunity you may get if you have had the disease in the past.

Measles

Measles (also referred to as rubeola) is highly infectious with symptoms appearing 7 to 14 days after contracting the virus. Typical symptoms include high fever, cough, runny nose, and watery eyes. A measles rash appears 3 to 5 days after the first symptoms. Measles may cause complications including ear infection, diarrhea, and pneumonia. Children younger than 5 and adults older than 20 are more likely to suffer complications.

Two doses of MMR vaccine usually give lifelong protection to measles, but in some cases the immune response of the vaccine may decline after 10 to 15 years.

Mumps

Mumps is a viral disease transmitted by air and by direct contact with symptoms including swollen salivary glands (located under the jaw), fever, headache, tiredness, and muscle pain. In complicated cases, the infection can go to the brain and spinal cord, causing meningitis and *encephalitis* (brain swelling). Inflammation of the testicles or ovaries can cause sterility.

Two doses of MMR offer 88 percent protection against mumps. However, immunity against mumps may decrease over time, and some people may no longer be protected against mumps later in life, but they're less likely to develop serious complications. After a person has been infected with mumps, they normally develop an active natural immunity against further infection for life-long.

Rubella

Rubella — also called ten-day measles or German measles — is a highly contagious airborne disease transmitted through tiny droplets in the air from an infected person's cough and sneeze. Typical symptoms of rubella are similar to other viral infections, including a low-grade fever, headache, mild pink eye, general discomfort, swollen and enlarged lymph nodes, cough, and runny nose. The main symptom of rubella is a red or pink spotty rash that starts on the face or behind the ears and spreads to the neck and body. The rashes takes 2 to 3 weeks to appear after the infection. Complications of rubella include heart problems, loss of hearing and eyesight, intellectual disability, and liver and spleen damage. Pregnant women who contract rubella are at risk for miscarriage or stillbirth, and their developing babies are at risk for severe birth defects.

People who receive an MMR vaccination are usually considered protected for life against rubella. After an infection, people have immunity to the disease for the rest of their lives.

Diphtheria

Symptoms of this infectious disease include sore throat, high fever, swollen glands in the neck, difficulty in breathing and swallowing, and weakness. A thick gray-white coating may cover the back of the throat, nose, and tongue. Diphtheria can occur more than once if the person isn't vaccinated.

Natural disease occurrence doesn't give a life-long immunity. According to a study, the effectiveness of the Tdap vaccine against diphtheria in children ages 5 to 9 exceeds approximately 75 percent.

Whooping cough

The first symptoms of whooping cough, a highly contagious respiratory infection, are similar to those of a cold, including a runny nose, red and watery eyes, a sore throat, and a slightly raised temperature. Intense coughing — sounds like "whoop," hence the name — bouts start about a week later and usually last a few minutes at a time and tend to be more common at night. Even if you had whooping cough, also referred to as *pertussis*, in the past, the bacteria can infect you again because immunity from the disease doesn't last a lifetime.

Tdap, the vaccine against tetanus, diphtheria, and pertussis protects about 7 out of 10 people in the first year. The effectiveness of the vaccine declines in each following year. About 3 or 4 out of 10 people are fully protected four years after getting Tdap.

Tetanus

A deadly disease, tetanus causes painful spasms, stiffness, and contractions, particularly in the jaw and neck muscles. These symptoms are followed by difficulty swallowing, abdominal muscle rigidity, and episodes of shortness of breathing or no breathing, sweating, nervous system dysfunction, eventually causing death. Tetanus bacteria enters the body through breaks in the skin — usually cuts or puncture wounds caused by contaminated objects.

Adolescents and adults receive either the Td or Tdap vaccines. These vaccines protect more than 95 percent of people from disease for approximately ten years. Currently, the CDC Advisory Committee on Immunization Practices recommends a booster shot every ten years. People who recover from tetanus don't have natural immunity and can be infected again.

Polio

Poliovirus, which is transmitted through contaminated water and food or contact with an infected person, infects through a person's throat and intestines, causing flu-like symptoms such as sore throat, fever, nausea, and headache. The infection can spread to the brain and spinal nerves, causing paralysis.

Two doses of IPV provide at least 90 percent protection, and three doses give almost 100 percent protection. Poliovirus infection can provide lifelong immunity against the disease. Although the disease has been eradicated from the United States and most parts of the world, a few cases of wild polio were reported in 2022 from Khyber Pakhtunkhwa and Punjab in Pakistan. Furthermore, the recent discovery of polio in New York City wastewater creates a new challenge for the polio eradication program.

Rotavirus

Rotavirus, the most common cause of watery diarrhea in children younger than 5, presents first as typical symptoms of a viral fever, such as moderate to high body temperature, cough, runny nose, and watery eyes. Diarrhea follows and is often accompanied with vomiting and dehydration.

Recovery from a first rotavirus infection usually doesn't lead to permanent immunity. The rotavirus vaccine is more than 85 percent effective at protecting against severe rotavirus infection in the first two years of life. Some babies who are vaccinated will still get rotavirus infection, but the disease is usually milder.

Covid-19

Covid-19 is a deadly, highly infectious viral disease with symptoms appearing 2 to 14 days after exposure to the virus. Most common symptoms include fever or chills, cough, muscle or body aches, headache, a new loss of taste or smell, congestion or runny nose, and diarrhea. If a person experiences any of the following warning signs, they need to seek emergency medical care immediately:

>> Trouble breathing

>> Falling oxygen saturation

>> Persistent chest pain or pressure

>> New confusion

>> Inability to wake or stay awake

>> Pale, gray, or blue-colored skin, lips, or nail beds

Available evidence shows that fully vaccinated individuals and those previously infected with SARS-COV-2 (the virus for Covid-19) have a low risk of subsequent infection for at least 6 months. The level of protection may not be the same for all Covid-19 variants and the types of available vaccines. The level of protection may also be decreased over time even in vaccinated people and among those who have had a previous infection, if the person is immunocompromised.

Chickenpox

The varicella-zoster virus causes chickenpox, which is an airborne disease and is also transmitted by droplet infections from an infected person. Chickenpox symptoms include an itchy, red rash that breaks out on the face, scalp, chest, back, and on the extremities. The rashes quickly fill with a clear fluid, rupture, and then turn into crusty blisters. Complications include infected blisters, bleeding disorders, encephalitis, pneumonia, and death (in rare cases).

Studies have shown that people vaccinated against varicella get antibodies for at least 10 to 20 years after vaccination. Most people who have had chickenpox will be immune to the disease for the rest of their lives. Very rarely, a second infection of chickenpox can happen. The virus remains inactive in nerve tissue and may reactivate later in life causing shingles (see the next section).

Shingles

Although shingles isn't life-threatening in fairly healthy adults, it does cause a painful skin rash that consists of blisters that typically scab over in 7 to 10 days. Before the appearance of the rash, the infected person may have itching, tingling, and pain in the area with the pain lasting even after the rash is gone. Most people who develop shingles have only one episode during their lifetime. However, a person can have shingles more than once.

Two doses of shingles vaccine provide strong protection against the disease. In one study, the vaccine was found 97 percent effective in preventing shingles in adults 50 to 69 years old with a healthy immune system.

Hib

Hib is caused by *Haemophilus influenzae* Type b infection. Symptoms vary from mild infection to ear infection to serious blood infection that cause severe headache, shortness of breath, pneumonia, meningitis, seizures, loss of consciousness, and death.

Hib conjugate vaccines are highly effective in producing immunity to Hib bacteria. More than 95 percent of infants develop protective antibody levels after receiving a primary series of two or three doses of Hib vaccine. Children who had Hib disease before 2 years of age may be at risk of getting Hib disease again. Children and adults who had Hib disease after 2 years of age are likely to be immune.

Preventing Disease for World Travelers

Vaccines protect travelers from serious diseases. Your career in epidemiology and public health may take you to different parts of the planet. Depending on where you go, you may come into contact with diseases that are rare in the United States like yellow fever. You may also be required to receive certain vaccines before you travel there. Even though you may not be required to be vaccinated before traveling to a country, you may still want to take preventive measures against any disease that is highly prevalent in the country of your destination, and more so, if you're staying there for a few months or longer. These sections give you the current recommended vaccines for travelers.

Vaccinating for cholera

Cholera is a disease that's highly prevalent in Afghanistan, Bangladesh, India, Nepal, Pakistan, Philippines, and other Southeast Asia countries. However, none of those countries, and in fact no country in the world, require you to take the cholera vaccine as a condition for entry.

The U.S. Food and Drug Administration (FDA) approved the use of a single dose oral cholera vaccine (CVD 103-HgR) in adults, 18 to 64 years old in June 2016. In clinical trials, CVD 103-HgR was 90 percent effective in preventing moderate or severe diarrhea from cholera in adults. Vaccine efficacy declined to 80 percent after three months.

In December 2020, results of vaccine effectiveness trials also showed promising results in children and adolescents. The FDA approved the use of a single-dose oral cholera vaccine (CVD 103-HgR) to children and adolescents between 2 and 17. The Advisory Committee on Immunization Practices (ACIP) recommends the oral cholera vaccine for travelers 2 to 64 years old traveling to areas of toxigenic *Vibrio cholerae* O1 transmission. The CDC defines areas of active cholera transmission where 100 or more cases have been reported within the past year.

Although a safe and effective vaccine is available for cholera, no countries require it for travel to the country. The reasons are based on the weight of the benefit over the potential risks.

>> Cholera is rare in travelers mainly because the dose of the bacteria to cause the disease (called the *infective dose*) is very high. Also, travelers usually stay in accommodations where clean drinking water is available.

>> The treatment is readily available and inexpensive.

>> Travelers are advised to adhere to proper hand washing and drinking clean water.

Protecting from malaria

Malaria-prone countries include Sub-Saharan Africa and India, which carry more than two-thirds of the global malaria burden. Six countries — Nigeria, the Democratic Republic of Congo, Uganda, Ivory Coast, Mozambique, and Niger — account for more than half of all malaria cases worldwide. In India, the states of Odisha, Jharkhand, Meghalaya, and Madhya Pradesh have the highest number of malaria cases. These states also have the highest number of *Plasmodium falciparum*, which causes the most dangerous type of malaria.

TIP

If you travel to malaria-prone countries (such as countries in Africa or Southeast Asia), you may use a medicine before travel, during your stay, and after returning from the country:

Three medicines — atovaquone-proguanil, doxycycline, and mefloquine — are most effective for prevention. Do the following:

>> Begin taking the medicine 1 to 2 days before travel.

>> Take daily during travel.

>> Take for 4 weeks after return.

Chapter 6 describes the strategies for controlling and preventing malaria in more detail.

USING REPELLANTS IN MOSQUITO NETS AND ON SKIN

Insect repellents can provide protection against malaria. In areas where mosquitoes feed in the early evening, the use of mosquito nets soaked with repellents between dusk and bedtime can effectively protect against mosquito bites, which has important implications in malaria vector-control programs. The CDC advocates the combined use of treated nets and insect repellents for most tourists travelling to high-risk areas.

The following mosquito repellents are commonly found to work:

- **DEET:** DEET (or diethyltoluamide) is a reliable and highly effective insect repellent and is sold under numerous brand names and comes in lotion, spray, and many other forms. Products with 10 to 35 percent DEET provide adequate protection under most circumstances.

Note: If you utilize DEET, make sure you use proper precautions, especially when using with children who can experience irritation or other reactions after swallowing or prolonged skin application. The American Academy of Pediatrics recommends that repellents used on children contain no more than 30 percent DEET.

- **IR-3535:** This is a non-DEET product. IR-3535 is used as an insect repellent against mosquitoes, deer ticks, and biting flies.

- **KBR 3023:** Also called *icaridin* or *picaridin*, it's a colorless and odorless broad-spectrum repellent that's effective against a number of insects including mosquitoes, ticks, fleas, gnats, and flies. It can be used directly on the skin and clothing.

- **Permethrin:** It's effective, both as a pesticide and a repellent. Permethrin only should be used for clothing, including nets, and shouldn't be used topically. It can retain its potency for at least two weeks, even after several launderings.

- **Lemon eucalyptus oil:** It's the synthetic form of an ingredient found in eucalyptus leaves and twigs. Lemon eucalyptus oil products shouldn't be used on children younger than 3.

Remember these application tips:

- **Do:** Use aerosol or pump sprays for treating clothing and skin except around the mouth or face. Wash repellents off the skin with soap and warm water when you return indoors.

- **Don't:** Apply near the eyes, lips, or mouth, or over cuts, wounds, or irritated skin.

Avoiding hepatitis

When travelling, you can reduce your risk of getting hepatitis if you first remember how hepatitis is transmitted:

>> Hepatitis A is transmitted through water and food.

>> Hepatitis B and hepatitis C are transmitted through unprotected sex, needle sharing, and contact with infected blood.

Vaccines are available for hepatitis A and hepatitis B. The preventive measures aim at breaking the transmission cycle:

>> Get vaccines for hepatitis A and hepatitis B.

>> Use a condom during sex.

>> Avoid multiple sex partners.

>> Don't share needles to take drugs.

>> Practice good personal hygiene such as hand washing with soap and warm water.

>> Avoid an infected person's personal items.

Knowing about the yellow fever vaccine

Yellow fever, a highly infectious viral disease, is transmitted through the bites of the *Aedes* mosquitoes. A safe and effective vaccine (YF-VAX) is available for yellow fever. A single dose of the vaccine gives lifelong protection. People 9 months to 59 years of age who are travelling to or living in areas at risk for yellow fever — mostly African nations — are highly recommended to take the yellow fever vaccine.

Chapter **13**

Recognizing Methods of Disease Surveillance

I n this chapter, you find the nuts and bolts of using surveillance in public health. Surveillance provides a means for determining whether health problems exist and, if so, whether they're increasing or decreasing over time and by place. In addition to communicable diseases, surveillance can also help in knowing the status of noncommunicable diseases or events. For example, surveillance systems may identify a higher-than-expected number of birth defects, a greater prevalence of teenage pregnancy, a decrease in fertility rates, or a decrease in breast-feeding of women within a specified population.

Without having a proper surveillance system in place, you can't know timely information about an emerging infection or the current status of an ongoing disease, which causes public health action to be paralyzed. Surveillance systems allow you to be aware of the changing nature of diseases or events in a population. Surveillance tools enable you as a public health expert in assessing the impact of a disease and combating a disease in your community.

Differentiating between Survey, Surveillance, and Monitoring

Knowing the difference between the terms *survey*, *surveillance*, and *monitoring* can be confusing. They're all used for collecting data — so you may wonder what makes them different. Here I explain in greater detail.

Survey — Making a single observation

A *survey* is a one-time observation where you measure and record something. For example, you're planning a baby shower for one of your friends. You're making a quick list of your closest friends who might come. Then you call them and ask a few questions about a suitable date, the venue, the décor, and the gift items they want to bring. This single process is called a survey.

REMEMBER

Here are several other popular methods of conducting a survey:

» **Online surveys:** This is one of the most popular types because it's quick, convenient, and less expensive. You can survey a large population in a short period of time with an online survey. Many business groups have online surveys for their products. Your doctor's office uses surveys as well. After your visit, you may get an online notification to provide feedback about your satisfaction level for the recent visit.

» **Paper surveys:** As the name suggests, this method uses the traditional paper and pencil approach. Usually this method is a more formal way of recording people's opinions. For example, after a census, you might get a printed paper copy of questions (called a *questionnaire*) by mail to ensure whether you or any of your family members participated in the census or not. The census itself is also a survey because it's used for enumerating people at one point of time.

» **Telephone surveys:** Researchers can conduct surveys over the phone. Sometimes, they use a technique called *random selection,* which means everybody has an equal chance of being selected. This kind of random selection method is used to reduce sampling bias. This provides equal odds for every person in the population to be chosen in the study. Telephone surveys were popular when people used their land-line phones. However, cellphone numbers aren't listed in a phonebook, which makes telephone survey difficult.

» **One-to-one interviews:** This method, also called *physical interviews,* is quite common in research. An interviewer goes to a person's house or to a class and asks a few questions using a questionnaire. This questionnaire can be self-administered, which means the respondent reads the questions and writes their answers. Ideally, this type of self-administered questionnaire should be short and easy to understand for the respondents. The other type of this interview is where the interviewer directly asks the respondent questions and they answer. One-to-one interviews are more accurate and have fewer missing values or dropouts; however, they are more time-consuming and expensive.

Surveillance — Tracking continuously

Surveillance means continuously collecting, analyzing, interpreting, and disseminating data. Surveillance is a cornerstone in public health because it provides accurate data about the endemic diseases in a population and also gives a signal when a disease appears in epidemic form.

REMEMBER

Public health surveillance is used for the following purposes:

>> **To quantify the disease burden:** By continuously monitoring disease events, you can identify the incidence (new cases), prevalence (the existing old plus new case), mortality (or deaths), and complications of a disease. You can also identify some risk factors, such as the age group, gender, race/ethnicity, and other characteristics that are most affecting the disease.

You can identify the burden of the disease in a population by comparing other disease burdens if you administer routine surveillance for several diseases in a population over time. For the same reason you can also monitor a time trend of a disease.

>> **To detect outbreaks or clusters:** You can detect a sudden increase in the number of cases only when you monitor the disease over time. In case of infectious diseases, such as measles, cholera, Covid-19, West Nile fever, and the like, epidemiologists use the term *epidemic,* which means an outbreak, when the disease appears as an unexpectedly large number in a population at a given time. For a noninfectious or noncommunicable disease and events, such as stroke, suicide, accidents, birth defects, cancers, and other events, which are chronic in nature, a sudden increase in the number of such cases is called a *cluster.* However, the term *cluster* also refers to a group of cases grouped in a place and time that are suspected to be greater than usual numbers.

>> **To help public health planning and actions:** The prompt recognition and reporting of cases to health authorities is a critical link in the public health chain of prevention and control. For certain diseases, a continuous monitoring of the pattern of the diseases is vital to make appropriate planning and take accurate interventions. For example, cases of several diseases are periodically notified to the CDC from the state level.

>> **To track the effectiveness of an intervention:** Public health planners and scientists execute many intervention measures in order to reduce the incidence and mortality from diseases and events. Covid-19 vaccine trials and the discovery

of several vaccines are recent examples of such public health interventions. These advances are only possible by the help of a properly conducted surveillance system to evaluate the effectiveness of the intervention measures.

>> **To evaluate disease eradication, elimination, and control:** Here I clarify these three terms with an example:

- **Eradication:** *Eradication* is a deliberate effort to permanently reduce a disease to zero in the world. Smallpox has been eradicated from the world.

- **Elimination:** *Elimination* means stopping the transmission of a disease in a locality or country but not worldwide. Polio has been eliminated from most parts of the world including the United States, and it's about to be eradicated from the world.

- **Control:** The term disease *control* refers to reducing the new infections and the number of people who become sick or die from a disease. A new disease, mpox (formerly known as monkeypox), appeared recently, still in sporadic forms in many countries. According to the World Health Organization (WHO), the disease is an "evolving threat of moderate public health concern" having a total of more than 83,000 confirmed cases and 66 deaths from 110 countries as of the writing of this chapter. The spread of mpox should be controlled so that it doesn't break out as an epidemic. A worldwide disease surveillance program can be helpful in monitoring a disease and evaluating the control measures.

>> **To gauge changes in environmental risk factors:** Public health surveillance also gauges changes in environmental factors, such as physical, biological, chemical, or psychological risks on human diseases, evaluates prevention and control programs for the risks, tracks long-term trends, plans for future resource allocation for the prevention and control, and suggests areas of future research.

Monitoring — Periodically checking

Monitoring refers to systematic reviewing, observing, or checking on the progress or quality of an activity (such as a study) over a period of time. There can be no planning without monitoring, and no monitoring without planning. Monitoring is a periodic tracking, whereas surveillance is a continuous process.

REMEMBER

Some methods of monitoring are as follows:

>> **Process monitoring:** Often referred to *activity monitoring*, process monitoring evaluates the input variables because they determine the outcomes in a study. For example, a machine tool operator performs routine monitoring

tasks; they visually detect missing and broken tools as well as chatter from the characteristic sounds the machine generates.

- **Compliance monitoring:** You need to monitor whether the people are following your intervention procedures. For example, you're offering a community intervention to assess the effect of iron supplementation on young children's health. You must monitor from time to time if the children are taking the medicine (iron) that you wanted them to take every day over a period of three months.

- **Context monitoring:** Also called *situation monitoring,* context monitoring tracks the overall setting in which the project operates. Context monitoring helps epidemiologists identify and measure risks, assumptions, or any unexpected situations that may arise at any point during the time the project is running.

- **Outcome monitoring:** Outcome monitoring can be done periodically throughout and also at the end of the study to evaluate the progress and the final outcome of a study. Some large programs, such as a statewide lead poisoning prevention program in children, or the breastfeeding program offered at a state health department are monitored periodically. However, national surveillance and monitoring of breastfeeding behavior are essential to improve the current low breastfeeding rates in low-income, poorly educated, women in the United States.

Defining the Types of Surveillance

Surveillance is often classified based how it's conducted. You can conduct surveillance by actively seeking reports from the data recorders, or you can wait for them to send it to you as part of their routine work. These sections examine the different types of surveillance.

Active surveillance

In *active surveillance,* you're taking steps to get the data promptly from the data source. This process can produce more complete data of better quality than data provided by other systems. In an active surveillance system, you are proactive and contact healthcare providers or laboratories requesting information about diseases. Often you ask for a report more often from healthcare workers than they would normally do. If necessary, you may offer incentives for additional work they do. In the event that some of the field level healthcare workers consistently fail to report or complete the forms incorrectly, you should discuss and provide feedback that's needed to improve their performance.

Active surveillance requires substantially more time and resources and is therefore less commonly used in emergencies. But it's often more complete than passive surveillance (refer to the next section for more information). It's often used when you suspect that an outbreak might start soon and you need more information, for which you want to keep a closer eye on the events. Community healthcare workers may be asked to do active case finding in the community in order to locate patients who don't go to healthcare facilities.

Passive surveillance

In the case of passive surveillance, you wait to get information from others. *Passive surveillance* often gathers disease data from all potential reporting healthcare workers. Health authorities don't remind healthcare workers to report diseases or provide feedback to individual healthcare workers.

REMEMBER

Passive surveillance is the most common type of surveillance in humanitarian emergencies. Furthermore, most surveillance for communicable diseases is passive. The surveillance coordinator may provide training to healthcare workers in how to complete the surveillance forms and may even send someone to periodically collect forms from health facilities. But little attention is given to individual health workers who report the information.

Although the data requested of each health worker is minimal, passive surveillance is often incomplete because healthcare workers have few incentives to report the data.

REAL LIFE
EXAMPLE

In Bangladesh, field-level healthcare workers called health assistants and community health workers collect all health-related data including new cases, deaths, and demographics at the village level. They go door-to-door to get the information. Then they report the data to the health administrator at the subdistrict level. The health administrator compiles and sends the data to the district level administrator called the civil surgeon. As an epidemiologist or an investigator, you get the compiled data from the civil surgeon for the district level cases and deaths. In addition, at the central level, epidemiologic surveillance teams collect the data. Sometimes it may be too late to wait for the passive surveillance system because you want to act to save lives.

Sentinel surveillance

Instead of attempting to gather surveillance data from all healthcare workers, a *sentinel surveillance system* selects, either randomly or intentionally, a small group of healthcare workers from whom to gather data. These healthcare workers then receive greater attention from health authorities than would be possible with surveillance that selects all healthcare workers.

Although sentinel surveillance requires more time and resources, it can often produce more detailed data on cases of illness because the healthcare workers have agreed to participate and may receive incentives. In fact, it may be the best type of surveillance if each case requires more intensive investigation to collect the necessary data. For example, sentinel influenza surveillance in the United States collects nasopharyngeal swabs from each patient at selected sites to identify the type of influenza virus. Collection of such data from all healthcare workers would be time consuming and nearly impossible.

Conducting Surveillance: The How-to

This section provides you a step-by-step guide for conducting a public health surveillance. The major areas focus on data collection, data analysis, dissemination, and future recommendations.

Planning a surveillance system begins with a clear understanding of the purpose of the surveillance. In public health, here are some examples where you may undertake a surveillance:

>> Assess the health status.

>> Determine public health priorities for the distribution of resources.

>> Identify the risk factors.

>> Identify cause, sources, mode of transmission, infectivity and virulence of the agent, and preventive methods.

>> Evaluate any intervention methods.

>> Conduct a research.

Follow this step-by-step guideline when planning and executing a surveillance system:

1. **Establish your objectives.**

   Determine what you want to achieve from conducting the surveillance.

2. **Develop all case definitions.**

   Use a uniform definition. Your team must use the same case definitions for the major variables. You want to be able to compare your results with others.

3. **Determine all data sources.**

   Data sources can vary, so select the data sources that can provide you the best possible information.

4. Create your team.

Depending on what your surveillance program needs, select the team members, which may include an epidemiologist, a few data collectors, a data analyst, a laboratory support person, and sometimes a medical doctor and/or a nurse.

5. Provide training.

All team members must have prior training on the case definitions, the data collection instruments, and the methods.

6. Determine the data collection mechanism you'll use.

Options include a cross-sectional study, retrospective case-control study, prospective cohort study, and intervention study. Select one that most suits the surveillance system based on the resources and the objectives.

7. Determine your data collection instruments.

If you use a questionnaire, develop it before beginning the surveillance. Sometimes, you may be able to use a data collection instrument that's already available and others have used it. You may also need to modify the instrument for the native language of the people and the purpose of the surveillance (see Chapter 17).

8. Pre-test the instruments in the field.

Conduct a small-scale test of the data collection instrument in the population before you actually use it.

9. Develop an analytic approach.

Having a thorough knowledge in statistical methods and data analysis procedures is important. If you don't, you need to have someone on your team who can provide statistical support.

10. Develop strategies for community involvement.

REMEMBER

Community engagement is the key to success. You need to build a good rapport with the community before beginning the surveillance procedures. Sometimes, cooperation from community leaders or religious leaders may be helpful. Community members may be trained on simple things such as sample collection or case finding.

11. Provide proper case management.

In the process of surveillance, you'll find new cases. Your team needs to provide proper case management and referral system if needed.

12. Disseminate the results and develop control strategies.

After the surveillance is completed, disseminate the findings to the public, health administrator, and health agencies so they develop further control strategies.

Chapter **14**

Investigating an Outbreak

The world is currently devastated by several epidemics, such as Covid-19 and HIV/AIDS. In epidemiology courses, you'll hear about two types of disease epidemics: small-scale outbreaks, such as a foodborne disease outbreak, that involve a select group of people and major epidemics that affect a large number of people.

What constitutes an epidemic? How can you find out the cause of an epidemic? This chapter answers these questions. As an epidemiologist your role is to investigate a disease outbreak or an epidemic and find out the possible causes or risk factors for the disease, to understand how to minimize the loss of lives by taking actions as quickly as possible, and to inform the general public about ways to control the disease and what actions they can take to prevent another outbreak.

An outbreak investigation involves several steps. The most important step is asking whether you're ready. Here I provide you with a step-by-step guide that can prepare you for an outbreak investigation.

Conducting an Epidemic Investigation

Just having a few cases of a disease isn't always an outbreak. However, epidemiologists would consider a single case of smallpox anywhere in the world a serious public health concern and a red flag because the disease has already been eradicated from the entire world. Epidemiologists may refer to this situation as an *impending epidemic,* which needs to be further investigated. The following sections help you with understanding the existence of an epidemic, the sources of the epidemic, and the ways to combat it.

Classifying epidemics

Here are the two types of sources of an epidemic (refer to Chapter 7 for more information):

>> **Common source epidemic:** An infectious agent or toxin causes this type of epidemic and spreads among a group of people from the same contaminated source, either food, water, or drink. Examples include a foodborne outbreak (such as salmonella infection) that spreads through contaminated food or a contaminated community water supply spreads the disease cholera.

To confirm that it's a common source epidemic, as an epidemiologist, you'd ask a few simple questions:

- Is the outbreak from a single source or a single point exposure?
- Is there continued exposure to a single source?

>> **Propagated source epidemic:** This type of epidemic spreads directly from person to person or through vectors or vehicles. Examples include an outbreak of hepatitis B virus infection or an epidemic due to shigellosis (also called blood dysentery).

To identify a propagated source epidemic, an epidemiologist would ask a few more questions:

- Is the disease spread from person to person?
- Is the outbreak from multiple sources and/or exposures?
- Is the outbreak airborne, behaviorally or chemically caused, and does it involve multiple events or exposures?
- Are the sources of infection not apparent?
- Is a vector involved in the transmission?
- Is an animal the reservoir of infection? (A *reservoir* is one where an agent lives, grows, and multiplies — see Chapter 5 for more information).

Understanding the threshold level of an outbreak

Several diseases, known as *epidemic-prone diseases*, can cause epidemics in many countries. They also appear in certain seasons of the year (which is called a *seasonal trend*) or they may show up in an epidemic form after a few year intervals (which is called a *secular trend*).

Here are some examples of epidemic-prone diseases:

>> **Cholera:** The waterborne disease cholera is extremely common in Southeast Asia Region and in African countries because of the lack of access to safe drinking water, sanitation, and hygiene. In Bangladesh, cholera appears in epidemic form every year, usually in two peaks, before and after the monsoon season. Figure 14-1 shows the epidemic of cholera appeared with higher average rainfall.

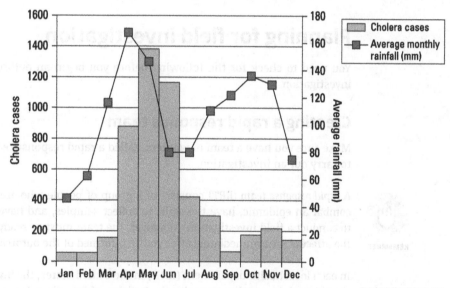

FIGURE 14-1: The seasonality of cholera epidemics.

© John Wiley & Sons, Inc.

>> **Blood dysentery:** The disease is called blood dysentery because people pass blood in the stool and have severe pain when defecating. The bacteria *Shigella* causes blood dysentery (also referred to as shigellosis). Two species of the bacteria are more commonly found in Asian countries: *Shigella dysenteriae* type 1 and *Shigella flexneri*. The disease caused by *Shigella dysenteriae* type 1 is more severe and life-threatening.

>> **Rotavirus diarrhea:** In developed countries and many developing countries, the main cause of diarrhea in children is rotavirus. Initially, rotavirus causes fever and vomiting followed by 3 to 7 days of watery diarrhea and crankiness. The disease becomes severe due to dehydration. Children with moderate-to-severe dehydration also become lethargic and must be treated for dehydration as soon as possible. In the temperate climates, rotavirus is more commonly seen during the fall and winter, whereas it occurs mostly in the autumn or spring in other parts of the world.

TECHNICAL STUFF

There is no magic number that constitutes an epidemic or what's called an *endemic state* of a disease. The number of cases of a disease that epidemiologists consider as an endemic for a particular country may be considered too big for another country. For example, in the hospital that I worked in Bangladesh, I used to see about 100 patients with diarrhea every day. At least five to six of them showed *Vibrio cholera* on a stool culture. A single case of cholera found in a New York or Washington D.C. hospital would cause a panic if epidemiologists suspected a cholera outbreak, whereas 100 cases of diarrhea and five cases of cholera found in Bangladesh may not be considered an epidemic there.

Planning for field investigation

You need to check for the following before you begin an outbreak or epidemic investigation.

Creating a rapid response team

Make sure you have a team of workers, called a rapid response team (RRT), ready to carry out an investigation.

REMEMBER

A *rapid response team (RRT)* consists of a group of people who are well-trained to combat an epidemic, have the skills to collect samples, and have the know-how to conduct a field investigation. Moreover, the team must be ready to move fast to the affected area immediately after you're informed of the outbreak.

In each local health department (LHD) in the United States, the investigation team should work in coordination with the Division of Infectious Disease Epidemiology (DIDE) for an infectious disease outbreak and the Chronic Disease Prevention Program at the State Health Department for a chronic disease outbreak. Remember, this is a coordinated effort to combat an outbreak.

TIP

Prepare the team as follows:

>> Identify the team members

>> Assign all responsibilities

>> Designate a team leader

>> Begin the investigation as early as possible

>> Communicate at all levels, including any relevant community members who the investigation team can start working with.

Having the adequate resources

Verify you have the resources to manage the patient load that you encounter during the epidemic. The two main types of resources are as follows:

>> **Personnel:** This highly trained skilled team should have at least a few field workers for data collection, one laboratory staff member to collect samples, a nurse, an epidemiologist, and sometimes a doctor for case management.

>> **Supplies:** Make sure you have a continuous flow of medicine, rehydration fluids, and cleaning supplies.

Digging Out Cases by Surveillance, Step-by-Step

Surveillance is a kind of detective work where you go door-to-door and scrutinize all the new and ongoing cases. The doctor and nurse(s) in the RRT treat all new cases either at the ill person's home or at a makeshift hospital (refer to the section, "Using Makeshift Hospitals," later in this chapter). The major complicated cases will be referred to a regular hospital. Here is more information about surveillance.

Establishing the existence of an outbreak

The following reasons are why you conduct surveillance:

>> **Identify patients and provide a quick treatment.** Do door-to-door case finding and provide their immediate treatment.

>> **Assess the magnitude of the epidemic.** Compare the current number of cases and deaths with those of the past (checking hospital records).

>> **Establish the existence of an outbreak.** Verify the diagnosis and the number of cases.

>> **Identify the pathogen involved and its drug sensitivity patterns.** This helps in selecting the right drugs for the treatment.

>> **Set up control measures and monitor the progress.** Refer to the section, "Implementing control measures," later in this chapter.

The following are the actions you take when conducting a surveillance:

>> **Counting numbers:** To help in assessing the risk and magnitude of an epidemic, you need to get the previous record of similar cases (if any) from other sources, such as the doctor's clinical records or hospital records.

>> **Preparing an epidemic curve.** You prepare a day-to-day record and plot all the cases and deaths before and after the outbreak, either using a bar chart or a line chart. This chart tells you when the outbreak started, when the peak was, when it started to decline, and when cases or deaths stopped. This chart shows a curve over time, which is called an *epidemic curve*. If the numbers exceed way beyond the expected numbers (or the endemic cases), you can estimate that there is an epidemic/outbreak.

>> **Identifying the pathogen.** Your job is to find out what's causing the outbreak. Collect stool samples (which include a rectal swab for diarrhea) and any food samples, if available. Lab tests will identify the pathogens that are causing the outbreak (refer to the next section). Sometimes isolating the causative agent from food sources or the water is difficult because the causative agent may not be present in sufficient numbers in the sources. For the purpose of treatment, you need to find the drug sensitivity pattern in case the common drugs aren't working. This is also done routinely in a lab.

Verifying the diagnosis with data

Use these two types of data to make and confirm the diagnosis:

>> **Clinical data:** This information includes the patient's history and examination findings.

>> **Laboratory data:** Sample specimens, such as stool, vomitus, blood, and environmental samples (water, food, and such) are tested in the lab for the presence or absence of any possible agents or organisms.

REMEMBER

The clinical and laboratory data confirms the diagnosis. For example, a person with watery diarrhea, rice-watery in color, with profuse vomiting, and the isolation of *Vibrio cholera* in their stool samples constitute a case definition of cholera.

Identifying new and ongoing cases

Some cases can only be diagnosed by house-to-house visits. The RRT team develops a questionnaire to collect data from all household members. All active cases must be managed promptly, preferably at the field level, using appropriate technologies and resources available in the field. The team refers complicated cases to a nearby hospital.

Intensifying the existing surveillance system

The RRT works with local health authorities (medical officers and other health professionals) and volunteers, recruited from the community to intensify the surveillance system. This type of surveillance targeted to a disease is known as *active surveillance*. The activities of the team are as follows:

>> **Review the reporting system.** The RRT team reviews the existing cases and deaths from hospital records.

>> **Follow the case definition.** The team prepares a case definition using the clinical and the laboratory data collected earlier. The team follows this case definition for investigating the epidemic.

>> **Provide more training to the RRT staff based on the experience gained from the ongoing investigation.** This is an important step in the investigation. Before launching further investigations, the team members and any local volunteers should be trained on the case definition, case finding techniques, and case management.

>> **Establish a daily reporting system of all cases and deaths.** All new cases and deaths should be analyzed and reported to the local health authority.

>> **Use line listing of cases and deaths and maintain a clinic/hospital record.** Line listing includes serial number, name, age, gender, address, date of attack, date of recovery or death, major symptoms, treatments given, and any complications.

Performing descriptive epidemiology

As the RRT gathers data, they conduct descriptive epidemiology, which includes comparing cases and deaths in terms of time, place, and person. The following sections provide characteristics of time, place, and person that they analyze:

>> **Time:** Determine each case (and death, if any) by the time of onset (or the time of death) using an epidemic curve. An epidemic curve shows time on the x-axis and number of cases (or deaths) on the y-axis (Refer to the section, "Establishing the existence of an outbreak," earlier in this chapter.

>> **Place:** Using a spot or dot map is useful in locating cases and deaths. It also gives clues about the cluster of cases and may help in determining the mode of transmission.

>> **Person:** All cases (and deaths) should be tabulated in terms of age, sex, race, religion, education, income, and other demographic characteristics.

The RRT can then use this information as it works to figure out the following:

>> **The type of epidemic:** Determine whether most cases of the epidemic occurred in a very short period of time or gradually over time.

>> **The source:** Identify the suspected sources of the epidemic by collecting samples and testing them for the agent.

Using analytical statistics to calculate the attack rates

Results of these analyses are vital to generate a hypothesis regarding the possible cause of the epidemic, the nature of transmission (common source or man-to-man transmission), the treatment outcome, and a possible time frame when the outbreak could be stopped. The team analyzes the data more to prove the hypothesis. Table 14-1 is a dummy table, having only symbols but no data in it. The team members collect and enter data using the dummy table and then they calculate attack rates, using this formula:

$$\text{Attack rate} = \frac{\text{Number of persons sick}}{\text{Total persons at risk}} \times 100$$

TABLE 14-1 **Calculating Attack Rates**

Food Item	Persons Who Ate Specific Food (Exposed)				Persons Who Didn't Eat Specific Food (Not exposed)			
	Sick	Not Sick	Total	Attack Rate (%)	Sick	Not Sick	Total	Attack Rate (%)
X	a_x	b_x	$a_x + b_x$	$\dfrac{a_x}{a_x + b_x}$	a_{0x}	b_{0x}	$a_{0x} + b_{0x}$	$\dfrac{a_{0x}}{a_{0x} + b_{0x}}$
Y	a_y	b_y	$a_y + b_y$	$\dfrac{a_y}{a_y + b_y}$	a_{0y}	b_{0y}	$a_{0y} + b_{0y}$	$\dfrac{a_{0y}}{a_{0y} + b_{0y}}$
Z	a_z	b_z	$a_z + b_z$	$\dfrac{a_z}{a_z + b_z}$	a_{0z}	b_{0z}	$a_{0z} + b_{0z}$	$\dfrac{a_{0z}}{a_{0z} + b_{0z}}$

REAL LIFE EXAMPLE

Suppose as an epidemiologist you're going to investigate a foodborne outbreak. The suspected source is a restaurant, where the following food items were served: rice, meat, and tomato salad. Some of the people got diarrhea, and some didn't; among those who were sick or remained well, some ate certain food items and some didn't eat them. Table 14-2 shows the distribution of the people among those who ate the food item and those who didn't eat them, and the people who were sick and those who weren't sick.

TABLE 14-2 **Distribution of Sick and Well People**

Food Item	Persons Who Ate Specific Food (Exposed)				Persons Who Did Not Eat Specific Food (Not Exposed)			
	Sick	Not Sick	Total	Attack Rate (%)	Sick	Not Sick	Total	Attack Rate (%)
Rice	62	31	$62 + 31 = 93$	$\dfrac{62}{93} \times 100 = 66.7$	2	0	$2 + 0 = 2$	$\dfrac{2}{2} \times 100 = 100$
Meat	63	25	$63 + 25 = 88$	$\dfrac{63}{88} \times 100 = 71.6$	1	6	$1 + 6 = 7$	$\dfrac{1}{7} \times 100 = 14.3$
Tomato salad	50	26	$50 + 26 = 76$	$\dfrac{50}{76} \times 100 = 65.8$	14	5	$14 + 5 = 19$	$\dfrac{14}{19} \times 100 = 73.7$

Now, calculate the risk of having diarrhea by eating each food item. Divide the attack rate of those who ate a specific food item with the attack rate of those who didn't eat the food item. This risk is called relative risk (RR).

$$RR = \frac{\text{Risk of the disease among the exposed (those who ate)}}{\text{Risk of the disease among the unexposed (those who didn't eat)}}$$

$$\text{RR for rice} = \frac{66.7}{100} = 0.67$$

$$\text{RR for meat} = \frac{71.6}{14.3} = 5.0$$

$$\text{RR for tomato salad} = \frac{65.8}{73.7} = 0.89$$

By analyzing the RRs for the three food items, the team finds that those individuals who ate meat had the highest risk (5.0). In other words, the risk of having diarrhea is 5 times among those who ate meat compared with the people who didn't eat meat. From this data, you may indicate that meat was probably the food item causing the disease outbreak. Further laboratory analysis of the food samples may identify the disease-causing agent.

Developing a hypothesis

Based on your investigation, you have some clues about the disease — whether it spreads from a common source, whether it's a food or drink, or whether it's transmitted from one person to another. Sometimes, a disease agent (a pathogen) can also be transmitted by a vector, such as mosquitoes. The symptoms of the disease help you come to a possible diagnosis.

With all this circumstantial evidence, you're ready to formulate a hypothesis. In the earlier example, your hypothesis is that eating meat might have caused the outbreak of diarrhea. Then you investigate it further to establish the cause and possible sources of the outbreak.

REMEMBER

A *hypothesis* is a statement of proposition or a proposed explanation made on the basis of limited evidence. Further studies are done to prove (or disprove) the hypothesis.

In the real-life example in the preceding section, based on the available data, you deduct a hypothesis about the food item that might have caused the outbreak. However, unless you investigate it further, you can't come to a conclusion. In general, in a diarrheal disease outbreak, there is a hypothesis for the agent that causes the disease and another hypothesis is how the disease is transmitted. Consider the following two hypotheses:

>> **Hypothesis 1:** Meat is the likely cause of the diarrheal disease outbreak.

>> **Hypothesis 2:** The causative bacteria contaminating meat is likely to be *Salmonella*.

Evaluating the hypothesis

You next want to investigate it further to gather more data. To evaluate the hypotheses, do the following:

>> For hypothesis 1, collect stool samples from several infected persons. Test the stool samples for common pathogens causing watery diarrhea.

>> For hypothesis 2, obtain samples of food items, such as rice, meat, and tomato salad, and test them for the common pathogens.

Implementing control measures

Because an outbreak is an emergency situation, you can't delay the control measures until the investigations are complete. Taking proper specific control measures may not be possible unless the investigations are complete with adequate knowledge of source/reservoir and mode of transmission. Basically you have to balance the two. Control/preventive measures for outbreaks are simultaneous ongoing procedures.

Analyze the available data from the surveillance of households, cases, and contacts. Doing so will help you find people who are at a high risk of the disease. In addition to active case management, you need to target high-risk groups in order to prioritize resource allocation. In the meantime, outreach programs and the use of mass media can help educate people in practicing preventive measures.

Reporting the findings

The information that the RRT gathers through the investigation is important to educate the appropriate people. Disseminate the data as quickly as possible to the following:

>> All people, particularly the community where the disease occurred the most

>> The authorities and stakeholders (public health authorities and nurses and doctors), in order to provide immediate steps in furthering control measures and for future disease prevention.

In the United States all data goes to the National Outbreak Reporting System (NORS).

CONTROLLING CHOLERA — A CASE STUDY

In July 1994, one of the worst cholera epidemics broke out among the nearly one million Rwandan refugees in Goma, eastern Zaire. An eight-member medical team from International Center for Diarrheal Disease Research, Bangladesh (Icddrb) went to combat the epidemic. During their two-week stay, the team, in collaboration with UNICEF and the Ministry of Health, Zaire, conducted an epidemiological assessment and set up a microbiology laboratory in Goma to identify the pathogens responsible for the epidemic and test the antibiotic sensitivity pattern of the isolated pathogens.

Deaths from cholera in the treatment centers were much higher than cases seen in the past, which was primarily due to *Vibrio cholerae* strains resistant to conventional antibiotics. In addition, an inappropriate use of rehydration therapy and inadequate experience of health workers failed to reduce deaths. The Icddrb medical team took over the operation of the treatment center at *Katindo* in Goma, which showed one of the highest case-fatality rates (CFR) (14.5 percent) before the arrival of the medical team. The team provided hands-on case management training, which included the use of intravenous fluid and antibiotics to health workers at the treatment center. At the end of the intervention, the fatality rate of cholera reduced from 14.5 percent to less than 1.0 percent.

Using Makeshift Hospitals

In an epidemic situation, the number of patients can be so overwhelming that a hospital with a limited number of patient beds can't provide adequate treatment. Remember, the number of patients attending a hospital in an epidemic situation is from four to ten times or more. That's when utilizing a makeshift hospital is important.

A *makeshift hospital* is a temporary facility which is used to treat patients in an emergency situation. For example, in a remote village that doesn't have enough hospital beds for patients in an epidemic, sometimes a school building is used for the purpose of patients' treatment.

Consider the following when setting up a makeshift hospital:

>> **Focus on location.** Based on the patient number and the need for rapid intervention, you need to establish the makeshift hospital in a place somewhere near the epicentre from where the most cases are reported. You may choose a school building or a temporary tent to accommodate patients.

>> **Maintain a buffer stock.** Verify you have enough medicine, intravenous fluid, cleaning supply, medical equipment like gloves and masks, and so on. Ensure you have enough reserve to manage about 50 to 100 more patients (depending on the rate of admission) all the time. This reserve of supplies is called a *buffer stock.*

>> **Involve community people.** You need more personnel because an epidemic is an emergency situation. Ask community members (such as young adults, school teachers, community leaders, religious leaders, and community healthcare workers) to volunteer. Train them on a few important tasks, such as educating people on hand washing, preparing oral rehydration solution at home, and collecting a stool sample.

HOW A MAKESHIFT HOSPITAL HELPED STOP AN OUTBREAK

REAL LIFE EXAMPLE

An epidemic of cholera was reported in several places in southern Bangladesh in February 1986. The local authorities reported 94 cases with 13 deaths from suspected cholera in seven days. The main mode of transportation for these rural places is by country boat, which makes reaching the main hospital difficult.

A team led by a doctor from a diarrheal disease hospital in a subdistrict (called *Upazilla*) immediately rushed to the affected areas. The team established a makeshift hospital in a local school building the next day after arriving with the help of community leaders. A number of local volunteers — the most important of whom were the relatives of the patients — offered assistance. They rendered nursing care and supplied food for the patients. The local administrator provided accommodation and other facilities for the physician and his assistants.

The local health providers who were unqualified to deal with this outbreak volunteered assistance with operating the makeshift hospital. The subdistrict large hospital provided the medicines and supplies at regular intervals. The team collected a sample of 24 rectal swabs that were confirmed as *Vibrio cholera,* the cause of the diarrhoeal outbreak. The team couldn't establish a common food or drink source to be the culprit. This local makeshift hospital was helpful in averting deaths of many patients who presented with severe dehydration, which could have caused death if the patients hadn't been treated immediately.

Walking through an Outbreak Investigation

Investigating a disease outbreak allows you to determine whether exposure to the source(s) of the infection is continuing or not. By identifying and eliminating the source of infection, you can prevent additional cases. For example, cans of mushrooms in a grocery store may contain some notorious bacteria (such as *Clostridium botulinum*). This bacteria and its toxin can affect people who are using the food at homes or in restaurants. Their recall and destruction can prevent further cases of the disease called botulism.

If you end up working in public health (or already are), studying some case studies can help you know what to do if an outbreak occurs in your area.

Here's an example:

In August 2021, an outbreak of pharyngitis (a throat infection) occurred in 325 of 690 inmates in Tampa, Florida. In a questionnaire of 185 randomly selected inmates, 47 percent reported a sore throat after lunch from August 16–22, 2021. Two food items were served at lunch — a beverage and egg salad sandwiches. Table 14-3 presents the data.

TABLE 14-3 **Food-Specific Attack Rates**

Item consumed	Ate (Exposed)				Did not eat (not exposed)			
	Sick	Well	Total	Attack Rate	Sick	Well	Total	Attack Rate
Beverage	179	85	264	68%	22	28	50	44%
Egg salad sandwiches	176	50	226	78%	22	51	73	30%

Calculate the attack rate for each of the suspected food items for those who ate (were exposed) and those who didn't eat (weren't exposed):

$$\text{Attack rate} = \frac{\text{Number of persons sick}}{\text{Total persons at risk}} \times 100$$

Among those who took beverage, attack rate $= \frac{179}{264} \times 100 = 68\%$

Among those who didn't take beverage, attack rate $= \frac{22}{50} \times 100 = 44\%$

Among those who ate egg salad sandwiches, attack rate $= \frac{176}{226} \times 100 = 78\%$

Among those who didn't eat egg salad sandwiches, attack rate $= \frac{22}{73} \times 100 = 30\%$

For both beverage and egg salad, attack rates are clearly higher among those who ate (or drank) the food item than among those who didn't eat or drink it. However, this table doesn't permit you to determine whether the beverage or the egg salad accounted for the outbreak.

In order to answer that question, do a different analysis called cross-tabulation. In Table 14-4, calculate cross-tabulation between egg salad and beverage consumed.

Calculate attack rates for the Table 14-4 data as follows:

Group 1: People who took beverage and ate egg salad

$$\text{Attack rate} = \frac{152}{201} \times 100 = 76\%$$

Group 2: People who took beverage but didn't eat egg salad

$$\text{Attack rate} = \frac{19}{72} \times 100 = 26\%$$

Group 3: People who didn't take beverage but ate egg salad

$$\text{Attack rate} = \frac{12}{15} \times 100 = 80\%$$

Group 4: People who didn't take beverage and also didn't eat egg salad

$$\text{Attack rate} = \frac{7}{28} \times 100 = 25\%$$

First, look at the data vertically by columns in Table 14-4. There is not much difference in attack rates between Group 1 versus Group 3 (76% versus 80%). Your first inference is: Among those who ate egg salad, the attack rates didn't differ between those who took beverage and those who didn't take it.

TABLE 14-4   **Cross-Table Analysis for Egg Salad and Beverage Consumed**

Item Consumed	Ate Egg Salad				Did Not Eat Egg Salad			
	Sick	Well	Total	Attack Rate	Sick	Well	Total	Attack Rate
Drank beverage	152	49	201	76%	19	53	72	26%
Didn't drink beverage	12	3	15	80%	7	21	28	25%

There is not much difference in attack rates between Group 2 versus Group 4 (26% versus 25%). Your second inference is: Among the non-eaters of egg salad, the attack rates didn't differ by drinking status.

Now look at the data horizontally (by rows), and you find a big difference in attack rates: Group 1 versus Group 2 (76% versus 26%). It tells that among those who drank the beverage, the attack rate among those who ate egg salad was higher than among those who didn't eat egg salad.

Again, if you compare attack rates between Group 3 versus Group 4 (80% versus 25%), you find a large difference. It tells that among those who didn't drink, the attack rate among those who ate egg salad was still higher than among those who didn't eat egg salad.

This analysis clearly implicated egg salad as the source of the outbreak. You may find further information about foodborne outbreak investigation from the following website: www.cdc.gov/foodsafety/outbreaks/investigatingoutbreaks/index.html.

MASS SUICIDE: AN EPIDEMIC?

A suicide epidemic is a large number of suicides taking place over a short period of time in a manner that resembles a disease epidemic. You can find many incidences of people taking their own life in a mass scale. Some are motivated by a religious cause or a common political view. Here are some of the mass suicides to investigate:

- **People's Temple Suicide (1978):** Jonestown, Guyana was the scene of one of the most disturbing tragedies in history. On November 18, 1978, 918 Americans, including 276 children, took their own life, including 909 members of the Temple. The charismatic cult leader Jim Jones instigated this mass suicide. He was recorded saying: "We didn't commit suicide; we committed an act of revolutionary suicide protesting the conditions of an inhumane world." The people in Jonestown died of an apparent cyanide poisoning, except two — Jones and his personal nurse. Jones died of an injury consistent with a self-inflicted gunshot wound. These poisonings followed the murder of five others, including Congressman Leo Ryan, by Temple members who were concerned about the dire situation and who were trying to negotiate with Jones.

- **Heaven's Gate Suicide (1997):** Thirty-nine followers of Heaven's Gate died in a mass suicide in Rancho Santa Fe, California in late March 1997. According to the teachings of their group, these followers believed that through this suicide their bodies would leave the human vessels and their souls would follow the comet Hale-Bopp. Some male members castrated their male organs in the belief that it would prepare them for genderless life after their suicide.

- **Adam House Suicide (2007):** Nine members of Adam's cult — all in one family in Mymensingh, Bangladesh — took their own life by throwing themselves under a train. They believed in a pure life like Adam and Eve and freeing themselves from any religion.

Chapter **15**

Identifying Disease by Screening

Screening programs are used in public health for the secondary prevention of disease morbidity and mortality. A screening test aims to find a disease before any symptoms appear. A number of screening tests are available to find out if an individual is at risk of a disease or a condition. A healthcare provider often initiates a screening test if early detection of a disease or condition can help in early intervention and reduce the disease burden in the community. As science advances, more and more screening tests are available. Scientists conduct research to find out screening tests that are less invasive and widely acceptable by the population.

This chapter explains how screening tests work and how their outcomes are interpreted. You can also discover some common diseases that screening tests can diagnose.

Defining Screening

Screening is a process of identifying apparently healthy people who may be at increased risk of a disease or condition. A healthcare provider ask the "apparently healthy" people to perform a screening test — most of the time, these screening tests are routing based on the age of the individual, or if the provider suspects risks of having a disease based on family history or the person's health conditions. After the provider suspects any abnormalities after the screening test, they may advise other confirmatory tests for the diagnosis and appropriate treatments.

Screening is a tool, not a diagnostic test; it helps in the early detection of a disease. Diagnostic tests are used in follow-up of positive screening test results. The following sections provide information about some common screening tests and a few important terms related to screening tests.

**REAL LIFE
EXAMPLE**

Prostate specific antigen (PSA) is a screening test for identifying men with prostate cancer. However, a negative PSA test doesn't mean that the individual doesn't have prostate cancer; similarly, a positive PSA test doesn't confirm prostatic cancer. A number of factors such as infection, benign enlargement of the prostate, ejaculation, and recent physical activity may cause a *false positive* result (meaning that the screening test tells the person has the disease but in reality they don't have the disease). After a screening test indicates an elevated PSA score, the patient undergoes another PSA test. Subsequently, a biopsy of the prostate can confirm the diagnosis. In this case, the biopsy test is called the *gold standard* (or the confirmatory test). Figure 15-1 shows a few steps of doing a screening test.

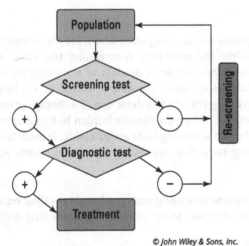

FIGURE 15-1:
A flow chart
showing steps of
screening and the
outcome.

© John Wiley & Sons, Inc.

Identifying the detectable
preclinical phase (DPCP)

The *detectable preclinical phase (DPCP)* is the time during which available screening tests can detect a disease before clinical symptoms appear. For example, one screening test for cervical cancer is called a Pap smear test, which can detect cancer cells of the cervix (the mouth of the uterus). At the beginning of cancer, the normal cells are changed to abnormal fast-growing cancer cells. These overgrown cells appear on the surface of the cervix where a qualified person can detect them during a Pap smear.

Suppose a woman starts growing cancer cells in the cervix of her uterus at age 40 and she starts showing clinical symptoms of cervical cancer at age 55. In that case, the DPCP during which Pap smear can be helpful is 15 years (55 − 40). If a screening test can detect the disease as soon as the pathology starts, the test is definitely highly effective. Therefore, in order for a screening test to be effective, the DPCP should be long. I discuss some other characteristics of a good screening test in the section, "Naming Ingredients of a Good Screening Test," later in this chapter.

Understanding lead time

Lead time is the time lapse between the detection of a disease using a screening test and the appearance of clinical symptoms. For example, if a Pap smear test is performed at age 50 and the clinical symptoms start at age 55, the lead time is 5 years (55 − 50 years).

Because no one knows when the disease starts producing symptoms, finding the actual lead time in an individual after a screening test isn't possible. However, you can estimate the lead time in a screening program by comparing the time of clinical diagnosis among the screened group and among the comparable unscreened group. In fact, lead time is considered a bias, when the screening test increases the perceived survival time. To prevent lead time bias (which is an error), an epidemiologist shouldn't compare survival rates; instead they should examine the disease mortality rates in a population. Chapter 10 discusses the calculation of mortality rates.

Naming Ingredients of a Good Screening Test

Certain characteristics of disease and screening tests are used to evaluate a screening test, which I discuss more here.

Focusing on disease characteristics

To ascertain qualities of a screening test, you should first know what type of disease the test is for. Consider the following:

>> **Disease burden is high.** The burden of a disease is high if it causes a large number of cases and deaths. In other words, the disease is serious in nature and therefore, it needs to be identified as early as possible.

>> **Early diagnosis enhances prognosis.** *Prognosis* indicates prediction of the likely outcome of a disease including sufferings, complications, recovery, or death. If treatments are available and an early intervention can improve prognosis, either by decreasing suffering, disease duration, or death, then having the screening test performed is helpful.

>> **DPCP is long.** An effective screening test is one that can detect the disease at an early stage of the disease, preferably when the pathological process starts. Refer to the section, "Identifying the detectable preclinical phase (DPCP)," earlier in this chapter.

>> **Prevalence is high.** The disease is widespread in the target population. Because of having a high level of prevalence, the disease should be screened for.

Noting effective test characteristics

A good screening test has the following features:

>> **Simple:** The test should be easy to do; paraprofessionals can conduct the test and don't need the supervision of a medical doctor.

>> **Rapid:** The test shouldn't take a long time to administer, and it yields results quickly.

>> **Valid:** The test should measure the truth. (The next section examines validity in greater detail.)

>> **Reliable:** The test should give similar results on repeated measures. (Refer to the next section for more information.)

>> **High sensitivity:** A screening text with high sensitivity means the test gives positive results most of the time when the disease is present.

>> **High specificity:** A screening test with high specificity refers to negative test results on most occasions when the disease is absent.

You can't expect 100 percent sensitivity and 100 percent specificity for a test because it's unrealistic to have a test with zero false negative and zero false positive cases. You have to compromise one with the other.

>> **Not cost prohibitive:** The cost of the test shouldn't be a prohibitive factor in performing the test.

>> **Convenient:** The test should be easily available to people.

>> **Less invasive:** Most people are more accepting to less invasive tests. For example, if urine samples can generate adequate information about the likelihood of a disease, most people prefer giving a urine sample compared to giving a blood sample.

>> **Safe:** The risk of doing a screening test shouldn't outweigh the benefits of the test.

>> **Acceptable:** The target population should be receptive to the test.

Explaining validity and reliability

An epidemiologist needs to know validity and reliability of a test because your job is to advise people on disease prevention. Also, when you conduct research, you'll want to ensure any instrument you use is valid and reliable:

>> **Validity:** *Validity,* also known as *accuracy,* is the ability of a measuring instrument to give a true measurement. For example, the true systolic blood pressure (BP) of a person is 140 mm of Hg. If a blood pressure instrument detects the systolic BP as 140, the instrument test is valid. Here are two types of validity:

- *Content validity* is often used to measure the validity of survey instruments. It means that the test or measurement accurately evaluates what the test or measurement is supposed to do.

- *Construct validity* means how well a test measures the concept it was designed to evaluate.

>> **Reliability:** *Reliability,* also known as *precision,* is the ability of a measuring instrument (or the screening test) to give consistent results on repeated use. Reliability also includes the accuracy of the observer(s).

For example, every time you measure a person's BP, the systolic BP is 130, but their true BP is 140. In this case, the instrument is reliable because it gives the same result every time, although the result isn't valid. An instrument's reliability depends on the regular monitoring of the quality of the instrument. Reliability of an observer depends on their skills and training.

Darts is a game in which small metal-shafted missiles with a pointed end are thrown at a circular target (dartboard) fixed to a wall. The target is to hit the center, called the bull's eye. Figure 15-2 illustrates the terms *validity* and *reliability* by using the example of a darts game.

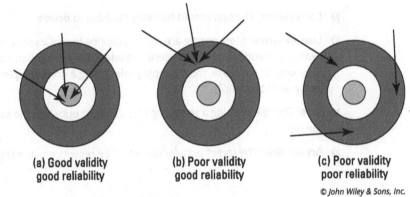

FIGURE 15-2:
Validity and
reliability of a
screening test.

(a) Good validity
good reliability

(b) Poor validity
good reliability

(c) Poor validity
poor reliability

© John Wiley & Sons, Inc.

Figure 15-2a shows that all the arrows hit the center. If all the test results of a screening test detect the true value, the test is valid and also reliable. In Figure 15-2b, all the arrows hit at one point, but they are away from the center. In this case, the test results are reliable but not valid because they don't hit the bull's eye. In Figure 15-2c, the arrows hit at different points, and are far away from the center. If the test results produce different values all the time, then the test is neither valid nor reliable.

Looking Closer at Some Common Screening Programs

Here I describe the details of a few screening tests that doctors use.

Mammogram

A popular screening test for breast cancer, a *mammogram* uses low-energy X-rays to examine human breast for the early detection of breast cancer. Other tests such as an ultrasound, ductography (also called galactography which is an X-ray exam of breast), MRI, and biopsy of breast tissue are extremely important diagnostic tests, which are used after an initial mammogram screening test.

The American Cancer Society recommends that a woman obtain her first baseline mammogram between the ages of 35 to 40. After 40, she should receive a yearly mammogram. The Canadian Task Force on Preventive Health Care and the European Cancer Observatory recommend mammography every two to three years between the ages of 50 and 69.

Researchers have more recently questioned the overall benefits of early detection of breast cancer by mammography. Consider the following:

>> False-negative results occur when mammograms appear normal even though breast cancer is present. Overall, screening mammograms miss about 20 percent of breast cancers that are present at the time of screening.

>> False-positive results occur when radiologists read the mammograms as abnormal but no cancer is actually present. False-positive mammogram results can lead to anxiety and other forms of psychological distress.

The additional testing required to rule out cancer can also be costly and time con-suming and can cause physical discomfort.

Breast self-exam

A *breast self-exam (BSE)* is another screening tool used for the early detection of breast cancer and other problems in the breast. Here are the American Cancer Society recommendations:

>> Women older than 20 should do a monthly BSE.

>> Women in their 20s and 30s should have a clinical breast exam every 3 years.

>> Women older than 40 should have a clinical breast exam yearly. Specially trained healthcare providers (doctors, nurse practitioners, and so on) should conduct clinical breast exams during a routine medical exam.

Pap smear

A *Pap smear* is a screening test used to detect precancerous cells and cancer of the cervix. The *cervix* is the lower part of the uterus that opens into the vagina. Named after a famous Greek doctor Georgios Papanikolaou, the test may also detect infections and other abnormalities in the cervix and the adjacent parts of the uterus. Regular Pap tests have led to a major decline in the number of cervical cancer cases and deaths. The timing of the test varies from country to country. In general, it starts about the age of 20 to 21 or 25 to 30 and continues until about the age 50 or 60. Pap smear screening should stop about age 65 unless a recent abnormal test or disease is present.

If the results of Pap smear is abnormal or shows minor changes in the cells of the cervix, the doctor will probably repeat the Pap test. If the test finds more abnormal cells, the doctor may advise further tests such as colposcopy to see the cells of the vagina and cervix in more detail, *endocervical curettage* (a sample of tissue is scraped from the lining of the cervical canal), or a biopsy.

Colonoscopy

A *colonoscopy* is the examination of the entire colon (large intestine) and the lower part of the small intestine with a camera on a flexible tube passed through the anus. The procedure looks for early signs of colorectal cancer and can help doctors diagnose any unexplained changes in bowel habits, abdominal pain, bleeding from the anus, and weight loss.

A colonoscopy can detect any inflamed tissue, ulcers, and abnormal growths. A colonoscopy is a primary routine screening test for colorectal cancer in people older than 45. A colonoscopy can detect any growth, such as a polyp in the colon, which a doctor can biopsy.

Prostate-specific antigen (PSA)

A *prostate-specific antigen (PSA)* is a protein produced by cells of the prostate gland. Men with prostate cancer often have an elevated amount of PSA in their blood. However, additional reasons can cause an elevated PSA level, and some men who have prostate cancer don't have elevated PSA. The most frequent benign (not cancerous) prostate conditions that cause an elevated PSA level are *prostatitis* (inflammation of the prostate) and benign enlargement of the prostate. Generally, PSA levels of 4.0 units (ng/ml) or lower are considered normal. A continuous rise in a man's PSA level over time may be suspicious and needs further follow-up to determine if the cause is prostate cancer.

Tuberculin test

The *tuberculin skin test* determines if someone has developed an immune response to the bacterium that causes tuberculosis (TB). This response can occur if someone currently has TB, or if they received the BCG vaccine against TB (which isn't performed in the United States). The TB skin test is also known as a PPD test.

TIP

A tuberculin skin test is used to find people who have TB, including:

» People who have been in close contact with someone known to have TB.

» Healthcare workers who are likely to be exposed to TB.

» People with TB symptoms, such as an ongoing cough, night sweats, and unexplained weight loss.

» People who have had an abnormal chest X-ray.

» People who have had a recent organ transplant or have an impaired immune system, such as those with HIV infection.

Fecal occult blood test

A *fecal occult blood* test checks for *occult* (not visibly apparent) blood in the stool. Positive tests may result from blood loss in the gastrointestinal tract and anywhere from the mouth to the end of the large intestine. The test doesn't directly detect colon cancer, but it's often used in clinical screening for that disease. Although many people believe that oral iron medications cause a false positive fecal blood test, they don't. Some healthcare providers may not be trained and erroneously notice the dark green or black appearance of iron in the stool and incorrectly read the test.

Screening newborn babies

Newborn screening is a public health program designed to screen infants shortly after birth for a list of treatable conditions. The number of diseases screened for can vary greatly between countries, states, or national governing bodies. In the United States, all babies get newborn screening for a number of blood tests, hearing tests, and heart screening tests:

» **Blood screening tests:** Babies with digestive and metabolic disorders don't break down food correctly. Of more than 20 to 25 different food-related tests, a few are listed here:

- **Beta-thalassemia:** This blood disorder reduces the production of hemoglobin. Hemoglobin helps in carrying oxygen to all cells in your body. The blood test is called *hemoglobin electrophoresis.*

- **Homocystinuria (HCY):** In this condition, the body can't process the amino acid (protein) methionine. If untreated, it can lead to mental retardation and even death.

- **Phenylketonuria (PKU):** Another essential amino acid for human body is phenylalanine. The body fails to digest this protein because of the absence of an enzyme called PAH. Babies with this disorder show cognitive defects.

- **Sickle cell anemia:** In this type of anemia, red blood cells turn into a sickle shape (Hb S) and die early, leading to low hemoglobin. In addition to a normal CBC (complete blood count), several tests are available for evaluating the type and amount of normal and abnormal hemoglobin.

>> **Hearing screening test:** A newborn baby is tested for hearing loss. A healthcare provider places tiny earphones in the baby's ears and checks the baby's response to sound using special computer graphs.

>> **Heart screening test:** Congenital heart diseases are screened for newborn babies. A provider uses a simple test called *pulse oximetry,* which checks the amount of oxygen in the baby's blood.

Evaluating Screening Tests

All screening tests are evaluated against a gold standard that refers to the most accurate test. For example, a colonoscopy remains the gold standard for colon cancer, a biopsy is the gold standard for breast cancer, isolation of *Mycobacterium tuberculosis* is the gold standard for the diagnosis of tuberculosis, and the coronary angiography remains the gold standard for evaluating coronary artery diseases. These sections discuss some math to help you evaluate a screening test.

Being familiar with key terms

Before evaluating a screening test, you should be familiar with a few terms by examining the conditions mentioned in Table 15-1 and the data presented in Table 15-2.

TABLE 15-1   **Common Terms Used in Screening**

Screening Test	Population With Disease	Without Disease
Positive	*True positive (TP):* Disease is present and the test is positive.	*False positive (FP):* Disease is absent, but the test is positive.
Negative	*False negative (FN):* Disease is present, but the test is negative.	*True negative (TN):* Disease is absent and the test is negative.

TABLE 15-2

Example of True Positive, False Positive, False Negative, and True Negative Using Hypothetical Numbers

Screening Test	Population	
	With Disease	Without Disease
Positive	50	100
Negative	20	500

REAL LIFE EXAMPLE

Table 15-2 shows some hypothetical numbers in four cells — each value refers to the following name:

>> **True positive (TP):** Sick people correctly diagnosed as sick = 50

>> **False positive (FP):** Healthy people incorrectly identified as sick = 100

>> **False negative (FN):** Sick people incorrectly identified as healthy = 20

>> **True negative (TN):** Healthy people correctly identified as healthy = 500

TP and TN produce correct results and FP and FN produce incorrect results.

Comprehending sensitivity

Sensitivity is the proportion of the people who are screening test positive among the people who have the disease. Sensitivity relates to the test's ability to identify positive results. A test with high sensitivity can be considered as a reliable indicator because it rarely misses true positives among those who are actually positive. Negative results in a high sensitivity test rule out the disease.

The letters in Table 15-3 demonstrate the numerators and denominators used in the formula:

$$\text{Sensitivity} = \frac{A}{A+C} \times 100$$

TABLE 15-3

Concept of Sensitivity, Specificity, and Predictive Values

Screening Test	Population		Total
	With Disease	Without Disease	
Positive	A	B	A+D
Negative	C	D	C+D
Total	A+C	B+D	A+B+C+D

Using the formula, calculate sensitivity for the data in Table 15-4.

TABLE 15-4

Data Illustrating Sensitivity, Specificity, and Predictive Values

	Population		
Screening Test	With Disease	Without Disease	Total
Positive	50 (A)	100 (B)	150 (A+B)
Negative	20 (C)	500 (D)	520 (C+D)
Total	70 (A+C)	600 (B+D)	670 (A+B+C+D)

REAL LIFE EXAMPLE

Based on data presented in Table 15-4, sensitivity of the test can be calculated as follows (The data is calculated in a percentage; therefore, they're multiplied by 100):

$$\text{Sensitivity} = \frac{50}{70} \times 100 = 71.4\%$$

Looking at specificity

Specificity is the proportion of the people who test negative among the people who don't have the disease. Specificity relates to the test's ability to identify negative results. Highly specific tests rarely miss negative outcomes, so they can be considered reliable when their result is positive. Therefore, a positive result from a test with high specificity means a high probability of the presence of disease (refer to Table 15-3):

$$\text{Specificity} = \frac{D}{B+D} \times 100$$

According to the data in Table 15-4, specificity can be calculated as follows:

$$\text{Specificity} = \frac{500}{600} \times 100 = 83.3\%$$

Predictive values

Unlike the statistics in the preceding sections, *predictive values* of a test depend greatly on the prevalence of disease as well as the accuracy of the test:

>> **Positive predictive value (PPV)** is the proportion of people who got the disease among those who screen test positive. Here's how to calculate PPV.

$$\text{Positive predictive value (PPV)} = \frac{TP}{TP + FP}$$

>> **Negative predictive value (NPV)** is the proportion of people who don't have the disease among those who test negative. Here's how to calculate NPV.

$$\text{Negative predictive value (NPV)} = \frac{TN}{TN + FN}$$

Based on the data from Table 15-5,

>> PPV = $60 \div 260 = 0.23$ or 23 percent

>> NPV = $1,400 \div 1,420 = 0.99$ or 99 percent

TABLE 15-5

Evaluation of Predictive Values of a Screening Test

Screening Test Results	Patients Diagnosed for a Disease		
	Disease Positive	Disease Negative	Total
Positive	60	200	260
Negative	20	1,400	1,420
Total	80	1,600	1,680

Total agreement of the test

Total agreement of a screening test is the sum of true positive and true negative. From the data of Table 15-5, the total agreement = 60 + 1,400 = 1,460. The total agreement results give you an overall idea how good the test results are in terms of the gold standard.

To calculate the percent agreement of the test, divide the total agreement by the total sample population for the test:

$$\text{Percent agreement} = \frac{1460}{1680} \times 100 = 86.9\%$$

This data shows that the screening test results and the gold standard test results are 86.9 percent similar, or they agree on about 87 out of 100 occasions.

Putting these statistics together in one example

REAL LIFE EXAMPLE

In 1,000 women tested for cervical cancer, Pap smear results show 496 positive results. Out of these 496 women, 480 had cervical cancer. Another 120 women tested negative but actually had the disease. Table 15-6 presents the data.

TABLE 15-6

Pap Smear Results of 1,000 Women Screened for Cervical Cancer

Pap Smear Results	Patients with Cervical Cancer		Total
	Present	Absent	
Positive	480	16	496
Negative	120	384	504
Total	600	400	1,000

The prevalence of cervical cancer $= \dfrac{600}{1000} = 0.6$ *or 60 percent*

The sensitivity of the test $= \dfrac{480}{600} = 0.8$ *or 80 percent*

The specificity of the test $= \dfrac{384}{400} = 0.96$ *or 96 percent*

$PPV = \dfrac{480}{496} = 0.968$ *or 96.8 percent*

$NPV = \dfrac{384}{504} = 0.762$ *or 76.2 percent*

Percent agreement of the test $= \dfrac{480 + 384}{1000} \times 100 = 86.4\%$

Predicting predictive value with changes in prevalence

REAL LIFE EXAMPLE

Table 15-7 and Table 15-8 show how the change in prevalence of disease directly influences predictive values. In other words, the predictive value increases with the increase of prevalence, and it decreases with the decease of prevalence.

For Table 15-8, prevalence $= \dfrac{500}{1000} \times 100 = 50\%$

$PPV = \dfrac{250}{500} \times 100 = 50\%$

For Table 15-8, prevalence $= \dfrac{200}{1000} \times 100 = 20\%$

$PPV = \dfrac{100}{500} \times 100 = 20\%$

TABLE 15-7

Relationship between Prevalence and Predictive Value

| Test Results | Patients with a disease | | |
	Present	Absent	Total
Positive	250	250	500
Negative	250	250	500
Total	500	500	1,000

TABLE 15-8

Relationship between Prevalence and Predictive Value

| Test Results | Patients with a Disease | | |
	Present	Absent	Total
Positive	100	400	500
Negative	100	400	500
Total	200	800	1,000

Data presented in Tables 15-7 and 15-8 shows that PPV increases with the increase of prevalence.

Explaining multiphasic screening

Multiphasic screening refers to the use of two or more screening tests together among large groups of people. For example, in the case of a diabetes screening, a random blood sugar test can be used as the first step to find out the people at risk of diabetes. As a second step, a glucose tolerance test can be used as another screening test among those who were found to be pre-diabetic in the first screening test.

Differentiating between mass screening and selective screening

Mass population screening refers to screening on a large scale of the total population, regardless of any prior information about the risk to the population. *Selective screening*, on the other hand, refers to targeted screening that is used for a subset of population who is known to be at a higher risk of a disease or a health condition based on family history, race, occupation, income, and some other sociodemographic and exposure factors.

Selecting a cutoff point

A good screening test correctly categorizes people as either having or not having the preclinical disease and identifies them as correctly testing positive or screening test negative. In a perfect condition, all screened people who have the preclinical disease are categorized as test positive, and all screened people who don't have the disease are listed as test negative. However, in reality you don't get 100 percent sensitivity and 100 percent specificity of a test.

Figure 15-3 demonstrates the effects of choosing various cutoff points between clearly positive and clearly negative test results. For example, fasting blood glucose, an indicator of diabetes, may be distributed normally in a population with a mean value of 100 mg/dL. A few healthy individuals (who don't have diabetes) may have incorrect results of elevated glucose levels, and some diseased individuals may show glucose levels at the lower range of abnormal levels. Thus, the two distribution curves may overlap.

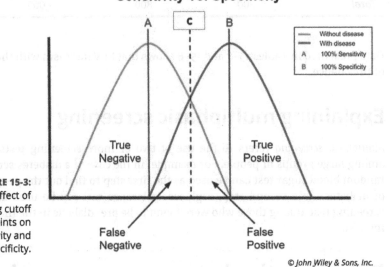

FIGURE 15-3: The effect of changing cutoff points on sensitivity and specificity.

© John Wiley & Sons, Inc.

Based on your decision whether you want to improve sensitivity or specificity, you may set the cutoff point somewhere between a normal and an abnormal value of fasting blood glucose (refer to Figure 15-3):

>> If you select the cutoff point at C, you maximize both sensitivity and specificity.

>> If you move the cutoff point to A by lowering the specific blood glucose level that's classified as abnormal, almost all the individuals who have the disease

will have the screening test positive. In that case, sensitivity will be close to 100 percent, and specificity will be decreased because many of the non-diseased individuals will be classified as diseased.

>> If you move the cutoff point of blood glucose at a higher level to B, specificity will be improved to almost 100 percent. In that case, sensitivity will be compromised because many diseased individuals will be misclassified as normal.

EVALUATING THE EFFECTIVENESS OF SCREENING AND BREAST CANCER MORTALITY

Several studies have been conducted in Canada, the United States, and Western Europe since the early 1960s to evaluate the effectiveness of breast cancer screening programs. Nearly 500,000 women were assigned to two groups: those who were screened and those who weren't screened but received the usual care, and both groups were followed up over time.

After 10 to 12 years of follow-up, about 30 percent of women aged 50 to 69 years had a lower risk of death due to breast cancer after they had been screened by mammography. In this group of women, the risk of false positive results by mammogram screening was 47.3 percent after 10 years.

In another group of women aged 40 to 49, the benefit of screening by mammogram was less obvious after five to seven years of follow-up and only marginally beneficial after 12 to 14 years of follow-up. Moreover, the risk of false-positive results was 56.2 percent in this age group after ten years of screening. This risk of false positive results lead to great emotional distress to the patient. Furthermore this risk of false positives also involves increased costs of outpatient care, screening, and other diagnostic tests such as biopsies. The National Institute of Health, therefore, suggested that a universal screening by mammogram isn't recommended for all women in their 40s.

Further studies conducted by two groups of scientists produced different results. One group found no survival benefits of using a mammogram to screen breast cancer in any women, including the older group of women. Another study observed a beneficial effect of a mammogram in reducing breast cancer mortality among women aged 40 to 74 years. These conflicting results on the beneficial effects of screening with a mammogram made scientists look for future research.

(continued)

(continued)

A study published in 2005 showed a 24 percent reduction in adjusted mortality rates from 48.3 to 38.0 per 100,000 women aged 30 to 79 years after mammogram screening and adjuvant therapies with tamoxifen and chemotherapy.

However, controversies continue. A new Canadian study of women aged 50 to 59 showed no additional benefits of reducing breast cancer mortality by mammography. The study involved about 40,000 women from 15 screening centers in six Canadian provinces.

A recent study outweighs the risks of overdiagnosis and unnecessary treatments due to early diagnosis of breast cancer by mammogram screening compared to its benefits of reducing breast cancer mortality. The latest study results don't support routine mammography at an early age. However, the American Cancer Society continues to recommend yearly mammography starting at age 40.

4

Examining a Study Finding

Assess whether an association is causal based on Bradford Hill's criteria.

Discover different methods of epidemiologic study design, their applications, and the pros and cons of the different study methods.

Apply concepts of epidemiologic methods and design different study designs, such as cross-sectional study, case-control study, cohort study, and ecological study.

Develop a questionnaire using both closed-ended and open-ended questions.

Understand how bias and confound affect your study results and how to minimize bias and confounding in research.

Examine the lack of ethical procedures in several past studies.

Apply ethical standards for the protection of the rights of the participants, preventing any harm or injuries, minimizing risks, and maximizing benefits to the study participants.

Chapter 16

Figuring Out Whether an Association Is Causal

I n order to find a causal relationship, first you need to dissect two factors:

» What is the outcome or the disease?

» What factors are associated with the outcome or the disease?

Not all factors found with a disease are causal. Sometimes a third factor can be there in the *causal pathway* (or a cause-and-effect relationship). For example, you're looking for an association between cigarette smoking and lung cancer. You assume that smoking is a cause of lung cancer. But you can't be sure because you found a third factor, which is drinking. How can you be sure that drinking isn't the real cause of the disease? This chapter provides you with the answers.

A second problem in the causal pathway is that sometimes one disease can be caused by more than one factor. When multiple factors are involved, you need to dissect which of the factors(s) are more important. That needs further statistical analysis.

A third problem is the type of research that you're doing. In some forms of research you really can't establish any causal relationship. Such studies are *ecological studies* and *cross-sectional studies*. I discuss different study designs and their pros and cons in Chapter 17. In this chapter, I emphasize fact findings using some criteria, which give you a better idea if the association could be causal. These criteria are known as *Hill's criteria*.

Establishing Causality

Epidemiologists often attempt to find out the cause of a disease. Why? Because once you know the *causative* factors (the formal term that means what causes something), then you can try to eliminate or reduce the risks or prevent the disease from happening in the future. Although it's tempting to think that a cause is a single condition or an event that leads to a disease or an outcome, in reality things aren't that simple. You need to establish, with sufficient evidence and justifications, that the factors that you found in association with the disease are, in fact, the causes of the disease.

The following sections discuss a few associations that could be trivial in nature and may not be causal. Subsequently, you get into some criteria that make an association causal.

Examining an association that may not be causal

Before you jump into causal factors, you must figure out what makes an association not causal. In your research, you're exploring what factors are causing heart disease in a young man in his 30s. He isn't a smoker or a heavy drinker. His bad cholesterol (LDL) levels in a recent blood work were found to be high, and he's overweight. He also has a strong family history of heart disease. You want to know which of these factors are more associated with the heart disease. Some of the factors may not show any strong evidence to support it's a cause of the disease. Why do you want to know this? By knowing the causal association, you can try to reduce those risk factors, which could help him be healthier.

Consider the following three scenarios where you find an association between two events:

>> **Scenario # 1:** People went to a Vegas casino show of superstar Lady Gaga. Two people had a car accident on their way home. By analyzing the fact

findings of these associations, you may come up with a few factors that might have caused the car accident. Ask yourself a few questions:

- Did a Lady Gaga song cause the car accident?

- Did the two people drink too much at the casino?

- Did the car have any mechanical problems?

- Did the weather like heavy rain or gusty wind make it difficult to see the road?

- Did a combination of these factors cause the accident?

» **Scenario # 2:** Every time you watch your favorite movie show on TV, your baby cries. Is this a casual association? Your baby may cry because of tons of reasons: feeling discomfort or irritation from a dirty diaper, having excessive gas, feeling cold, being hungry, needing comforted, and so on. All babies cry, and some babies cry a lot.

On average, a baby cries between one to two hours to as much as five to six hours per day. Should you not be concerned when your baby cries? Of course, however, relating your baby's cry with watching your favorite movie may or may not be related. If your baby feels emotionally lonely when nobody else is nearby, they may cry just to get attention. All you have to do is find out the real cause.

» **Scenario #3:** A frog croaks and rain is coming. Parts of Appalachia believe that if you hear a frog croaking exactly at midnight, it means rain is on the way. Examine the fact in greater detail. Croaking is an innate behavior of frogs. Male frogs croak to get the attention of a female frog. Croaking is especially common during a frog's mating season in the spring *after* it rains. Can a few frogs croaking bring rain? You must establish an observation with sufficient facts that enables a causal relationship.

Identifying confounders that affect a causal link

A potential *confounder* is a variable that's associated with the exposure or the causative factor and also is associated with the outcome or the disease. A confounding variable is a kind of nuisance variable, which blocks you from finding the actual cause. A confounder competes with the real factor that causes the disease. Here are some examples of confounders:

» **Age:** Older people get heart disease (an outcome) more often than younger people. If you examine more facts, you also know that older people are more likely to be less active or inactive (an exposure factor). In this case, age is a confounder because older age is associated with both exposure (sedentary lifestyle) and the outcome (heart disease).

» **Drinking:** Many studies report the beneficial effect of moderate amount of drinking in reducing cardiovascular diseases (CVD). The question is whether the effect of drinking is causal or not. If you suspect that drinking isn't a real cause of CVD but may be a confounder, you'll need to use some of the following steps: using restrictions, matching, stratification, and conducting multivariate data analysis. I discuss all these methods in Chapter 18.

If you go into more depth into reported epidemiologic studies, you'll find that the frequency of alcohol consumption, the drinking pattern (steady or binge drinking), and the type of beverage confound the effect of alcohol on CVD. In addition, certain factors such as regular exercise, a healthy diet, higher socioeconomic status, and better overall health can be other confounders because they're more common among regular drinkers and wine drinkers. Therefore, you need to resolve several questions to establish a causal relationship.

Seeing examples of a causal effect

Here are a couple examples of causal effect.

BMI and type 2 diabetes

An increase in body fat is generally associated with an increase in the risk of metabolic diseases (such as type 2 diabetes mellitus), hypertension, and increased cholesterol. Among several causes of type 2 diabetes, evidence shows the risk of high body mass index (BMI) associated with type 2 diabetes — see Figure 16-1.

Cigarette smoking and lung cancer

Lung cancer is now the most common type of cancer in the world. Approximately 2.09 million new diagnoses of lung cancer occur each year with about 1.76 million cancer deaths worldwide. The American Cancer Society estimates about 236,740 new cases of lung cancer (117,910 in men and 118,830 in women) with about 130,180 deaths from lung cancer (68,820 in men and 61,360 in women) in the United States in 2022.

Smoking is a strong known cause of lung cancer. Figure 16-2 shows the cumulative risk of lung cancer among cigarette smokers who continued smoking versus those smokers who stopped smoking at different ages of life and those individuals who never smoked.

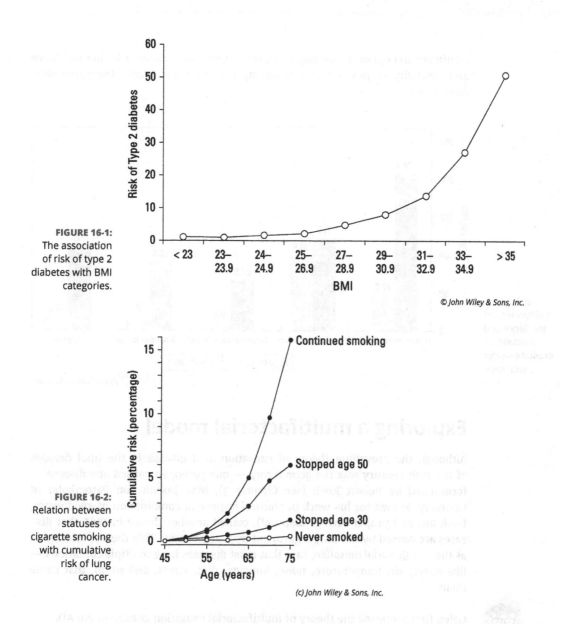

FIGURE 16-1: The association of risk of type 2 diabetes with BMI categories.

© John Wiley & Sons, Inc.

FIGURE 16-2: Relation between statuses of cigarette smoking with cumulative risk of lung cancer.

(c) John Wiley & Sons, Inc.

Prostate cancer and race

Black men are about two times more likely to have prostate cancer than White men. Although there's no clear reason for these differences, several factors can impact cancer risk and outcomes in Blacks. Race in the United States is correlated with socioeconomic status, and lower socioeconomic status is correlated with increased cancer risk and poorer outcomes. Furthermore, Black men may also be harmed by racial bias in preventive care — they're less likely than White men to be offered the option of having a PSA test. Figure 16-3 shows a higher incidence and mortality of prostate cancer among non-Hispanic Blacks compared with other races.

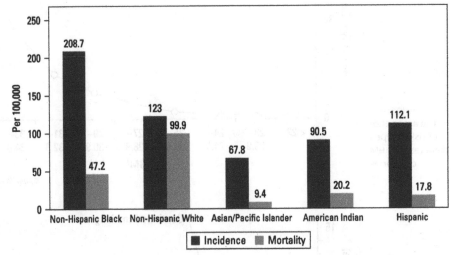

FIGURE 16-3:
Comparison of incidence and mortality of prostate cancer with race.

(c) John Wiley & Sons, Inc.

Exploring a multifactorial model

Although the prevailing theory of causation of a disease in the final decades of the 19th century was the *germ theory* — one pathogen caused one disease — formulated by Robert Koch (see Chapter 3), Max Joseph von Pettenkofer of Germany, known for his work in *practical hygiene* (a combination of good water, fresh air, and proper sewage disposal), coined another theory in 1865 that diseases are caused by not only a germ but by many causes. This theory, referred to as the *multifactorial causation*, says that most diseases have multiple conditions — like water, air, temperature, noise, housing, diet, stress, and so on, that cause them.

TECHNICAL STUFF

Galen first proposed the theory of multifactorial causation at around 150 AD.

Improvements in public health and medicine in the early 1970s brought about a decline in infectious diseases but an increase in chronic diseases in many countries. This is known as *epidemiologic transition* (mentioned in Chapter 8). As a result of these disease pattern changes, chronic and noncommunicable diseases such as heart disease, cancers, stroke, diabetes, and hypertension are on a rise in modern industrialized societies. Moreover, the latter doesn't fit with the single cause of germ theory. On the other hand, some infectious diseases, although primarily caused by a germ, can be multifactorial. For example, tuberculosis is an infectious disease, caused by a bacteria called *Mycobacterium tuberculosis*, but several factors including poverty, overcrowding, and malnutrition contribute to the occurrence of tuberculosis. Almost all noncommunicable diseases (such as heart disease, cancer, diabetes, and so on) are multifactorial.

REAL LIFE EXAMPLE

Consider this example: Myocardial infarction is a life-threatening complication of heart disease. In fact, it's the number one leading cause of death in the United States. Arteries of the heart (also called *coronary arteries*) narrow down due to plaque deposits (referred to as *arterial blocks*). The plaque causes a complete blockage, cutting off the blood and oxygen supply. Because the heart muscles don't get any blood supply, they die. If the heart's muscle cells begin to suffer damage and start to die, the condition is called myocardial infarction, or in plain English, a heart attack. Irreversible damage of heart muscles begins within 30 minutes of blockage. The result: The lack of oxygen causes heart muscles to no longer work as they should. The heart fails to pump blood properly to other parts of the body, resulting in heart failure.

If a person knows the causes and risk factors of myocardial infarction, they can try to reduce the risks that are modifiable. Many such modifiable risk factors include unhealthy lifestyle choices such as smoking, heavy drinking, lack of exercise, poor diet, inadequate sleep, and stress, which may result in obesity, high cholesterol, high blood pressure, and diabetes (see Figure 16-4). However, some other risk factors such as age, gender, race, and genetic susceptibility aren't modifiable.

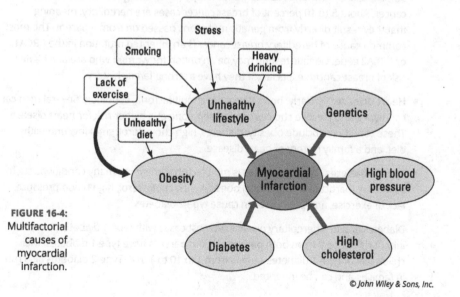

FIGURE 16-4: Multifactorial causes of myocardial infarction.

© John Wiley & Sons, Inc.

Therefore, myocardial infarction is a multifactorial disease. Detecting the risk factors, making smart choices related to one's health, and changing one's lifestyle may reduce many complications of heart disease, including a heart attack.

INHERITING A MULTIFACTORIAL DISEASE

Researchers are discovering that nearly all conditions and diseases have a genetic component. An inherited medical condition caused by a DNA abnormality is a genetic disorder. Many chronic diseases having multifactorial causes may have a genetic component. Therefore, multifactorial conditions tend to run in families.

A person's risk for a multifactorial trait or condition depends on how closely related they are to a family member with the trait or condition. Family members, such as parents, siblings, and children, share about half of one's genes. A person is at a greater risk of a disease if their parents or siblings have it, whereas they're at a lower risk if someone like a cousin has it. However, because more than one factor causes multifactorial diseases, determining a person's real risk of getting a disease or passing it on to their children is difficult.

Here are some diseases that are caused by multiple factors, and one of which is a genetic cause:

- **Breast cancer:** Multiple factors, including smoking, alcohol intake, obesity, radiation exposure, hormone replacement therapy (HRT), and genetics can cause breast cancer. About 5 to 10 percent of breast cancer cases are hereditary, meaning that they result directly from genetic mutations passed on from a parent. The most common cause of hereditary breast cancer is an inherited mutation in the BRCA1 or BRCA2 gene. Genetic testing may be an option for women who are at a higher risk of breast cancer, especially if they have a strong family history.

- **Heart disease:** Similarly, heart disease is a multifactorial condition. Several medical conditions and lifestyle choices can put someone at a higher risk for heart disease. These conditions include obesity, diabetes, high cholesterol, smoking, unhealthy diet, and a family history of heart disease.

- **Type 2 diabetes:** Type 2 diabetes is multifactorial, meaning many conditions such as obesity (particularly abdominal obesity), high cholesterol, high blood pressure, lack of exercise, and poor diet can cause type 2 diabetes.

  Diabetes is also a hereditary disease. In most cases with type 1 diabetes, people inherit risk factors from both parents. If both parents have type 1 diabetes, their child's risk of type 1 diabetes ranges from 1 in 10 to 1 in 4. Type 2 diabetes also runs in families and can be inherited.

Scientists have found certain genes linked with type 1 diabetes in certain races. For example, most White people with type 1 diabetes have genes called *HLA-DR3* or *HLA-DR4*, which are linked to autoimmune disease. African Americans are at risk of type 1 diabetes if they carry *HLA-DR7* gene, and Japanese having *HLA-DR9* gene are at risk.

Several other health disorders are caused by a combination of multiple factors and genetics. These disorders include

- Alzheimer's disease
- Arthritis
- Asthma
- Birth defects (cleft lip and cleft palate and neural tube defects)
- Cancers of the prostate, bowel, ovaries, and skin
- Hypertension
- Skin conditions such as psoriasis, and eczema

Understanding Hill's Criteria for Causality

An English epidemiologist Sir Austin Bradford Hill suggested some criteria for assessing causality in 1965. I don't have any magic number for how many of these criteria you have to meet to call an association causal. The more you meet these criteria, the more likely that the association between an exposure (or the risk factor) and the disease (or the outcome) is likely to be causal. Chapter 4 discusses the idea of Hill's criteria for a causal association. Here I examine those criteria in more detail.

Examining strength of association

The stronger the association between exposure and disease, the more likely it is to be causal. In other words, the more of the Hill's criteria that fit with your case, the better you can establish that the association of the factor in question is a causal factor.

English surgeon Percivall Pott illustrated strength of association. In 1775, Pott found that young boys who were sweeping chimneys developed testicular cancer almost exclusively — about 200 times more than people of other occupations. He determined a link of environmental toxic substances that caused cancer. His research helped in preventing scrotal cancers by having chimney sweeps wear protective clothing.

REMEMBER

Advances in statistical theory and the computational processing power have allowed scientists to delineate strong versus weak associations. Some of the epidemiological measurements that you may check to know how strong or how weak the association is include the following:

» **Odds ratio (OR):** This is the odds of having a disease among the exposed population compared to the unexposed population. Refer to Chapter 17 for more specifics.

» **Relative risk or risk ratio (RR):** This refers to how much higher the risk is among the exposed group compared to the unexposed group. Check out Chapter 17 for more information.

» **Standardized mortality ratio (SMR):** It's the ratio between the observed number of deaths and the expected number of deaths, given that you use a standard population. Refer to Chapter 10.

» **Statistical significance (p-value):** It indicates whether the evidence that you gathered from a sample is statistically different from the real value in the population or not. If the p-value is less than or equal to 0.05, it means that the data is statistically significant. Check out Chapter 15 for more details.

REAL LIFE EXAMPLE

Check out this example where I use relative risk (RR) to identify the association of food items with a recent episode of gastroenteritis (see Table 16-1).

TABLE 16-1   ## Use of Relative Risk to Identify an Association

Food Item Consumed	Consumers (Percentage %)	Nonconsumers (Percentage %)	Relative Risk (RR)
Shrimp salad	$8/12$ (67%)	$5/35$ (43%)	1.6
Olives	$19/32$ (59%)	$5/18$ (28%)	2.1
Fried chicken	$19/42$ (45%)	$1/4$ (25%)	1.8
Barbecued chicken	$16/16$ (100%)	$6/30$ (20%)	5.0
Beans	$12/26$ (46%)	$12/22$ (55%)	0.8
Potato salad	$17/37$ (46%)	$8/14$ (57%)	0.8
Tomato	$5/21$ (24%)	$18/28$ (64%)	0.4

The value of RR explains how much higher (or lower) the risk is for the food items among the consumers compared to the nonconsumers — take the example of the first food item of shrimp salad — divide 8 by 12 and multiply by $100 \left[\left(\frac{8}{12} \right) \times 100 \right] = 67$ percent. This tells you that 8 out of 12 people or 67 percent who ate shrimp salad had gastroenteritis. If you move to Column 3, 15 out of 35 (43 percent) who didn't eat shrimp salad also had gastroenteritis. In Column 4, you calculate RR by dividing the data in Column 2 by the data in Column 3, which is as follows: 67 divided by 43 = 1.6.

Based on this data, four food items had a higher risk of gastroenteritis among consumers compared with nonconsumers; those items are shrimp salad (RR = 1.6), olives (RR = 2.1), fried chicken (RR = 1.8), and barbecued chicken (RR = 5.0). Here, 100 percent of consumers versus 20 percent of nonconsumers had symptoms of gastroenteritis after eating barbecued chicken yielding a RR of 5.0, which is higher than the risk of any other food items. In this case, the association of barbecued chicken with gastroenteritis is likely to be causal. In plain English, that means barbecued chicken is probably the culprit.

However, a statistical association isn't always enough to measure the strength of association. You need to get into the depth of the study and ask these types of questions:

>> How many samples were studied? The more samples are included in your study, the stronger (or more valid) your conclusions are drawn from the data.

>> Are they representative samples of the population? If you use a proper sampling technique (such as random sampling), the data is likely to represent the population.

REMEMBER

Furthermore, make sure you compare the weight of the evidence in the literature. For the assessment of the weight, you need to compare previously published studies. If most of the study results are in the same direction (for example, the use of hormone replacement therapy is strongly associated with breast cancer), then you infer that the weight of the association is strong. The results of the two studies are consistent (see the section, "Striving for consistency," later in this chapter).

Sometimes you need rigorous statistical methods to analyze the data more efficiently to know the real strength of association. Example of a rigorous statistical method is *multivariate regression analysis*, in which many variables are taken into consideration to predict a dependent variable. A *dependent variable* is one that depends on one or more variables. Suppose you wanted to find out what factors cause a high blood pressure. Here blood pressure is a *dependent variable*. You can find the association of blood pressure with stress, age, and gender, all separately. Analyzing them separately is important, but not a rigorous method of analysis.

Alternatively, you can do another analysis to see the combined effect of stress, age, and gender on blood pressure. The latter is called a *multiple regression analysis*, which is a rigorous analysis and a more sophisticated statistical test.

Consider this example: In a published report of testing lung function after exposure to certain flavoring chemicals, a group of scientists showed a 2.8 times greater annual decline in lung function. Later, another group of scientists reanalyzed the same data set using a more sophisticated statistical test and didn't find any statistically significant associations between the chemical exposure and compromised lung function. This explains why a rigorous analysis is important.

Considering dose-response

Dose-response refers to an increase (or decrease) in the intensity, duration, or total level of exposure to a risk factor. There's a progressive increase (or decrease) in the risk of the disease or the outcome. This kind of response is a *direct effect* — that means changes in E (exposure) and D (disease) go in the same direction. On the other hand, the changes of E and D can go in the opposite directions. In this case, when the dose of the exposure (or the risk) increases, the disease (or the outcome) decreases, and vice versa.

Figure 16-5 illustrates this phenomenon. With an increasing dose of a substance, the effect (or the outcome) of a variable (suppose a disease) gradually increases. However, for an initial period, there's no change — this period is called the *time of no effect*. After the gradual increase of the effect with an increasing dose, there's a plateau in the curve, meaning the effect has reached its maximum level and there's no more change in the effect even with an increasing dose.

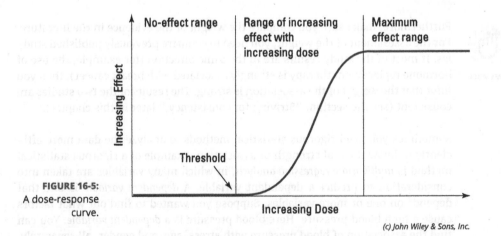

FIGURE 16-5:
A dose-response curve.

(c) John Wiley & Sons, Inc.

A CASE STUDY SHOWING DOSE-RESPONSE RELATIONSHIP

REAL LIFE EXAMPLE

Arsenic is a naturally occurring chemical found in combination with either inorganic or organic substances in soils, sediments, and groundwater:

- Organic arsenic compounds are found mainly in fish and shellfish.

- People are most likely exposed to inorganic arsenic through drinking water and through various foods to a lesser extent.

People in Bangladesh and West Bengal, India, were exposed to arsenic from thousands of contaminated underground drinking water sources called tube wells. A *tube well* is a water pump well that consists of a long tube bored into the ground and sunk to the water table. Between 33 and 77 million people in Bangladesh have been exposed to arsenic in the drinking water — a catastrophe that the World Health Organization (WHO) has called "the largest mass poisoning in history." In Bangladesh, arsenic contamination was first reported in early 1996 from southwestern districts bordering India.

The research team which I led had investigated clinical features and complications of 150 arsenic-exposed patients who attended an outpatient dermatology department in a major district hospital in southern Bangladesh in 2000. The majority of patients (82 percent) had a moderate to severe form of rain-drop appearance of the skin. This particular kind of skin lesion is due to pigmentation and depigmentation of the skin. It's a typical skin lesion found in the case of arsenic poisoning. The team collected water samples from the patients' households or nearby tube wells. Thirty-one percent of the water samples had arsenic concentrations ten times higher than the permissible limit of 0.05 mg/L in Bangladesh and 50 times higher than the WHO guideline value of 0.01 mg/L. The higher concentration of arsenic in water was associated with the more severe illnesses — meaning that the association showed a dose-response relationship.

Sometimes you can use a correlation chart to demonstrate the relationship between an exposure and an outcome. In a *correlation chart*, you show how close two variables are in a plot. Figure 16-6 presents the results of an ecological study of dietary fat intake and a long-term risk of coronary heart disease (CHD).

The CHD death rates strongly correlated with dietary intakes of saturated fat, with a correlation coefficient value of 0.92 (the perfect correlation coefficient is 1). The relationship was *direct*, meaning that the risk of CHD increased with the increased intake of dietary fat intake. The country names in Figure 16-6 are abbreviated; for example, both the average fat intake and the CHD death rate were highest in East Finland (EF), and both were lowest in Tanushimaru (TA), Japan.

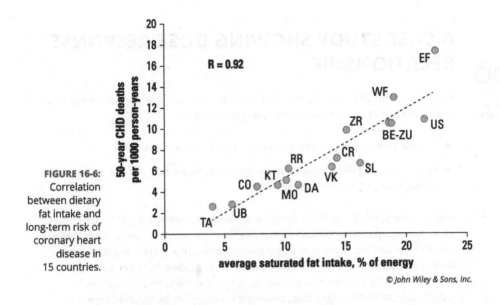

FIGURE 16-6:
Correlation
between dietary
fat intake and
long-term risk of
coronary heart
disease in
15 countries.

© John Wiley & Sons, Inc.

Grasping temporality

Temporality is a key criterion of the Hill's suggested criteria for causality. In this case, the exposure (E) to the causal factor *must* come first and then the disease (D). For instance, if asbestos is the cause of lung cancer, an exposure to asbestos must precede the incidence of lung cancer. Lack of temporality rules out causality. In other words, if E doesn't come before D, the association isn't causal. Sometimes you may come up with a situation where it isn't easy to find out what causes what. Refer this issue to the nearby sidebar for an example.

Focusing on specificity

Sometimes establishing the causal relationship is easy to do if the exposure (E) is specific to the disease (D). *Specificity* means the causal factor (such as a bacteria) is specific to cause only one disease and that the disease should result from only this causal factor. An example of such a one-to-one relationship is the bacteria *Shigella* that causes blood dysentery (or shigellosis).

WARNING

However, specificity remains one of the weakest criteria because most of the time one organism can cause more than one disease, and at the same time, a disease may be multifactorial in addition to the particular organism being one of the several causes.

FIGURING OUT WHAT CAUSES WHAT ISN'T EASY

This particular example illustrates the fact that denoting a variable as a cause of an outcome could be confusing. Pulmonary embolism (PE) and atrial fibrillation (AF) may coexist. PE is an acute emergency condition, which occurs when a blood clot gets stuck in an artery in the lung, blocking blood flow to part of the lung. Symptoms of PE include sudden onset of shortness of breath, which worsens with exertion, chest pain, and cough (often with bloody sputum). If PEs aren't treated quickly, they can cause heart or lung damage and even death. AF is an irregular and often very rapid heart rhythm (arrhythmia). AF isn't usually life-threatening or considered serious, but AF can be dangerous if a person has diabetes, high blood pressure, or other diseases of the heart.

Which of these conditions comes first? The general wisdom is that PE causes AF. However, AF can also lead to blood clots in the heart. Establishing whether PE is the cause of AF or the other way around is difficult. From a systematic review of 1,347 published articles, the direction and extent of this association isn't conclusive. As part of the complications of PE, one can develop cardiac arrhythmias as well as atrial and ventricular fibrillations. The underlying mechanism how AF occurs in the presence of PE is possibly due to an increased pressure in the right ventricle of the heart or due to the action of inflammatory cytokines. PE and AF also share many common risk factors, including old age, obesity, heart failure, and inflammatory conditions. AF, in turn, may lead to clot formation in the right atrial appendage and thereby PE.

For example, consider smoking as a risk factor or an exposure. Smoking can cause lung cancer, but smoking isn't a specific exposure factor for lung cancer because smoking causes many other diseases, such as other cancers, heart disease, stroke, diabetes, Buerger's disease (also known as *thromboangiitis obliterans*, TAO), and lung diseases including chronic obstructive pulmonary disease (COPD), emphysema, and chronic bronchitis. On the other hand, smoking is one of the causes of heart disease; however, many other risk factors, including diabetes, obesity, hypertension, high cholesterol, unhealthy food habits, and lack of exercise, can cause heart disease.

Striving for consistency

The term *consistency* means your study results are similar to others, even though studies were conducted in different countries, different populations, and at different points of time.

REPEATING STUDIES TO REACH CONSISTENCY

Rotavirus diarrhea is the most common cause of watery diarrhea in small children. Because of frequent loose bowel movements and vomiting, the child gets dehydrated. The only available treatment for rotavirus diarrhea is hydrating and replacing the loss of water and electrolytes from the body. I led a team to conduct a double-blind clinical trial of an immunological treatment for rotavirus diarrhea. The term *double-blind* means neither the patients nor the investigators know which patient gets the study medicine and which patient gets a placebo or a control medicine (a medicine other than what's being tested). The study medicine used colostrum from immunized cows against rotavirus, referred to as hyperimmune bovine colostrum or in short HBC. The placebo group of children received colostrum from unimmunized cows. Both the medicines (colostrum with antibody and colostrum without antibody against rotavirus) looked alike and also tasted similar.

After 48 hours of treatment, 50 percent of the patients treated with HBC recovered, whereas 100 percent of the placebo group still continued having diarrhea. The treatment with HBC was successful in early recovery of children with rotavirus diarrhea compared with the control group.

Following this study, another group of scientists repeated the study in children infected with rotavirus. They showed consistency that HBC works for rotavirus diarrhea in children.

However, in another study of children suffering from a different disease called shigellosis, the medicine didn't work. Therefore, in the case of shigellosis, the study results weren't consistent.

Repeating a study isn't bad because it can suggest that findings from one study aren't just a chance but a reality. The nearby sidebar shows an example where repeating a study showed consistent results.

Explaining biological plausibility

The statistically significant association established between exposure (E) and the disease (D) in your study should be *plausible* (or explainable) in terms of known biological facts about the *pathophysiology* (or mechanism) of the disease. In other words, you should be able to explain why a certain exposure and a disease are related to each other.

REAL LIFE EXAMPLE

Most people die in bed. Is it plausible that sleeping in bed causes death? I hope that's not the case! Sleeping in the bed and dying aren't causal facts because the existing knowledge doesn't support any reason behind the association.

What about this example? Many people in Nigeria are reported not getting better on a conventional anti-malarial treatment for their fever. After a thorough investigation, the scientists found that most blood samples from patients who weren't improving on the conventional treatment showed a parasitic infection due to *Plasmodium falciparum*. Moreover, this parasite was found resistant to the common medicines used for the treatment of malaria. Hence, the events of patients not responding to conventional treatments and the isolation of multi-drug resistant *Plasmodium falciparum* parasite are related, and the association of treatment failure and drug-resistance are plausible and proven in laboratory tests.

Contemplating coherence

Coherence means an association is causal when the available evidence concerning factors such as the natural history, biology, and epidemiology of the disease stick together or form a cohesive whole.

REAL LIFE EXAMPLE

The rise of smoking in Western countries during the early and mid-20th century was accompanied by a corresponding increase in lung cancer mortality. The two events are coherent because one would expect the two events to occur given the current knowledge about smoking.

Conducting more experimentation

You developed a hypothesis about a possible link of exposure and the disease. Suppose that particular hypothesis needs some pathophysiologic (or mechanistic) studies, which can't be tested by conventional epidemiologic studies. For further mechanistic studies, you may require more experimental epidemiologic studies, natural experiments, *in vitro* laboratory experiments, or studies in animal models in support of a causal hypothesis. Both clinical trials and community-based intervention trials are examples of experimental epidemiologic studies. I discuss experimental studies in greater detail in Chapter 17.

Finding analogies

Hill suggested that epidemiologists use *analogies*, or similarities between observed associations and any other associations. Analogy is perhaps one of the weaker of the criteria because analogies are speculative in nature and are dependent upon the subjective opinion of the researcher. For example, if one pharmaceutical drug (such as thalidomide) causes severe birth defects, you would be ready to accept similar evidence of birth defects with another drug.

WARNING

Failure to establish analogy doesn't preclude a causal association. That means you don't have to prove that there are similarities between two events.

Making Rothman's Causal Pie

In 1976, Kenneth Rothman proposed the conceptual model of causation known as the *sufficient-component cause model*, which is popularly called *Rothman's causal pie*. Today, many chronic diseases of multifactorial origin can be better explained by Rothman's causal pie.

According to Rothman, the causal factors of a disease can be classified as one of the following:

>> Sufficient cause

>> Necessary cause

>> Component cause

>> Contributory cause

Refer to www.cdc.gov/csels/dsepd/ss1978/lesson1/section8.html to see what Rothman's causal pie looks like.

In this link, you may find three pie charts, each having five pieces of the pie. Collectively these five pieces are sufficient to cause a disease. Therefore, each pie is a *sufficient cause*. Each sufficient cause has five pieces, meaning five *component causes*. If you look at each piece of the pie carefully, you can find that one piece is common to all — the letter A. That letter is called a *necessary cause*.

A *contributory cause* is neither necessary nor sufficient for causing a disease. A *contributory cause* (such as X, not shown in these figures) increases the likelihood of getting a disease.

The following sections break down these four factors in plain English.

Knowing what a sufficient cause means

In a multifactorial model, no single factor can cause a disease. Rather, several factors may act in consort to form a sufficient cause, and a particular disease might have several different sufficient causes. The complete pie, which might be considered a *causal pathway*, is called a sufficient cause. In the link to Rothman's pie, you find three pies — each of them represent a sufficient cause, which means each of the sufficient causes can produce the same disease.

REAL LIFE EXAMPLE

Type 2 diabetes is a chronic disease of multifactorial origin. Factors, such as obesity, family history of diabetes, lack of physical exercise, race and ethnicity, age, elevated blood lipids, and so on, are collectively called a sufficient cause of diabetes.

Understanding a necessary cause

The factors that must be present for the disease to occur are called necessary causes. A component that appears in every pie or pathway is called a necessary cause, because without it, disease doesn't occur.

REAL LIFE EXAMPLE

Consider these examples of a necessary cause:

>> The tubercle bacillus, *Mycobaterium tuberculosis,* is necessary to cause, because it must be present to cause tuberculosis.

>> When you isolate *Vibrio cholera* from stool samples, you confirm that it's cholera. *Vibrio cholera* is a necessary cause in the causal pathway.

Defining component causes

In Rothman's pie, each piece of the pie is a component cause of a disease. These components individually can't produce a disease; however, they collectively cause the disease.

Getting into contributory cause

Contributory causes are factors that aren't capable of producing a disease themselves but provide favorable conditions for the disease to occur. Contributory causes for a diarrheal disease can include the following:

>> Lack of pure drinking water

>> Low levels of education

>> Malnutrition

>> Poor living conditions

>> Poor sanitation

>> Poverty

>> Unhealthy food habits

Chapter **17**

Investigating the Types of Epidemiologic Studies

Epidemiology uses several study methods when conducting research to find out more about a disease or an event that's creating a public health problem in a population. When you hear about a disease, several questions may come to your mind. Basically you're curious and want to know more about the disease. You may want to know who's mostly affected by the disease, who's at risk of getting the disease, how serious the disease is, whether it's severe enough to cause death, how the disease spreads, how people may be informed whether they're likely to get the disease in the future, and so on. To answer these questions, you can conduct several types of epidemiologic research, which are collectively called *descriptive studies.*

As a public health professional, you may want to provide some health education or other type of intervention so that the disease can be controlled. Furthermore, you want to find out if your intervention works, which is another type of epidemiologic study called an *experimental study.*

For example, recently, you may have heard about an epidemic of mpox (formerly known as monkeypox). Based on the latest information published by the World Health Organization (WHO), the number of new cases reported for the first week of January 2023 came down compared to the preceding week. However, most cases (79.8 percent) have been reported from the Americas (including North America,

Central America, South America, and the Caribbean). You might be interested to know whether the disease has already shown up in your state. If so, how many people are affected? Is there a particular group of people who get the disease more often than others? How effective is mpox vaccine? Based on your research questions, you select an appropriate study design.

REMEMBER

Selecting the correct epidemiologic study is the most important step to discover the correct answers to your research questions or your hypothesis. The correct method of conducting the study is another equally important step. You can also choose between two or more study methods, depending on how much time and resources you may have or how accurate you desire the results to be. The type of study method you use also depends on the source of data and the availability of data that you have for conducting research.

This chapter walks you through step-by-step the different types of epidemiologic studies that are available, when you can use them, and how to use them. Near the end of the chapter, I guide you on designing a data collection instrument, called a *questionnaire*.

Looking At the Anatomy of Epidemiologic Studies

You basically have two kinds of epidemiologic studies:

>> **Descriptive:** Descriptive epidemiologic studies are used mainly to generate a *hypothesis* (a statement that you anticipate about possible outcome of a study). If you want to answer questions addressing what, when, where, and who, then you use a descriptive study.

>> **Analytical:** Analytical epidemiologic studies help in testing the hypothesis. Even if you don't have a hypothesis, you probably have some research questions. If you want to know why and how, then you use this type.

Chapter 2 introduces the terms descriptive and analytical epidemiology with examples whereas Chapter 7 discusses descriptive epidemiology in more detail. Here I provide more information about descriptive and analytical epidemiologic studies.

Figure 17-1 gives you an overview of the different types of epidemiological studies.

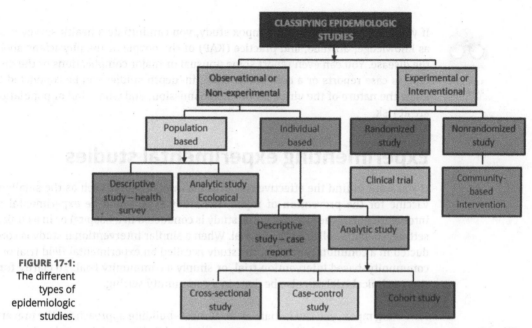

FIGURE 17-1:
The different
types of
epidemiologic
studies.

© Amal Mitra

Look at the two arms of the flow chart. On the left side, you find a group of studies called *observational* or non-experimental studies. On the right side of the arms, you find another group of studies known as *experimental* or interventional studies. Under the observational studies, you may find examples of descriptive studies — they include health survey and case report. Other studies, namely ecological studies, cross-sectional studies, case-control studies, clinical trials, and community-based intervention studies are examples of analytical studies. On the other hand, experimental studies are also analytical in nature.

The next sections describe some of these studies in more detail.

Observing observational studies

Observational studies can be either descriptive (to answer what, when, where, and who), or analytic in nature (such as identifying risk factors or finding an association between two or more variables). You can do a study among a group in a population (such as a census or a health survey), and also you can do it at an individual level (such as a case report or a case series).

If you take the example of the mpox study, you can initiate a health survey such as knowledge, attitude, and practice (KAP) of the people or the physicians about the disease. You can even report some unusual or major complications of the disease as case reports or a case series. More in-depth studies can be conducted to know the nature of the virus, mode of transmission, and what kind of population are at risk.

Experimenting experimental studies

If you want to find the effectiveness of some interventions, such as the smallpox vaccine for the prevention of mpox, the study type would be experimental or interventional. If the interventional study is conducted in a hospital or in a clinical setting, then it's called a clinical trial. When a similar interventional study is conducted in a community setting, the study is called an experimental field trial or a community-based intervention trial, or simply a community trial. To clarify further, a clinical trial can also be done in a community setting.

Revisiting mpox, you can initiate an awareness-building approach for the prevention of mpox transmission in a community — in other words, you're doing an *intervention*. You can also find out if the smallpox vaccine works or not in the case of mpox. For a vaccine trial, the several steps or phases are

1. **Conduct a laboratory-based study of the composition of the vaccine to know how it works.**

2. **Conduct a small-scale study on the effectiveness of the vaccine in a few volunteers.**

3. **Do the same study in a small number of patients to find the efficacy and side effects of the vaccine through a clinical trial.**

4. **Find the effectiveness, side effects, and the acceptance of the vaccine among a large group of people in the community.**

Using the hierarchy of study design

Of the different types of studies, scientists rank them from the highest quality to the lowest quality of studies. Figure 17-2 shows a list of studies from most reliable or from the highest quality to least reliable or studies of the lowest quality.

You may find that a systematic review with meta-analysis tops the list, followed by randomized controlled trials or RCTs, cohort studies, case-control studies, and cross-sectional studies. Case reports, case studies, and other types of documentations such as editorial and an expert opinion are also important, but they're at the lowest level of the scale based on the study quality and risk of bias.

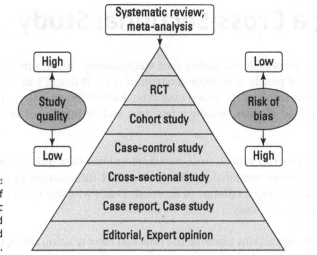

FIGURE 17-2: Hierarchy of epidemiologic studies based on quality and risk of bias.

Systematic review; meta-analysis

High — Study quality — Low

RCT
Cohort study
Case-control study
Cross-sectional study
Case report, Case study
Editorial, Expert opinion

Low — Risk of bias — High

© John Wiley & Sons, Inc.

Differentiating between retrospective and prospective studies

In a *retrospective* study, you look back and find out the cause or the risk factors of the disease in question. With mpox, in a retrospective study, you select some people who already have had mpox — they're the cases; you select another group of people who didn't have mpox — they're the controls. Then you look back at their history or check their medical records and get the information about what happened before they became infected or not infected with the disease. You gather relevant information and compare the exposure or the risk factor not only among the group of people who had the disease but also among the people who didn't have the disease.

Meanwhile, in a *prospective* study, also called a *longitudinal study,* you follow and observe a group of subjects over a period of time to gather information and record the development of the disease (or outcome). For a prospective study, you start with an *exposure factor* (a causative factor or a risk factor for a disease). This type of epidemiologic study follows groups of individuals over time who are alike in many ways but differ by a certain characteristic.

For example, you want to find whether exposure to secondhand smoke can cause asthma. In this case, secondhand smoke is the exposure factor. You take a group of people who are exposed to secondhand smoke and another group of people of similar age (similar cohort) who aren't exposed to secondhand smoke. You follow up with them in a certain time frame, such as five years (make sure it's long enough to be effective). At the end of the follow-up period, you find out whether anybody in the exposed group and the nonexposed group developed asthma.

Conducting a Cross-Sectional Study

A *cross-sectional study* is a widely used epidemiologic study, sort of like a snapshot of a group of people at a single moment of time. It doesn't look in the past, and neither does it follow the group over time. Rather data is collected generally over a short period of time, usually a few days and definitely not several months or years.

However, you can repeat cross-sectional studies in a quick successive time if needed. In cross-sectional studies, you collect information to calculate a rate, called a *prevalence*, of a disease or an event. That's why this type of research is also called a *prevalence study*.

The following sections examine the pros and cons to using this type of study and describe how you conduct one.

REAL LIFE EXAMPLE

A group of scientists conducted a cross-sectional study in Malaysia's Bachok district located at the southeastern border of Thailand from October 2008 to August 2009. The study, which involved 306 people ages 18 to 70 years, studied metabolic syndrome, which is a combination of health problems that include a large waistline, increased blood pressure, high blood sugar, high levels of triglycerides (one type of cholesterol), and decreased levels of HDL (also called "good cholesterol"). These conditions increase the risk of type 2 diabetes, heart disease, and stroke.

The survey used a structured questionnaire to collect information on demographics, lifestyle, and medical history. Body measurements, such as weight, height, body mass index, waist and hip circumference, and blood pressure were measured. A doctor or nurses took blood samples and analyzed them for lipid profile and fasting blood sugar. The overall prevalence of metabolic syndrome was 37.5 percent and was higher among females (42.9 percent). A significant higher proportion of women who were unemployed or older homemakers were associated with metabolic syndrome.

This cross-sectional study suggested weight management and preventive community-based programs involving the homemakers, the unemployed, and adults with poor education to prevent and manage metabolic syndrome. Cross-sectional studies can provide descriptive information that helps in developing strategies for further health interventions or in conducting more research.

Identifying the pros and cons

No research is always good or always bad, and most studies have advantages and disadvantages. Table 17-1 identifies the pros and cons of a cross-sectional study.

TABLE 17-1   **Pros and Cons of a Cross-Sectional Study**

Pros	Cons
Efficient for time and resources.	Can't establish whether the disease or the risk factor happened first.
Individual level data.	Doesn't help to determine causal relationships.
Ability to control for multiple confounders.	Not good for rare diseases.
Can assess multiple risk factors.	Not good for diseases of short duration.
Used to prove or disprove an assumption.	Not used to analyze behavior.
Can calculate prevalence; can also calculate prevalence odds ratio.	Can't calculate incidence.
Data can be used to develop a hypothesis.	An independent study must be done to prove a hypothesis.

Formulating a cross-sectional study

In cross-sectional study, you collect data of a disease or an event (outcome) and possible causes or the risk factors (exposure factors) — all at the same time. A cross-sectional study selects the participants based on the inclusion and exclusion criteria set for the study. After the participants have been selected for the study, you carry out the study to collect data for the exposures and the outcomes. After you gather the data, you analyze it to find any associations or risk factors between the exposures and the outcomes.

Figure 17-3 is a schematic diagram of a cross-sectional model where you're collecting data from a sample. The sample is a cross-section of the population. Look at the four arrows of the figure pointing toward the four factors — disease or no disease, and exposure or no exposure. In a cross-sectional study, you get data for these four factors — all at the same time of your data collection.

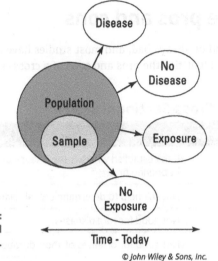

FIGURE 17-3:
A cross-sectional study model.

© John Wiley & Sons, Inc.

IS SHISHA SMOKING SAFER THAN CIGARETTE SMOKING? A CROSS-SECTIONAL STUDY

REAL LIFE EXAMPLE

While I was working in a medical university in Kuwait, my students and I had four to five months to compare whether smoking shisha — also referred to as *hookah, waterpipe, narghile, galyan,* or *hubble-bubble,* in young people in Kuwait — is safer than cigarette smoking. Shisha has been a traditional method of smoking in the Middle East, the Indian subcontinent, and some other parts of the world for several decades. The waterpipe heats the tobacco used in shisha smoking with charcoal, filters the smoke in a bowl of water, and then directs it to a rubber pipe for inhalation.

My students decided to conduct a cross-sectional study. The study sample was young university students because any result generated from this study could possibly be generalized to young adults of the country. Some of these students conducting the study were health-related majors. When they later became doctors or nurses, they could rely on their current experience and behavior to influence their future patients and the health message they give those patients could have a greater impact.

We studied students enrolled in health-related and non-health related professions from three private universities in Kuwait and at Kuwait University, which is a public university. The investigators developed a short questionnaire to gather information from the subjects about their demographics, personal history of smoking, types of smoking, any self-reported health complaints (present or in the past), sleep patterns, and lifestyle. They also asked about any family history of smoking and any major illnesses that family members had. In addition to the self-administered questionnaire, the study measured the participants' lung function using a portable instrument called a peak expiratory flow rate (PEFR) meter. This instrument measured how forcefully they could blow air out of their mouth after taking a deep breath. The study also measured the subjects' height and weight to calculate the body mass index (BMI).

The most common self-reported medical conditions among smokers were frequent respiratory infections, persistent cough, shortness of breath, chest pain, and fast heartbeat — all were significantly more frequent in smokers (shisha and/or cigarette) than in nonsmokers. Fewer shisha smokers than cigarette smokers complained of persistent cough, chest pain, and rapid heart rate. The PEFR values were significantly lower among smokers (shisha and/or cigarette) than nonsmokers. However, there was no significant difference in PEFR between shisha smokers and cigarette smokers. In conclusion, our study didn't show enough evidence suggesting that shisha smoking is safer than cigarette smoking.

Plotting a Case-Control Study

A case-control study is one of the most popular analytic studies because it's easy to do and you can get a great deal of valid information compared with a cross-sectional study (see the previous section). Here, I describe how to conduct a case-control study.

In a case-control study, you start with a group of cases and controls and look back to identify the association of exposure (or risk) factors between them. Hence, this study is a perfect example of retrospective study. However, you can also conduct a case-control study prospectively or conduct one in future time. A case-control study can help in testing a hypothesis about an association between a risk factor and a disease. However, some other study designs such as a cohort study or a clinical trial are more rigorous in proving a hypothesis.

Selecting a suitable control

Although conducting a case-control study takes less time to do compared to a cohort study, selecting a suitable control still takes time. Suppose you want to do a case-control study to know what causes the high incidence of lung cancers in your community. In this example, cases are known patients with lung cancer. You have several different possibilities in selecting a control. Consider these options:

>> **Cancer control:** The control should be people who don't have lung cancer, but they have any other forms of cancer.

>> **No cancer but other disease control:** The control should be people who don't have lung cancer, but they suffer from a disease other than forms of cancer.

>> **Healthy control:** The control should be people who are healthy and have no other diseases.

Before you can decide which control is better, you need to contemplate three other issues:

>> **A risk factor:** Take smoking. A healthy control remains healthy because of many reasons including a healthy lifestyle. If they're a lifetime nonsmoker, comparing the risk between a group with lung cancer and the healthy controls can yield a huge difference between the two groups. On the other hand, smoking not only causes lung cancer but also causes other cancers and many other diseases. Therefore, if your comparison group has other cancers or other diseases, the observed difference in the risk of smoking between the cases and controls may not be as high as that of a healthy control.

>> **The location:** Another issue is where you should select a control. Refer to the section, "Sources of controls," later in this chapter for more details.

>> **Demographics:** The third issue is whether you should match the controls with age, gender, or any other factor. Remember, matching may be important but overmatching is a problem. For example, you want to match cases and controls by age. If you select one six-year-old child as a case, you can match the age with a control of similar age but may not be exactly the same age — for example, the control age is ± 2 years of the case age. If you match cases with control for several variables (such as age, gender, income, location), the situation is called *overmatching*.

Sources of cases

You can get cases from several sources — depending on the type of case. In this study where the cases are lung cancer, you should try to get cases from as many sources as possible so that you don't miss any. The sources for a cancer case are as follows:

>> Cases diagnosed in a hospital or clinic

>> Cases entered into a disease registry — for example, a cancer registry, a registry of birth defects, a death registry, and others

>> Cases found through mass screening — for example, screening for cervical cancer with Pap smears of all women older than 25, blood pressure screening

of all adults in a community by using home measurement of BP; cataract screening in an eye camp, and others

>> Cases identified through a prior cohort study — for example, lung cancers in an occupational asbestos cohort

Sources of controls

Selecting controls is more difficult than selecting cases. Your selection of a suitable control makes a difference in the results of your study. Here are the three types of control groups you can consider:

>> **Hospital controls:** Hospital controls aren't generally recommended because of several issues:

- Hospital controls also may have diseases resulting from the exposure of interest — for example, the exposure (smoking) is related to the disease of interest (cancer) and to heart and lung diseases which the controls may be suffering from.

- Hospital controls may not be representative of the exposure prevalence in the source population of cases — for example, hospitals may have a higher prevalence of admitted patients who are smokers.

>> **Neighborhood or relative controls:** This type of control is recommended provided they don't share the exposure of interest (such as smoking in cases of cancers).

>> **Population controls:** They're the most desirable method of control selection. Non-cases are sampled from the source population giving rise to cases. Sampling randomly from census block groups or a registry such as the Department of Motor Vehicles (of adults who are able to drive) are examples of ways to find and recruit population-based controls.

REMEMBER

Consider a few other general heads-ups while conducting a case–control study:

>> You can do a case-control study only after you have selected cases and appropriate controls.

>> If your comparison group isn't suitable, you may have artificially inflated results between cases and controls.

>> Controls aren't always healthy.

>> Cases can also include subjects who died when you use controls who survived. Refer to the nearby sidebar for an example of deceased persons as cases and survivors as controls.

USING DEATHS AS CASES AND SURVIVORS AS CONTROLS

While working in a rural hospital in Bangladesh, I encountered a number of children who died from common health problems, one being blood dysentery (also called shigellosis). I wanted to know why some children died and others didn't. If I knew that answer, maybe I could try a better treatment for those affected or be better prepared for similar types of ailments in addition to blood dysentery. From hospital records, my team selected children who had died with a diagnosis of blood dysentery as the cases for our study. Using the hospital registry of all admitted patients, the team found a child who matched the age of the case but didn't die. They selected two such patients who survived and were of similar age as controls for each case.

After the selection process of cases and controls, the team recorded the demographic factors such as gender, mother's education, family income, smokers in the family, duration of illness, and accompanying other illnesses of the child, such as febrile illness, malnutrition, pneumonia, history of measles, and immunization. The hospital records provided some of this information; the rest was collected by interviewing family members.

The team visited the dead children's households and interviewed the mother or anyone who took care of the child when they were sick. After a careful investigation, the investigators identified the following:

- Girls died more often than boys.

- The cases were sicker for a longer time before they were admitted to the hospital.

- The cases had accompanying lower respiratory infection (or pneumonia) and severe malnutrition compared to those who survived.

Number of controls

In research publications, you may come across many case-control studies where the number of controls compared to cases are sometimes the same and sometimes they're different. In many studies you may find that the scientists used one control for each case. In the nearby sidebar, I used two controls who survived the disease for each case who died. In some studies, you may find more than two controls per case, so what's the rule?

REMEMBER

Don't have fewer controls than cases. If your total cases are 50, you must have at least 50 controls or more. Having more controls than cases increases the validity (also called *statistical power*) of the study. The ratio of cases and controls can be 1:2, 1:3 or 1:4, which means that the number of controls should be two to four times the cases. In mathematical calculations, scientists have shown that the more control you have, the more the power of the study is. However, if you increase the controls beyond four, the study doesn't gain much statistical power, so four is the optimal magic number.

Counting the pros and cons

Conducting a case-control study has a number of advantages and disadvantages. Table 17-2 lists some of the pros and cons.

TABLE 17-2   **Pros and Cons of a Case-Control Study**

Pros	Cons
The most efficient design for rare diseases or rare events (such as death and suicide).	Not suitable for rare exposures.
Requires a much smaller study sample than cohort studies.	Although this study can establish correlation, it can't establish causation.
Allows more intensive evaluation of exposures of cases and controls.	Selection of controls can be a problem.
Considerably less time and cost to carry out the study.	Missing data because you're replying on data that was collected earlier; there's chance of missing information in the data.
Confounding (an unwanted or noise variable) can be controlled in the design phase. By the process of matching a confounder, you can avoid its effect in the study results.	May be subject to recall bias if exposure is measured by interviews and if recall of exposure differs between cases and controls.
Can assess multiple risk factors.	Can't provide any information about the incidence or prevalence of a disease.
Used to prove or disprove an assumption.	Can't calculate a rate or risk because the denominator isn't defined.
Used to calculate odds ratio.	Because you can't calculate incidence or risk, you also can't calculate risk difference or risk ratio.
Data produces valid information to support a hypothesis.	More robust studies are needed to prove a hypothesis.

Putting together a case-control study

To conduct a case-control study, focus on these two common ingredients:

>> Disease or outcome

>> Exposure of risk factors

Here's what you need to do to put together a case-control study:

1. **Assign cases and controls.**

   The cases are who you want to study — the people who have a disease. The controls are the people who don't have the disease. Refer to the section, "Selecting a suitable control," earlier in this chapter where I discuss how to select a suitable control, how many controls to select per case, and from where you should select your controls.

2. **Collect data from the exposure factors.**

   Investigate to determine which subjects in each group (cases and controls) had the exposure(s), comparing the frequency of the exposure in the case group to the control group.

   Gather information from at least three areas:

   - **Demographic information:** Age, sex, race, ethnicity, occupation, income, education, and any other social factor that may influence the outcome

   - **Risk factors:** What you're looking for in your study in terms of associated risk factors

   - **Any variables that could potentially confound with your variable(s) of interest:** A *confounder* is a variable that can affect the results and create a problem in getting a true association between the exposure and disease. You should take measures to avoid or eliminate its effect. See Chapter 18 for more information.

Figure 17-4 illustrates a case-control model. You find that at the time when you begin the study, you have two groups:

>> Disease

>> No disease

You look to find out how many of the cases (the disease group) and the controls (the no disease group) had any exposure or risk factor in the past.

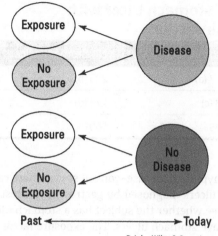

FIGURE 17-4:
A case-control
study model.

Past ◄————————► Today

© John Wiley & Sons, Inc.

WARNING

Bias is an issue in case–control studies. As I discuss in Chapter 18, several factors can create bias when collecting the exposure data. To avoid bias, you can take several precautionary measures:

>> Collect the data the same way for both groups.

>> Because you already know the outcome, be aware of potential researcher bias in getting data from the past records.

>> Take special care to be objective in the search for past risk factors.

>> If possibly, always try to mask the information about the outcome (disease or no disease) from the person who's collecting data about exposures or risk factors or who's interviewing patients.

>> Be aware that people who suffer from a disease (cases) are more likely to relate the past events (or exposure) with the disease.

>> Make sure you don't ask about events that happened too long ago. When you interview someone about potential risk factors including history of smoking, specific food items, or exposure to certain event, a person who doesn't have the disease (control) may not recall all the events correctly — this is called *recall bias.*

The time period of the past record is variable, depending on what source you use for the exposure factors. For instance, if you collect data from a hospital record, you can access it quickly, whereas getting the data by using a telephone survey or from visiting door-to-door takes more time (sometimes a couple of days). In either case, you arrange the data in a 2 x 2 contingency table as shown in Table 17-3 — this study investigates the link between stomach ulcers with a *Helicobacter pylori* infection among 625 subjects.

TABLE 17-3   The Association of Stomach Ulcer with *Helicobacter Pylori* Infection

Exposure	Stomach Ulcers	No Stomach Ulcers	Total
Helicobacter pylori (*H. pylori*) infections	107 (a)	225 (b)	332
No *H. pylori* infections	18 (c)	275 (d)	293
Total	125	500	625

This data comes from a hypothetical case-control study where cases are subjects who developed stomach ulcers diagnosed by gastroscopy, a test to directly look inside the stomach and see whether the subject has a stomach ulcer. Controls are individuals who didn't have stomach ulcers. The exposure factor in this case was a bacterial infection with *Helicobacter pylori*. A blood antibody test was conducted because this bacteria can cause stomach ulcers.

This study had a total of 125 cases with a diagnosis of stomach ulcers. You wanted to conduct a study with more power by having four times the number of controls than the cases, which would mean you'd need 500 controls (4×125). After getting all the data, you arrange them in the table and analyze the data for any association between the exposure and the disease.

Measuring association

The epidemiologic measurement for a case-control study is called an *odds ratio* (*OR*). As you may find in the earlier Table 17-3, the data is denoted by a, b, c, and d, where $a = 107$, $b = 225$, $c = 18$, and $d = 275$. The formula for calculating OR is as follows:

$$OR = \frac{ad}{bc}$$

$$OR = \frac{107 \times 275}{225 \times 18} = \frac{29425}{4050} = 7.3$$

In this study, you find that odds of getting stomach ulcers among those who had *H. pylori* infections is 7.3 times higher than those who didn't have *H. pylori* infections.

Nesting a nested case-control study

A *nested case-control*, which is referred to as a case-control study nested within a cohort study, is a retrospective study. Here are the major advantages of doing a nested case-control study (compared to a cohort study — which I discuss in the section, "Leading a Cohort Study," later in this chapter):

>> They reduce time and cost.

>> They require a smaller sample.

>> They're efficient because not all subjects of the parent cohort require diagnostic testing.

>> They reduce selection bias because cases and controls are selected from the same population.

>> They reduce information bias because risk factor exposure can be assessed with the investigator being blind to case status.

One disadvantage of nested case-control study is that it reduces power because the sample size is reduced. How much power is reduced can be calculated from the following formula:

$$\text{Power reduced (from the parent cohort)} = \frac{1}{(c+1)}$$

where, c = number of controls per each case

For example, if you use two controls per case, power will be reduced by $\frac{1}{(2+1)} = \frac{1}{3}$ or $one-third$.

If you use three controls per case, power will be reduced by $\frac{1}{(3+1)} = \frac{1}{4}$ or $one-fourth$.

From the cost-benefit analysis, nested case-control is a better design than a regular case-control study, and a more cost-efficient design compared to a cohort study.

In this study, participants come from the cohort study; the investigator is blind to the information about the exposure variable until the cases and controls have been selected. I provide detailed information about a cohort study in the next section.

REAL LIFE EXAMPLE

Here's a hypothetical example of nested case-control study. In a prospective cohort study (refer to the section, "Identifying the three types of cohorts," later in this chapter, 90,000 women were being followed for more than ten years to study the determinants of cardiovascular disease (CVD) and cancer. The women were interviewed a couple of times about exposure factors. The blood and environmental samples were collected, analyzed, and frozen for future use, following proper ethical procedures and consent from the women.

You want to test a hypothesis that past exposure to pesticides such as DDT is a risk factor for breast cancer for women older than 45. To do so, follow these steps:

1. **Select the cases and controls.**

   Using a time frame of ten years, you find that 1,500 women in the cohort have developed breast cancer. They are your cases. You choose women not having breast cancer (but they're more likely to have other diseases) as your controls. To increase the statistical power, you select four controls for each case from the cancer registry of women.

2. **Look at the exposure data among cases and controls.**

   By doing so, you discover a total of 13,500 women at some point of their life were exposed to DDT.

3. **Construct a 2 x 2 contingency table for data analysis as Table 17-4 demonstrates.**

TABLE 17-4 **Breast Cancer Occurrence among Women with or without DDT Exposure**

	Breast Cancer	No Breast Cancer	Total
DDT Exposed	560	12,940	13,500
Unexposed	940	75,560	76,500
Total	1,500	88,500	90,000

4. **Calculate relative risk.**

   Relative risk is a ratio of the risk among exposed and the risk among unexposed populations.

   Risk of breast cancer among women who were exposed to DDT $= \frac{560}{13500} = 0.04$

   Risk of breast cancer among women who were not exposed to DDT

   $= \frac{940}{76500} = 0.01$

   Relative risk (RR) $= \frac{0.04}{0.01} = 4.0$

   You can interpret that women exposed to DDT had four times the risk of breast cancer compared to the women who weren't exposed to DDT.

Leading a Cohort Study

The word *cohort* means a group of people that have some common characteristics. These common characteristics can be that they live in a same place, they were born in a similar time frame, such as the people born in New York City in 1975, or they have the same occupation or job. A cohort study is an example of a prospective or longitudinal (forward) study. Here I describe the types of cohort studies, the pros and cons of cohort study, and how to construct a cohort study.

Identifying the three types of cohorts

Here are the three types of cohort studies.

Prospective cohort

Prospective means that the study relates to the future, so the prospective cohort is a longitudinal or forward-looking study. This study begins by identifying the exposure status of participants. You follow the participants over time and record the incidences (new occurrences) of the outcome (or disease).

Therefore, in prospective cohort study, you begin with two groups:

>> Exposure

>> No exposure

In this case exposure means some risk factors that can cause a disease. For example, smoking is one important exposure factor for lung cancer. In a cohort study, you'll have one group who are smokers and another group for nonsmokers. You then follow them for a defined period of time (for example, five years), and record the number of people who developed the disease of interest. In this example, look for those who develop lung cancer and those who don't in five years of follow-up.

Retrospective cohort

A *retrospective cohort* study means you look in the past. In a retrospective cohort study, the study period starts before the current study started. The follow-up period of a cohort happens in the past among those who participated in another study. You have the same two groups — one group has the exposure of interest and another doesn't have it. Rather than following them over time, find out how many of the two had developed the disease and how many didn't in the past. The follow-up period happens before the present study starts.

Mixed cohort

In a *mixed cohort study*, the exposure period is in the past but the period of disease development occurs in the future, in respect to the starting point of the present study. In simple words, you get historical data to determine the exposure and non-exposure from the past record, and then follow up over time in the future to observe and record the disease incidence.

Recognizing the pros and cons

Cohort studies aren't without any problems. Table 17-5 provides a list of pros and cons.

TABLE 17-5   Pros and Cons of a Cohort Study

Pros	Cons
The most efficient design for rare exposures.	Not suitable for rare diseases.
Can establish a causal relationship.	Requires a much larger study sample than other studies.
More detailed data are recorded over time.	Cost and time are more than the other study designs.
Multiple outcomes can be measured.	Lost to follow-up.
Confounding can be controlled.	Poor response rate.
Can control certain biases (such as recall bias and interviewer bias).	Can't provide any information about incidence or prevalence of a disease.
Used to prove or disprove an assumption.	Compliance is a major issue during follow-up.
Calculate incidence, relative risk, attributable risks.	Ethical issues are more rigorous.
Data produce valid information to test a hypothesis.	Missing data.

Devising a prospective cohort study

The framework for a prospective cohort study is just the opposite of what you do in a case-control study, which I discuss in the section, "Putting together a case-control study," earlier in this chapter.

In a prospective cohort study (see Figure 17-5), you follow people exposed to a risk factor and those not exposed to the same risk factor over time. The subjects either contract the disease or don't. Also, record how many of them die or survive. In other words, the outcome measurement depends on your study objective — the outcome can be a disease, or an event, or death.

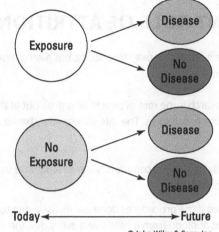

FIGURE 17-5:
A prospective cohort study model.

Today ←————————————→ Future

© John Wiley & Sons, Inc.

REAL LIFE EXAMPLE

Here you can find an outcome measure of a cohort study that's other than a disease. Sleep-disordered breathing is a serious health problem. The symptoms of sleep disorders range from disturbed sleep to inadequate sleep to breathing problems including gasping due to shortage of breath during sleep. Sleep disorders can cause a number of negative outcomes including high blood pressure, atrial fibrillation (or irregular heartbeats), worsening heart failure (the heart fails to pump out blood properly), worsening kidney disease, and others. A group of scientists studied more than 6,000 men and women and followed them for more than eight years. The outcome measure of this study was the death rate due to any cause. The breathing difficulties were categorized in four groups according to the degree of severity. The death rate from any cause in the cohort was significantly higher among those who had moderate-to-severe breathing difficulties compared to those who had mild breathing problems.

An important thing to note that men with a neck size of 17 inches or more or a woman with a neck size of 16 inches or more could be at risk for obstructive sleep apnea (a severe form of sleep disorder causing loss of breath).

With this study, the follow-up period was more than eight years. If the outcome measure is cancer, the follow-up period could be even longer. One issue with longer follow-up is a chance of attrition — which includes people dropping out, dying, or losing track of people who are in the study. In a cohort study, you must keep a record of all people who dropped out of the study or died. It's a red flag if a large number of people drop out because of question of bias in the study results. In addition, scientists will question why the study has such a large attrition rate. Sometimes attrition happens because of a large disruption of people due to a natural calamity, such as war, cyclone, or other disasters. It happened to one of my own research projects in Mississippi (see the nearby sidebar).

THE 20 PERCENT RULE OF ATTRITION

A general rule is that 5 percent attrition is okay for a study, but having more than 20 percent attrition is a concern.

The *attrition rate* in heath research is the rate of people who drop out of the study before they complete the study procedures. The rate varies widely based on a number of factors:

- The attrition rate is usually higher in a community-based follow-up study compared with a hospital-based clinical trial.

- The attrition rate increases if the procedures done are invasive and too many. For example, if you draw a lot of blood from a child's vein every day, the mother may not want to keep the child in the study, which requires daily visits to the hospital after they child is discharged.

- People may not want to spend time answering a self-addressed questionnaire interview.

- If you have sensitive questions in the questionnaire, people may not want to answer them. You may find a lot of missing data and attrition.

- If the study population is less educated, the attrition rate can be higher.

- Day-to-day workers more than likely can't stay in a study if it's too long because they need to go to their job.

One of my community-based intervention studies conducted in Mississippi that involved many health centers had another reason for higher attrition. The study subjects were women of low income who were enrolled in a government-supported nutrition supplementation program. My study started in 2004 was interrupted by Hurricane Katrina that hit Mississippi on August 29 and devastated the area. Many homes were destroyed, uprooting people and shutting down clinics and hospitals. As a result, the study lost many participants, causing a large attrition rate for the follow-up.

Figuring Out an Ecological Study

An *ecological study*, also called a *correlational study*, is a population-based observational study. This study, which I detail in the following sections, generally describes the association between a certain risk factor and a disease. You can also use this study when you want to compare the health event between many countries in a single study.

Knowing what ecological fallacy is

When conducting an ecological study, interpret the data with caution. *Ecological fallacy* refers to an inference drawn based on aggregate data for a group instead of individual-level data. Because of the lack of individual-level data, an ecological study showing that the incidence of breast cancer increases with the dietary intakes of fat in many countries means the country-level aggregated data can't establish a causal relationship. The fallacy of this kind of study is that conclusions are inappropriately inferred about individuals, whereas the results arise from aggregated data of a country population.

REMEMBER

To avoid ecological fallacy, researchers having no individual data should first find out what's occurring at the individual level. Taking the example of fat intake and breast cancer incidence, researchers should identify individual-level fat intakes and then correlate that fat intake with the aggregated amount of fat intake of the country. Finally, the researchers should conclude whether anything occurring at the group level adds to the relationship between fat intake and breast cancer incidence.

Focusing on the pros and cons

Table 17-6 lists the pros and cons of ecological studies.

TABLE 17-6 **Pros and Cons of an Ecological Study**

Pros	Cons
Can study a large population at a given time.	A universal case definition is needed for cross-country comparison.
Large geographical studies can generate a hypothesis.	Other study designs are needed to prove the hypothesis.
Make geographical comparisons between disease incidence and/or mortality and the prevalence of risk factors.	A causal relationship can't be established.
Many useful observations have emerged from geographical analysis.	Care is needed for their interpretations to avoid ecological fallacy.

Looking at examples of ecological studies

Several well-known ecological studies have provided valuable information on the relationship between fat intake and breast cancer across different countries. In such studies, scientists showed a linear relationship between per capita fat intake and breast cancer mortality, meaning that the more fat a woman eats, the more likely she is to die from breast cancer. This study used data from 40 countries about the estimated daily fat intake per person and death rate from breast cancer. Among all countries, the fat intake and breast cancer death rates were the lowest in countries such as Thailand, Japan, Taiwan, El Salvador, and the Philippines, whereas both were the highest in some developed countries such as the Netherlands, Denmark, United Kingdom, New Zealand, United States, Switzerland, Ireland, and Belgium.

In another ecological study, a similar direct relationship was observed between the increased per capita (per person) supplies of fat calories and the increased incidence of breast cancer dietary fat intake with increased mortality from breast cancer, using data from 21 countries. Both the breast cancer incidence and per capita fat supply were highest in the United States and lowest in Japan. The other countries with a high rate of breast cancer incidence and also high amount of fat intake were Switzerland, Denmark, Germany, Canada, France, New Zealand, and the United Kingdom.

Developing a Questionnaire

Questionnaires provide an efficient way to collect data. In epidemiologic studies, questionnaire-based data collection method is used for several reasons:

>> You can administer a questionnaire simultaneously to hundreds of people.

>> You can easily tabulate or score the responses from a questionnaire and then easily analyze that data.

>> You can physically verify any missing data.

>> You can administer questionnaires anonymously. Therefore, they're useful for collecting information on sensitive matters or even illegal or unsocial activities if required

>> A questionnaire-based data collection doesn't cost a lot of money.

This section discusses how to plan, develop, and execute a questionnaire-based data collection.

REAL LIFE EXAMPLE

For example, if you want to know why minority female students are falling behind in science, technology, engineering, and math (STEM) education, you can select a few community colleges, prepare a well-designed questionnaire, administer it to hundreds of seniors, and do the data analysis.

Creating an efficient questionnaire

Here I give you a few tips for preparing an efficient questionnaire:

>> Prepare a written list of specific objectives for the research.

>> Take advantage of the insights of your friends, your mentor, or others by asking them whether the objectives are realistic and measurable.

>> Review the literature and get any sample questionnaire used for the same purpose.

>> Plan time from the point of preparing a draft questionnaire, pretesting it, and collecting data.

>> Avoid using negatives in statements.

>> Avoid acronyms.

>> Use "I don't know" sparingly as a choice.

>> Make the choices mutually exclusive.

>> Don't make it too lengthy.

Using closed and open-ended questions

When writing your questionnaire, focus on writing most of them to be *closed-ended*. In a closed-ended question, the answers are embedded within a set of multiple-choice answers, (such as A, B, C, D, or All of the above), or you choose your answers from a scale of 1 to 5, or the closed-ended questions can be answered with Yes or No. Meanwhile, write one or two of your last questions to be *open-ended*, which focus on questions that allow someone to give a free-form answer. In open-ended questions, you may ask about the respondent's own views or opinion.

Here is an example of a closed-ended question:

How supportive were your teachers during your first year of schooling in the college?

Very supportive

Moderately supportive

Somewhat supportive

Very unsupportive

Here's an example of an open-ended question:

Mention briefly how the student-teacher relation can be improved in a school environment:

Knowing what else to include

Here are a few other important parts of a good questionnaire:

» **Demographic questions:** Age, gender, race/ethnicity, occupation, income, county name, and so on.

» **Variables of interest:** The variables you want to know based on your research objectives and research questions.

» **Confounders:** Data from any other variable that can affect your results.

» **Variables of a higher scale:** Use age instead of age-group. If you get the actual age, you can always make groups, but you can't get the real age from a grouped data, such as an age-group.

» **Concluding courtesy statement:** End the questionnaire thanking the respondent for their time in answering the questions.

Chapter 18

Encountering Bias and Confounding

Research is susceptible to errors, and the results of a study can be faulty if you're not careful. One of the reasons that errors can happen is because of the presence of bias. Bias can be introduced at any stage of a study, including the stages of designing the study, conducting the study and collecting the data, analyzing the study's data, or even during preparing the manuscript, including the citation and publication of the study results. In epidemiologic studies, bias occurs less commonly because the investigator is prejudiced; rather it happens because of ignorance or unavoidable decisions made during the course of a study. You can avoid some of the biases if you're careful enough and you know how to avoid biases. This chapter explains what biases are, how you can avoid them, and how you identify biases in studies.

Furthermore, a study can produce erroneous results in the presence of confounding. A *confounder* is an extraneous variable that can mix up the study's results. A confounder is sometimes called a *nuisance variable* because the results are faulty because you didn't control for it. This chapter also discusses how to identify a confounder and how to control for one in a study.

Defining Bias

Bias is a systematic error that happens during the course of a study. Bias results are an incorrect or invalid estimate of the measurement between the exposure factors and the disease. Bias can occur in any type of epidemiologic study; however, retrospective studies (such as case–control study) are more susceptible to bias than prospective studies (such as cohort study or clinical trials), mainly because of differences in the timing of the study.

REMEMBER

When evaluating a study for the presence of bias, you must make the three following actions:

» **Identify the source of bias.** Bias comes in many forms — for example, sampling bias occurs when the sample doesn't represent the population from which the data are collected. Bias can occur when the researchers have an interest in the outcome. You first have to identify the source because doing so will help you assess the strength and the direction of the bias.

» **Estimate the magnitude or strength of the problem.** This means how strong the association is between the exposure and the disease.

REAL LIFE
EXAMPLE

Suppose a true risk (risk ratio) of a sedentary lifestyle (an exposure) that causes heart disease is 2.8, which means that your risk of heart disease is 2.8 times higher if you have a sedentary lifestyle compared to someone who isn't sedentary (they actively exercise on a regular basis). If the strength of bias is small, it might alter the estimate of the true risk ratio slightly, say to 2.6 or 2.9, but it can't alter the results drastically. Even though some amount of bias is present because the strength of bias is so weak, it can't pull the results to make any incorrect conclusion.

» **Assess its direction.** Bias can go in either direction — helping your hypothesis or going against your hypothesis.

REAL LIFE
EXAMPLE

In statistics, you'll come across a term called *null effect,* also referred to as the *null hypothesis,* which means there's no difference in the outcome. Bias can pull the results of the outcome (such as risk ratio) either toward or away from the null. Stated another way, an existence of bias can either underestimate or overestimate the true measure of the association.

Clarifying What Confounding Means

The term *confounding* refers to a situation in which a noncausal association between a given exposure and an outcome is observed as a result of the influence of a third factor (or a variable), usually designated as a confounding variable or simply a confounder.

The variable that's considered a confounder must meet several criteria:

>> **Be associated with the exposure (or risk factor) of the disease:** That means the confounding variable (for example, drinking alcohol) must be more or less common in the exposed population (for example, smokers) than the comparable population (for example, nonsmokers).

>> **Be an independent cause or predictor of the disease:** That means that the association between the confounding variable (in this case, drinking alcohol) and the disease (for example, bladder cancer) is present among both the exposed (smokers) and unexposed population (nonsmokers).

>> **Can't be an intermediate step:** This means that the confounding variable (for example, drinking alcohol) can't be an intermediate step or a modifier in the causal pathway between the exposure (for example, smoking) and the disease (for example, bladder cancer). In other words, when a variable is found to work as modifier in the causal pathway, the variable is no more called a confounder.

Reviewing Bias-Affecting Research Findings

Bias can occur at many different stages of a study starting from the beginning to the end where you publish the results. Two most important types of bias are selection bias and information bias. I discuss different types of bias under these two broad headings in the following sections.

Examining and avoiding selection bias

Selection bias can occur at different stages of epidemiologic studies, such as during study subject selection and during the follow-up of subjects.

Selection bias most commonly happens in retrospective studies, such as a case-control study and a retrospective cohort study. It can also happen in prospective or longitudinal studies, such as a prospective cohort study or an experimental study. Refer to Chapter 17 where I explain these types of studies in more detail.

Selection bias can happen in several different ways, including the following:

>> **At the time of subject selection:** Cases and controls are two groups of people that are selected at the beginning of a case-control study. This bias in subject selection occurs in the case of a retrospective case-control study and at the beginning of a retrospective cohort study. Here are two examples:

- **Control selection bias:** In a case-control study, selection bias occurs when subjects for the control group aren't truly representative of the population that produced the cases. Remember, the controls are selected to estimate the exposure potential among them compared to exposure potential of the cases. Ideally, cases and controls should be selected from a similar population so that other extraneous factors don't affect the results. If cases and controls come from different populations (for example, cases selected from one hospital that caters to populations from one area and controls selected from a different area), selection bias can happen.

- **Self-selection bias:** In statistics, self-selection bias arises in any situation in which individuals select themselves into a group. For example, very often survey respondents are allowed to decide entirely for themselves whether or not they want to participate in a survey. Hence, the people who choose to take part in a study and the people who choose not to may have a number of differences between them, such as motivation, socioeconomic status, or prior experience. For example, a larger proportion of people with the exposure (smoking) and the disease (bladder cancer) participating in the case group compared to the control group can cause erroneous results.

>> **At the time of follow-up:** Called *loss to follow-up bias,* this type of bias occurs in retrospective and prospective cohort studies and in experimental studies. If a large amount of subjects drop out, bias may occur.

You can take a number of measures to avoid selection bias:

>> **Randomization:** The best way to avoid selection bias is to use simple random sampling for the subjects. The method of randomization ensures that the two groups are comparable in terms of observable and unobservable characteristics.

For example, when designing a clinical trial, randomly select the samples and distribute them in treatment groups (either study treatment or control) by using a random digit chart or random computer-generated numbers. A clinical trial that uses randomization procedures ensures that the baseline characteristics of the samples are uniformly distributed to the treatment and the control groups without any bias. This type of study design is called *randomized controlled trial (RCT).* RCT is a prospective experimental study (check out Chapter 17). You can also use this similar procedure for a sample selection in a cohort study or a case-control study. However, selection bias can still occur and make erroneous results if the sample size is small. Thus, make sure you pay extra attention in estimating the sample size required for the study.

>> **Selection of cases and controls:** Whenever possible, study subjects (both cases and controls) should be chosen from defined reference populations.

>> **Retention:** Successful methods should be adopted to retain and trace study subjects in order to prevent them from being lost to follow-up.

>> **No self-selection:** To avoid self-selection bias, don't allow individuals the ability to select themselves to be included in a survey. Ideally, you should utilize a probability sampling method. Probability sampling (such as random sampling) allows everyone in the population an equal chance to be selected, whereas a nonprobability sampling method (such as convenience sampling) allows you to get sample data easily from a conveniently available sample.

BERKSON'S BIAS — A KIND OF SELECTION BIAS

In 1946, Joseph Berkson described bias in the assessment of the relationship between an exposure and a disease due to conducting the study in a clinic where attendance was affected by both exposure and disease. Berkson's bias, also referred to as *collider bias,* is a special type of *selection bias.* It can arise when the sample is selected from a subpopulation and not the general public. Berkson first recognized this type of bias in case-control studies when both cases and controls are sampled from a hospital rather than from the community.

When you select samples from a hospital for a case-control study design (see Chapter 17 for more information), you select two groups:

- **Cases with a disease (of interest):** In other words, people who have a disease being studied

- **Controls:** Controls are patients who don't have the disease

You may assume that the chance of admission to the hospital for a disease doesn't depend on the presence or absence of the risk factor. This may not be the case, especially if the risk factor is another disease. That's because people are more likely to be hospitalized if they have two diseases rather than only one. In this case, an exposure and an outcome have a shared common cause (or colliding) that isn't controlled for.

Eyeing and avoiding information bias

Information bias is when an error arises from either imperfect definitions of study variables or flawed data collection procedures. These errors may result in misclassification of exposure and/or outcome status for a significant proportion of study participants.

For example, when you're asking about smoking status, make it clear whether you're asking about current smoking status or whether the person has smoked at any time in their life. You also may want to be more specific, such as how many cigarettes a person smokes each day and for how long they've smoked that amount.

In the following sections, I discuss several types of information bias and ways of controlling it. The two main categories of information bias related to exposure identification are recall bias and interviewer bias.

Recall bias

Recall bias is a type of information bias. It occurs when there are different levels of accuracy in providing information about past events. Recall bias occurs most often in case-control studies because you're naming the events that happened in the past in this type of study.

Suppose your goal is to identify the relationship between smoking status and lung cancer. In a case-control study, if the cases with lung cancer remember and report their smoking status more accurately than the controls (those without lung cancer), the process results in a recall bias.

Recall bias can happen in retrospective cohort studies. If you want to conduct a retrospective cohort study using the same topic of the relationship between smoking and lung cancer, one group will be the people who are exposed to smoking (the exposure group) and the other group will be people who don't smoke and aren't exposed to smoking. You then consider the disease events during the study period (for example, five years) in the past. Ask them whether they developed lung cancer (or any other cancer) during the study period. If, for some reason, the smokers remember or report their disease occurrences more often and more accurately during the five years of observation compared to the nonsmokers, a recall bias occurs.

Recall bias can also occur is a cross-sectional study if the study asks participants about past exposures.

TIP

To avoid recall biases, use these methods to control or prevent them:

>> **Verify responses.** You can easily use this simple method by reviewing hospital records to confirm medical diagnoses. Furthermore, you can contact physicians or pharmacies to double-check information. For example, you're studying the relationship between any past uses of hormone replacement therapy (HRT) with breast cancer. You can contact physicians or pharmacies to verify the kind of HRT that has been used and for how long for cases (those with breast cancer) and controls (those with no breast cancer). For retrospective cohort studies, you confirm the disease occurrences. You must differentiate between the ongoing cases and the new occurrences of breast cancer.

>> **Use objectives criteria.** Using objective criteria is more reliable than subjective criteria. Consider that participants often underreport self-reported diagnosis of high blood pressure. You should try to verify the diagnosis from the doctor's notes or by actually measuring the blood pressure in the field.

>> **Use a suitable study design.** Case-control studies most often suffer from information bias because you reply on getting the records from past records. Sometimes the information regarding a particular risk factor can be missing. A better study design is a nested case-control study compared to a retrospective case-control design.

A nested case-control allows for exposure data to be restored in the past from another prospective study. Typically, in a nested case-control design, the information about the exposure and some other confounders (or unwanted or nuisance variables) are collected earlier before the start of the nested case-control study. The participants of a nested case-control study come from a cohort. In the cohort, when a disease occurs, those subjects are called cases, and those who don't have the disease within a given time are called controls. Thus, the problem of getting accurate information of the exposure is almost next to impossible. Chapter 17 discusses the nested case-control design along with other epidemiologic study designs in more detail.

Interviewer bias

Interviewer bias is a type of *observational bias.* Human mistakes can't be ruled out in any study. Unless the study is *blinded* (or masked), the interviewer may often be biased if they know the study's objective while getting any information by using a data collection instrument. This type of bias introduced due to the interviewer is called interviewer bias. *Interviewer bias* refers to the systematic differences in soliciting, recording, or interpreting information that occurs in studies using in-person or telephone interviews. Interviewer bias can occur during data collection. The data collection instrument can be as simple as a survey questionnaire or a measurement tool, such as machines used for measuring height, weight, blood pressure, and so on. In a questionnaire–based study, the most common mistake is the interpretation of a question. Ways to prevent interviewer–induced bias is through proper training and monitoring.

To avoid interviewer bias, do the following:

>> Pretest the questionnaire for any ambiguity or unclear questions.

>> Provide training to the field workers and assistants who collect the data.

>> Monitor and provide surprise field visits to assess the accuracy of data recordings and take remedial measures for any identified inaccuracies.

>> Standardize data collection instruments according to the population you study or use standardized questionnaires. Refer to the next section for more details about instrument bias.

>> Use a detailed operation manual (such as a laboratory manual or training manual).

>> Train people on a code of ethics. Chapter 19 discusses ethics in greater detail.

>> Keep the interviewers blind of the research objectives and your hypothesis.

>> Conduct single-blinded or double-blinded method, wherever applicable. Refer to the section, "Blinding," later in this chapter for how to do a blind study.

Recognizing and avoiding instrument bias

Instrument bias is one of the most common sources of measurement bias in quantitative experiments. In a quantitative experiment, a faulty scale can cause an instrument bias and invalidate the entire experiment. In qualitative research, the scope for bias is wider and more subtle, and the researcher must be constantly aware of the problems. A good instrument will produce consistent and valid data.

An instrument's *reliability* is estimated using a correlation coefficient of one type or another — for example, if a blood pressure–measuring instrument consistently gives the same result, the instrument is called reliable. Meanwhile, the *validity* of the instrument's results is the extent to which a test measures what it claims to measure — for example, if a person's true systolic blood pressure is 130, and the instrument measures it at 130, the result is valid. A test method is said to be accurate when the test value approaches the absolute "true" value of the substance being measured.

Here's what you can do to steer clear of instrument bias:

>> Calibrate instruments before using them.

>> Take multiple samples to eliminate any obviously flawed or aberrant results.

>> Ensure that labs perform routine quality control tests, usually every day, and in many cases, several times a day. Quality control tests usually include normal and abnormal samples to ensure that the equipment, the technicians, and the reagents used in the test are meeting established standards.

>> Institute a frequent quality control program in all laboratory measurements. Repeat a random sample of test results to ensure the tests are valid and reliable.

>> In addition to a quality control program, laboratories must participate in proficiency testing programs, in which an external agency (for example, the CDC) sends what are called *challenge samples* to be tested, and the lab must report results back to that agency.

REMEMBER

A process of internal and external validity is the key to quality research. *Internal validity* refers to a process that you use to monitor validity of the study using your research team or the institution. With *external validity,* qualified people outside the lab or study verify and access the process and outcome of the study. External validity helps in the generalizability of the study.

REMEMBER

A measurement error has nothing to do with the instrument in some instances. Rather the error is because the person using the instrument lacks the knowledge, skills, and experience in using it. Such variations may also result in instrument bias. To avoid these types of errors, hire properly trained people or arrange regular training for the research team or your workers before and during the data collection process.

Understanding response bias

Response bias is a general term for a wide range of tendencies for participants to respond inaccurately or falsely to questions. These biases are prevalent in research when a participant self-reports, such as structured interviews or surveys. On many occasions, response bias occurs when a person selects an answer to a question that they're aware is incorrect, but they make this choice because they're uncomfortable reporting their honest answer. People answer inaccurately for a number of reasons:

>> They misunderstand or misread the question.

>> They refuse to answer the question honestly.

>> They don't want to answer any way that could embarrass their family (or influential people).

>> They're constrained for time, particularly if the interview is long.

THE PLACEBO EFFECT

The *placebo effect* is a bias that occurs due to the participants' false perception that they're benefitting from the study even though they're given a placebo (an inert substance) and not the actual test drug. Researchers have observed that the study participants who receive a placebo instead of the test drug improve over the course of the experiment. A *placebo*, often a sugar pill (or a substance that has no therapeutic effect), is used to mimic the active product of a medicine (or a procedure) being studied in a clinical trial. The unexpected but beneficial effect produced by the placebo is the placebo effect, also referred to as the *halo effect* or *Hawthorne effect*. The benefit is probably because the participants believe because they were told that they will improve. The apparent improvement of the participants in the placebo group may stem from the attention they received by participating in the study.

The term *Hawthorne effect* originates from the Western Electric Company's Hawthorne Works Plant in Chicago where in the late 1920s and early 1930s researchers tried to study the effects of altered workplace lighting on worker productivity. Workers' productivity improved not only when the lighting was increased, but also when the lighting was dimmed. In fact, the changes in workplace conditions didn't affect productivity. What did change was the workers knew they were being observed.

Consider this real-world example of the placebo effect: Patients with radiotherapy often complain of nausea. In a randomized control study of cancer patients with radiotherapy-induced nausea, one group of participants were given acupuncture and another group was provided with sham acupuncture. The participants in both groups were asked whether they thought that the treatment was effective. Surprisingly 95 percent of the acupuncture treatment group and 96 percent of the sham group reported that the treatment was very helpful, and similar proportions in each group reported that the occurrence of vomiting and the use of anti-vomiting medicines decreased.

In epidemiological terms, the improvement of participants in a placebo treatment group is most likely because participants either consciously or subconsciously change their behavior or mindset just because they're being studied.

Here are some types of response bias to watch out for:

>> **Social desirability bias** is related to a desire to conform to the sentiment of a group. One way to avoid this bias is not to conduct several studies using the same cohort of people.

>> **Extreme responding bias** is only selecting answers at either end of a positive-negative spectrum. You can avoid the problem by pre-testing your questionnaire.

>> **Neutral responding bias** is selecting all neutral answers. Although avoiding this bias is difficult, you can steer clear of making your questionnaire too lengthy, which might help.

>> **Acquiescence bias** is when the participant only chooses answers in agreement. You should use a different pattern of questions to avoid this issue.

>> **Dissent bias** is when the participant only chooses answers in disagreement. Consider using a different pattern of questions to avoid this issue.

Noticing and avoiding lead time bias

Lead time is the time between making an early diagnosis with a screening test and noticing when the clinical symptoms start to appear.

Lead time bias can overestimate the benefit of screening test programs. When evaluating the effectiveness of a screening test, lead time bias happens if the disease survival is counted from the time of the screening tests, instead of the biological onset or the actual beginning of the disease pathology. Survival may then be increased from the time of the early screening until the time of recovery. Lead time bias is only applied when estimating survival (or time-to-event) from the time of diagnosis.

TIP

To avoid lead time bias, calculate the mortality risk or rate among all screened and control subjects rather than the cumulative probability of survival (or cumulative case-fatality probability) from diagnosis among cases only. For example, to avoid lead time bias, use the survival rate of breast cancer and don't compare breast cancer survival between screened and not screened women.

Another problem arises when you estimate the lead time for individual patients. Knowing when the diagnosis would have been made is impossible if screening tests hadn't been carried out. Thus the use of an average lead time is justifiable.

Identifying and avoiding publication bias

Publications ignore negative findings in scientific studies, which shouldn't be the case. In fact, the chance of publication of a study is stronger when you have positive results. This is called *publication bias.*

Negative results generally means the study didn't find an effective therapy. Consequently, when other researchers conduct systematic reviews and meta-analysis, they hardly find any studies with negative findings because many of the previous studies with negative results weren't published. In that case, the meta-analysis results are distorted in favor of positive findings. Clinical trials with negative findings or with serious side effects often don't get published. Just imagine, what's happening to truth in science!

Sometimes, you aren't getting the true picture of the effectiveness of a therapy or drug. Consider this hypothetical scenario: In a small study researchers find that a drug works against the disease in question. However, another researcher conducts a larger study and finds that the drug doesn't work and also that the drug causes some unacceptable side effects. If that earlier study has been published and the latter hasn't been published because of having negative findings, what does that mean for science? This publication bias is dangerous if the results are only revealed and published when they're positive. However, publication bias isn't always the case because sometimes negative studies also get published.

If a study methodology is sound and valid, its results should be published, including negative ones. In fact, the International Committee of Medical Journal Editors recommends that researchers should publish negative data in order to prevent publication bias and potential waste of time and money because of duplication. Furthermore, the Committee on Publication Ethics states that journals shouldn't refuse to publish negative findings.

Steering Clear of Bias in the Initial Stages of Research

Understanding bias and steering clear of it at all levels of research is crucial. Bias can damage your research if you allow it, distorting the data and observations. Bias and confounding are potential problems that interfere with the association between the exposure and the disease. Therefore, you need to control for both bias and confounding in research.

How can you control bias? The following sections discuss the possible ways to avoid bias in the design phase and during statistical analysis.

Designing the study

The most common type of bias that can be avoided in the design phase of your study is selection bias. The best way to avoid selection bias is to use randomization. Refer to the section, "Examining and avoiding selection bias," earlier in this chapter for more specifics.

WARNING

Don't compromise with the required sample size when designing your study. It's not the question of time or resource constraints that will decide your sample size; utilize the objectives and the variables of interest to calculate the required sample size. If you need, consult with a statistician for the sample size estimation.

Here are a few other factors to focus on to avoid bias in the design phase:

>> Have measurable objectives.

>> Evaluate your hypothesis.

>> Use properly formulated, clearly articulated, and easy-to-understand study questionnaires. A questionnaire is an extremely important tool in data collection.

>> Use defined protocols for all procedures and a lab manual for any lab work.

>> Conduct an internal and external validity of the procedures used in the study, including the data collection instruments (refer to the section, "Recognizing and avoiding instrument bias," earlier in this chapter.)

To avoid information (or observer) bias at the time of data collection and data analysis, you may follow procedures during the design stage, such as:

>> Use multiple people to code and enter the data.

>> Provide training to the study volunteers or research assistants so that they're consistent and unbiased in collecting data.

>> Use a periodic monitoring and evaluation system for data collection, avoiding missing data and dropouts. A large dropout rate in your study can produce bias.

>> Share the statistical analytical duties with the team.

>> Discuss study results internally in periodic research staff meetings.

>> Include an external evaluation system (for example, an external evaluator or a community advisory committee) in your study project.

Blinding

By using a blinding method, you can avoid bias. *Blinding* comes in a few forms:

>> **Double-blinding:** Both the study participants and the researchers don't know the identity of the treatment during the entire study period.

>> **Single-blinding:** Only the participants don't know whether they're receiving the study treatment (such as an antibiotic that's being tested) or a placebo (check out the nearby sidebar about the placebo effect).

>> **Triple-blinding:** The participants, investigators, and those who are in data analyses — three parties in the study — all are kept blind of the identity of the treatment groups (study or placebo) until the data analysis has been completed.

In some clinical trials, it isn't possible to make the product blinded, such as a food product. Still, to avoid bias, researchers follow at least randomization procedure in subject selection.

Controlling for Confounders

Chapter 16 discusses how to identify a confounder that affects a causal link. Getting rid of confounders to demonstrate the real causal effect between an exposure and an outcome is important, and the process needs to start at the design phase. However, the effect of confounding can also be controlled in the data analysis phase or as a combination of the design phase and the analysis phase. I discuss both phases here.

Addressing during the design phase

The following are the processes of addressing confounders during the design phase.

Assigning treatment by randomization

Randomization ensures that the subjects are distributed to the groups in an unbiased fashion. It also results in a balanced distribution of known and unknown confounding variables if the sample size is large enough. Use randomization when assigning two or more treatment groups to study subjects. Refer to the section, "Examining and avoiding selection bias," earlier in this chapter for more information about randomization.

Utilizing restriction

Restriction means that the admissibility criteria for the study subjects are limited. For example, age is a potential confounder in many studies. In that case, you can reduce confounding effect of age by restricting a study to individuals within a narrow age range, such as 19 to 45 years. You can also restrict the study only for a certain race or gender.

However, the more you restrict, the more you lose your ability to generalize your study findings. Furthermore, from an ethical standpoint you have to justify why you include some groups and exclude others.

Matching

Matching ensures the identical distribution of confounders between cases and controls in a case-control study and between exposed and unexposed individuals in a cohort study. Suppose you find from readings that age and overweight or obesity are potential confounders in studies showing the effect of exercise on the risk of female breast cancer. By the process of matching in a cohort study, you can enroll a 35-year-old female with a normal body mass index (BMI) in the exposed group (an exerciser) and an age-matched female with a normal BMI in the unexposed group (a non-exerciser).

WARNING

Overmatching is always a problem because you lose the ability to find the effect of the variable(s) that you have matched between cases and controls. For example, if your controls are age-matched with cases, you can't show whether age is a risk factor for the disease.

Focusing on confounders during analysis

Here are the ways you can control confounders during the analysis phase.

Utilizing standardization

Chapter 10 discusses the methods of standardizing rates. *Standardization* is a method of statistical analysis to compute and compare adjusted rates of diseases that indicate how the groups would have differed if they had had the same distribution of confounders. For example, if age is considered a confounder in a study, the observed rate of a variable (such as mortality rate from the disease) in the study population is compared to the expected rate if the study population had had the same age distribution as the standard population.

Using stratification

Stratification is a process by which you can detect and control for confounders. By using stratification, you make the groups homogenous (the same) between cases and controls for a case-control study and between the exposed and the unexposed groups in a cohort study. Each group is known as *stratum*. Then measures of association between exposure and disease are analyzed separately for each stratum.

The homogenous groups or stratum should be free of confounding by statistical analysis after stratification.

When you use stratified analysis, you have the option of reporting either by stratum-specific results or by using a standardized or pooled summary result. Pooling should be considered only if stratum-specific estimates are similar to one another.

Conducting multivariate analyses

Researchers rely heavily on *multivariate analyses* to find out the potential predictors of a dependent variable. Multiple regression (such as linear regression and logistic regression) is an advanced statistic that is used to adjust for confounding variables. For example, suppose you want to find out which factors significantly predict (or increase the risk of) blood pressure out of the following variables — age, gender, race, stress, exercise, body weight, and so on. After multiple regressions analysis, you can find out the effect of major risk factors (called predictors) of blood pressure, after controlling for the confounders.

Chapter 19

Focusing On Ethics in Health Research

I n the mid-20th century and earlier, some researchers conducted studies that weren't ethical. For example, the Nazis forcefully enrolled people in research and treated them with unproven drugs. In the United States, the Public Health Service Act of 1985 ratified the establishment of Institutional Review Boards (IRBs), partly in response to many unethical procedures associated with Nazi experiments and other subsequent studies such as the Tuskegee Syphilis Study.

This chapter discusses the evolution of ethics in human research. I also examine what the different codes and reports are that ensure research is ethical, what those ethical principles are, and what elements are necessary in constructing a consent form.

Comprehending the Evolution of Ethical Norms in Research

Sparked from disturbing stories of many unethical studies conducted in German concentration camps from 1933–1945 and in many health institutions thereafter, the process of developing ethical norms began and took several years. The establishment of review boards sought to eliminate fraud and misconduct in human research.

Although standard guidelines are now available for conducting good clinical practice and following ethical procedures in human research, an international harmonized framework for managing research fraud and misconduct still makes research a highly vulnerable area for fraud.

These sections examine several examples of unethical studies based on the current ethical norms, known as the Nuremberg Code of Medical Ethics, the Helsinki Declaration, and the Belmont Report for code of ethics.

Looking into cases of scientific misconduct

According to the Office of Research Integrity (ORI), scientific misconduct means falsification, fabrication, or plagiarism in preparing, performing, or reviewing research, or in reporting research results. The following explains what that means in plain English:

» **Fabrication:** Making up data or results and recording or reporting them.

» **Falsification:** Manipulating research materials, equipment, or processes, or deliberately changing or omitting data or results such that the research isn't accurately represented in the research record.

» **Plagiarism:** The appropriation of another person's ideas, processes, results, or words without giving appropriate credit. Plagiarism is, perhaps, the most common form of research misconduct.

The prevalence of scientists who have been involved in scientific misconduct is a small number — only 1 to 2 percent. However, the implications of scientific misconduct can be grave because many people trust what the science is telling them about the facts of a disease or what they should do to be healthy. Any departure from the facts by scientific misconduct may be damaging to the image and the faith of the people in scientific reports.

REMEMBER

Preventing scientific misconduct isn't easy. To prevent it, you first need to educate people (both the researcher and the public) how important it is to conduct research. As an individual, it's your responsibility to provide true information, and at the same time, as a researcher you must be honest in every step of the research from the initiation to the publication of the results. At the institutional level, it's the responsibilities of the Institutional Review Board (IRB) members in following policies governing academic research, executing the set procedures properly, and assuring quality research. Everybody involved in research must have training on ethical norms and procedures.

Examining some unethical practices in the past

The history of human research has many examples of studies that were conducted in unethical manner. The following examines some of the most disturbing medical research studies conducted on humans.

The Nazi medical experiments

The Nazis encouraged population growth in the Aryans, who they considered to be "Good Nazis." These so-called "Good Nazis" had blonde hair and blue eyes. According to the Nazis, these Good Nazis were super men, the only race fit to survive. Blacks, Hispanics, Jews, gypsies, homosexuals, and anyone else should die. The Nazis looked at their race as superior and conducted many unethical experiments on these racial enemies, including the following:

>> **Sterilization experiments:** Their goal was to develop an efficient and inexpensive procedure for mass sterilization.

>> **Euthanasia experiments:** Theses experiments focused on finding an easy and painless death, called *euthanasia,* and many other unethical medical experiments.

>> **Experiments to test drugs and treatments:** Scientists used concentration camp inmates to test the effectiveness of vaccines for the prevention and treatment of infectious diseases including infectious hepatitis, malaria, tuberculosis, typhoid fever, and typhus fever. They conducted experiments in bone grafting and tested newly developed sulfanilamide drugs. Prisoners were exposed to poisonous gases such as phosgene and mustard gas in order to test antidotes against them.

>> **Experiments on twins:** Scientists measured living data taken from twins. Then they killed the twins by a single injection of chloroform in the heart. The organs were sent to research centers for further research.

The Nazi experiments violated numerous human rights:

>> The selection of subjects was racially biased.

>> The subjects couldn't refuse to participate.

>> Involved subjects were frequently killed or sustained permanent physical, mental, and social damages as a result of the procedures.

The Tuskegee Syphilis Study

Often referenced as a classic example of unethical research conducted on humans, the Tuskegee Syphilis Study, also referred to as the Tuskegee Study of Untreated Syphilis in the Negro Male or the Tuskegee Experiment, studied syphilis in Black men in Tuskegee, Alabama.

In 1932 the U.S. Public Health Service initiated the study with the aim to determine the natural course of untreated syphilis in adult Black men. The study group consisted of 600 Black men; of them, 399 men had syphilis, and they were untreated. The control group had 201 men who didn't have syphilis. The subjects were examined periodically, and study results were published every four to six years. By 1936, initial results suggested that men with syphilis developed more complications than the control group. Ten years later the death rate of those with syphilis was twice as high as it was for the control group.

Although penicillin was found to be an effective treatment, information about the antibiotic was withheld from the subjects. In fact, deliberate steps were taken to keep the subjects from receiving the treatment.

The study continued for 40 years with no efforts made to stop the study. In 1969, the Centers for Disease Control and Prevention (CDC) decided that the study should continue. In 1972, an account of the study in the *Washington Star* sparked public outrage, and the study stopped.

The Tuskegee Syphilis Study researchers violated several ethical standards, such as

>> They never obtained informed consent from the participants. *Informed consent* is taking consent from the individual after they're informed about the study; refer to the section, "Using Informed Consent," later in this chapter for more information.

>> They didn't tell participants that they were part of an experiment.

>> They never mentioned the contagious nature of the disease to the families of infected cases, so sexual partners and children were infected.

>> Participants were misinformed about one of the diagnostic tests, called spinal taps — the test was mentioned as "a special free treatment".

>> The selection was biased. They enrolled only disadvantaged, rural Black men.

>> They didn't offer participants available treatments, even after penicillin was discovered and became widely available. As a result, some women contracted syphilis from men who participated in the study.

>> They intended to promote fear of syphilis and gain further support for the study by publishing data, such as reduced life expectancy of the patients with syphilis.

The Willowbrook study

The study period was from the mid-1950s to the early 1970s among mentally retarded children housed at the Willowbrook State School in Staten Island, New York.

The Willowbrook study attempted to understand the natural history of infectious hepatitis and subsequently to test the effects of gamma globulin in preventing or decreasing the severity of the disease.

The selection procedures and several other methods conducted in the Willowbrook study were unethical for a number of reasons:

>> The study subjects were mentally retarded children — people with diminished autonomy.

>> Researchers deliberately infected all the previously uninfected study children with the hepatitis virus to produce antibodies. These antibodies would protect the children from future outbreaks.

>> Researchers fed stool extracts from infected individuals to the early group in the study. They injected the latter group with the protective antibodies prepared from the virus.

>> Parents were forced to give permission for their child to be in the study in order to gain their child's admission to the institution.

The researchers defended injecting the children with the virus by saying that:

>> Because the vast majority of the children would acquire hepatitis anyway while at Willowbrook, they said it would be better for the children to be infected under carefully controlled research conditions.

>> The study authorities mentioned that they provided many benefits to the subjects, such as a cleaner environment, better supervision, and a higher nurse-patient ratio.

The Jewish Chronic Disease Hospital study

In 1963, chronically ill and debilitated non-cancer patients at the Jewish Chronic Disease Hospital in New York were injected with live human cancer cells. The aim of the study was to determine the patients' rejection responses to injected cancer cells.

Here are some ethical procedures that the study violated:

>> The researchers didn't notify the patients that they were taking part in research and that the injections they received were live cancer cells.

>> The researchers never presented the study to the institutional research committee for review.

>> The researchers didn't notify the physicians who were caring for the patients that the study was being conducted.

>> The study subjects had the risk of injury, disability, or even death.

Responding to unethical studies

In response to the unethical and inhumane studies conducted in Nazi Germany and elsewhere, the world community started enacting different codes to ensure scientific research was ethical. The following sections examine some of the big steps taken to ensure research is ethical and humane.

The Nuremberg Code of Ethics

The people involved in the Nazi experiments were brought to trial before the Nuremberg trials. The mistreatment of human subjects in the studies I discuss in the section, "The Nazi medical experiments," earlier in this chapter led to the development of the famous *Nuremberg Code of Medical Ethics* in 1949. The code includes guidelines for the following:

>> Participants have to give voluntary consent.

>> Any time after being enrolled, participants can withdraw for any reason.

>> The participants aren't to be harmed by participating in the study.

>> The risks of participating should be minimum, and the benefits must overweigh the risks.

The Declaration of Helsinki

In response to reports of unethical studies, The World Medical Assembly in 1964 adopted The Declaration of Helsinki, which has since been amended several times.

The Declaration differentiates therapeutic research from nontherapeutic research:

>> **Therapeutic research:** It provides the patient an opportunity to receive an experimental treatment that might have beneficial results.

>> **Nontherapeutic research:** It's conducted to generate knowledge for a discipline, and the results might benefit future patients but probably won't directly benefit the research subjects. Greater care is needed to protect subjects from harm in nontherapeutic research.

The Declaration also states that researchers have to strongly justify exposing a healthy volunteer to substantial risk of harm just to gain new scientific information. Furthermore, the researcher must protect the research subject's life and health.

The National Commission for the Protection for Human Subjects

The National Commission for the Protection of Human Subjects of Biomedical and Behavioral Research was formed in 1978, and the organization established these three ethical principles:

>> **The principle of respect for persons:** People have the right to self-determination and the freedom to participate or not participate in research.

>> **The principle of beneficence:** Researchers are encouraged to do only good to the study subjects and do no harm to them.

>> **The principle of justice:** All human subjects should be treated fairly.

The commission required researchers to provide justification for the use of subjects with diminished autonomy. Researchers agree to treat the following people with additional protection:

>> **Children:** When children aged 7 or older are involved in research, the regulations require the written assent of the child as well as the written permission of the parent(s). *Assent* is the agreement of someone not able to give legal consent to participate in the activity.

>> **People who are legally and mentally incompetent:** Approval from the prospective subject and their legally authorized representative is required.

>> **Terminally ill subjects:** A terminal illness is a disease or health condition that can't be cured and is likely to result in the patient's death.

> » **Individuals confined to institutions:** An *institutionalized individual* means someone who is in an inpatient unit in a nursing facility or in a medical institution. In most cases, they're involuntarily confined or detained because of a civil or criminal statute.

The Belmont Report

The National Commission for the Protection of Human Subjects of Biomedical and Behavioral Research prepared The Belmont Report, which was published in April 1979. This ten-page document identifies basic ethical principles for conducting research that involve human subjects. It also sets forth guidelines to assure these principles are followed throughout the research process.

The report is made readily available to scientists, members of IRB, and federal employees. The commission recommended that The Belmont Report be adopted in its entirety as a policy. In this report, the three core principles identified as basic ethical principles are as follows. They're basically the same as the next section where I discuss these three terms:

» Respect for persons

» Beneficence

» Justice

Grasping the Importance of a Code of Ethics

Three basic principles are particularly relevant in the ethics of research involving humans. This section elaborates on them.

Respecting persons

The Belmont Report recognizes two separate moral requirements: the requirement to acknowledge autonomy of people and the requirement to protect those with diminished autonomy. In most cases of research involving human subjects, respect for people demands that subjects enter into the research voluntarily and with adequate information. On the other hand, people with diminished autonomy (such as prisoners) need extra protection.

Ensuring beneficence

People are treated in an ethical manner not only by respecting their decisions and protecting them from harm, but also by making efforts to secure their well-being. In the report, the term *beneficence* has two aspects:

>> Don't harm.

>> Maximize possible benefits and minimize possible harms.

Providing justice

Ideally, everybody should have an equal chance to be selected in your study, irrespective of gender, race, age, income, and others. You need to offer proper justification in excluding certain group(s) from your study. While selecting research subjects, don't select a certain group of people (for example, only Black males as was the case in the Tuskegee Syphilis Study) because of their easy availability.

REMEMBER

You must give proper reason if you don't select people of all genders and people from all races in your research.

Using Informed Consent

Informed consent is usually a written document that both parties — the participant and the investigator — sign. Sometimes, instead of a written informed consent, many clinical investigators use the consent document as a guide for the verbal explanation of the study.

The IRB regulation requires that the person signing the consent document receive a copy of the form. That's to ensure the person can review the information with others, before and after deciding to participate in the study. In addition, with the form handy, the participant can review the project scope, including the lab procedure, schedules for the procedures, and the contact persons if they have any questions about the study procedures. To be effective, the process of informed consent should provide ample opportunity for the participant and the investigator to exchange information and ask questions.

A verbal approval doesn't satisfy the requirement for a signed consent document. However, it's acceptable to send the informed consent document to the legally authorized representative (LAR) by an email or a regular mail and conduct the consent interview by telephone when the LAR can read the consent as it's discussed. In some exceptional cases, when the participant isn't physically capable of signing a document, the LAR can sign the consent after reading it to the participant and return it to the investigator. Depending on the data collection methods and procedures, the IRB may waive the use of an informed consent for the project.

These sections provide information about some important elements of a consent form, examples where an IRB approval may be waived or expedited, a guide for an IRB application.

Including this essential information

The proposal format for requesting IRB approval varies with the institutional requirements; however, the essential elements of a consent form are the same. They are as follows:

>> **Assurance of anonymity and confidentiality:** The participant's identity should be kept anonymous. Any data provided by the participant must be kept in a safe and locked place so that only the investigators in the study have access to them.

>> **Compensation:** Compensation is a predetermined form of payment provided to research participants for their time and inconvenience participating in a research activity. Compensation can be monetary, travel reimbursements, or electronic gift cards. Only a reasonable amount of compensation is allowed. For example, in a community-based study participants are paid $25 for the initial screening visit and $75 for a day-long session. However, this amount depends on the procedure done on the participant.

>> **Offer to answer question:** Participants should be able to ask questions about the aim of the study, the procedures, and any other research-related questions. The phone number of the principal investigator should be included in the information sheet given to the participants.

>> **Noncoercive disclaimer:** *Noncoercive* means not using threats or force to achieve compliance. Participation is voluntary; refusal to participate doesn't involve any penalty or loss of benefits to which the subject is otherwise entitled.

>> **Option to withdraw:** Participants can withdraw from the study any time after enrollment.

>> **Consent to incomplete disclosure:** Participants may have the option not to answer some questions.

For further information, check out this site for an IRB application and guidelines: www.jsums.edu/research/forms-and-applications/.

Using an expedited review

Based on the nature of a study, the process of IRB can be done quickly without having a full-committee meeting. This kind of review is usually expedited for a student project, a brief survey, a brief questionnaire-based descriptive study in a limited pilot study, or studies of similar nature. This type of review is called an *expedited review*. An expedited review is offered when the research involves "no more than minimum risk".

The IRB may also use the expedited review procedure to review minor changes in previously approved research during the period covered by the original approval. Under an expedited review procedure, the IRB chairperson or one or more experienced members of the IRB that the chairperson designates can review the research.

Waiving the informed consent

Any human research project must be submitted to the IRB for approval. Based on the procedures mentioned in the project proposal, the IRB may waive the requirements of the full committee meeting, and the IRB chair or their representative can decide on the project approval. This method of the review process is called an expedited review, which I discuss in the preceding section.

In some circumstances the IRB may consider waiving the requirement for some or all of the elements of informed consent:

>> The research involves no more than minimal risk to the subjects.

>> The waiver or alteration won't adversely affect the rights and welfare of the subjects.

>> The research couldn't practically be carried out without the waiver or alteration.

>> Whenever appropriate, the subjects will be provided with additional pertinent information after participation.

An example of a type of study that may qualify for a full waiver of consent is a review of publicly available data or secondary data using online sources. When a professor involves their students in class to conduct a survey as part of their class work, the professor needs to submit it to the IRB for clearance. In the event that the survey is conducted by using a questionnaire, the professor must include the questionnaire along with a short description of the procedures involved in the research. The IRB committee may do an expedited review without going for the full committee review based on the research.

UNDERSTANDING THE INS AND OUTS OF YOUR INSTITUTIONAL REVIEW BOARD

An Institutional Review Board (IRB) is an administrative unit within an institution that's responsible for protecting the rights and welfare of human subjects recruited to participate in research activities. An IRB consists of a minimum of five members of varying backgrounds, and IRB members should have the professional background and experience to provide appropriate ethical and scientific review of the research protocols.

At least one member of the IRB should be outside the institution and one member should be a non-scientific person. However, the IRB regulations prohibit any member from participating in the IRB's initial or continuing review panel of any project in which the member has a conflicting interest. In special cases, the IRB can co-opt any person who has the experience about the rights and privileges of the special group of participants in the study. For example, my university IRB received a research project on prisoners' health. Nobody in the IRB Committee at that time had adequate knowledge dealing with prisoners' rights. To review that research project, the IRB had to hire one prisoner as a temporary board member.

In many occasions, the IRB members deal with some diseases that need the expertise of a medical doctor or a clinical investigator. Depending on situations the IRB members may need to consult with some professionals. The board has several consultants who advise the IRB and are involved in protocol review.

Ideally, all research projects must be submitted to the IRB, even if it's a student project. The Board will decide which project needs to be sent to the full committee, which project deserves an expedited review, and which one is exempt from IRB review. The principal investigator (PI) of a project should submit an IRB application following the institutional guidelines. The project application submitted to the IRB should have the following sections:

- The title of the project

- Contact information

- Aim of the project

- Methods and procedures

- If there are any invasive procedures, such as bloodwork, you must clearly mention how much blood will be drawn, how often blood will be taken, who will draw the blood, where it will be processed and analyzed, and all methods for the prevention of risks.

- If you use a data collection instrument, such as a questionnaire, a copy of the questionnaire must be included. Mention whether you'll ask any sensitive questions, how much time participants will need to answer the questions, and how the questionnaire will be administered (self-administered or by an interviewer).

In addition to the preceding descriptions, other important ethical issues to be addressed are as follows:

- **Principle of confidentiality:** Specify how you'll maintain the confidentiality of the participants' information.

- **Principle of autonomy:** Describe the right of the participants about their participation — whether it's completely voluntary or not. Mention that the participant can withdraw from the study any time after being enrolled.

- **Principle of beneficence:** Mention the direct and indirect benefits that the results will provide for the participants.

- **Principle of nonmaleficence:** Specify any risk involved for participating; if there's any risk, describe how'd you minimize the risk and maximize the benefits.

- **Alternative treatments:** Disclose if any alternative treatment options are available so that participants will be able to make an informed decision whether they participate in your study or not.

- **Provision for informed consent and assent for young children (ages 7 or older):** Informed consent can be verbal or written based on the institutional requirement. For young children ages 7 or older, they should be given an assent.

- **CITI training certification:** The Collaborative IRB Training Initiative (CITI) is an educational program for the protection of human subjects in research. CITI was developed by experts in the IRB community and is focused on different aspects of bioethics and human subject research. Most institutions require a CITI certification of all investigators involved in the study, including research assistants or graduate assistants.

5

The Part of Tens

Chapter **20**

Ten Careers with a Degree in Epidemiology

Think about the world where infections are common visitors and new diseases are rampant. Epidemiology is a special field of public health that trains you in several areas, such as finding causes and assessing risk factors of diseases, investigating epidemics, monitoring trends of diseases, designing studies, analyzing data, and describing health status of a population.

With a degree in epidemiology, you'll gain skills in using statistical software and dealing with real-life data. With this knowledge and training, you have the option of taking an entry-level position in data collection and data management, conducting research, or working in the public or private sector. You may also build up your future career in a number of areas as an epidemiologist. This chapter highlights ten career opportunities for you.

Epidemiologist

A number of epidemiologist positions are available in different disciplines and health facilities. The requirements of an epidemiologist in any given facility can be quite specific and different from one another. For example, epidemiologists' positions in different disciplines include environmental, social, injury, cancer, hospital, clinical trial research, and so on.

To give you an idea of what to expect, here's a job summary of an epidemiologist's position in a hospital setting:

» Detects and analyzes the distribution of infectious diseases and/or chronic diseases, both potential and real, affecting all age groups within the hospital environment, and implements the appropriate control measures

» With minimal guidance, manages all aspects of population health data analysis and finds conclusions of the data

» Conducts epidemiologic investigations used in the prevention and/or control of infectious and chronic diseases

» Independently conducts complex statistical analysis and reporting within established time frames

» Fulfills a critical role in evaluating public health data for community health improvement initiatives and outcome measurement

» Helps in study design, sampling, questionnaire design, and sample size estimation of health research

As an epidemiologist at the health department, you have tons of job opportunities. Here is a job summary in a health department:

» Carries out a range of epidemiologic and surveillance activities

» Identifies and analyzes public health issues and their impact on public policies, scientific studies, or surveys

» Creates an action plan for a potential health crisis

» Analyzes study or implements project activities

» Identifies and evaluates a wide range of health conditions

» Performs statistical analyses as part of a segment of a nationwide data collection and analysis program

» Utilizes statistical techniques commonly used in epidemiologic evaluations to interpret and analyze health phenomenon

» Provides scientific advice and technical assistance for various public, private, and/or nonprofit and/or health-related agencies and organizations

» Develops and coordinates the sharing of health-related educational or informational materials

» Prepares reports and responses to inquiries.

Environmental Epidemiologist

An environmental epidemiologist focus on environmental factors that cause a disease. Here are the responsibilities for an environmental epidemiologist listed by the Bureau of Environmental Surveillance and Policy (BESP), Division of Environmental Health, within The New York City Department of Health and Mental Hygiene (DOHMH):

>> Analyzes and interprets data from health outcomes related to extreme weather events such as heat waves and other environmental hazards; relevant data types include emergency department syndromic surveillance data, hospital discharge data, poison control center data, weather, and air quality data

>> Maintains, improves, and trains others in implementing surveillance data analysis and quality control protocols

>> Maintains data use and institutional review board agreements for relevant data

>> Participates in environmental surveillance emergency preparedness and response activities

>> Develops and contributes to the development of presentations, scientific and public reports, web content, and other products to disseminate surveillance and epidemiologic study findings within and outside the agency

Surveillance Data Analyst and Epidemiologist

A surveillance data and epidemiologist helps the state health officer and other health personnel in the ongoing surveillance programs and with data management.

A surveillance data analyst and epidemiologist is required to carry out the following duties:

>> Collects, analyzes, and interprets public health data

>> Conducts disease surveillance

>> Applies analytical tools to public health surveillance and data reporting activities

>> Applies epidemiological principles of infectious disease

>> Communicates with different disciplines

>> Writes reports

Infection Control Officer

An epidemiologist gathers knowledge on infectious diseases and control of infections. They can be valuable as an infection control officer at a hospital. Here are the essential responsibilities of an infection control officer:

>> Assists with the day-to-day activities of the infection control/hospital epidemiology division

>> Utilizes epidemiologic tools to identify patients and personnel at risk of infection and variation in the levels of nosocomial infections

>> Identifies clusters or outbreaks of infections, or single cases of unusual infections

>> Assists in designing collection, analyzing, and presentation of data

>> Assists in the maintenance of ongoing formal and informal educational programs for all hospital employees

>> Acts as a departmental resource in the development, implementation, and interpretation of infection control policies and guidelines

Research Scientist

An epidemiologist develops special skills and knowledge in conducting scientific research. During your coursework, you'll learn basic tools on how to develop a research project using different epidemiologic techniques, identify a population for a study, conduct a survey, collect data, and analyze data in a meaningful way. There are no limits and boundaries to the research areas. You may choose areas from infectious diseases to noncommunicable and chronic diseases, to cancer studies, to tobacco prevention, or health disparities.

REMEMBER

If your passion is to make a change in the health of the population, you can do it as a public health researcher. Epidemiology is a good field that trains you to become a health researcher.

Research Associate

Imagine you're just beginning your career as an epidemiologist. You may consider the position of a research associate. Many world-class scientists invite people to help them in their research (I was once a research assistant!). This type of position is a great opportunity to learn research from them. You'll get the opportunity to conduct small-scale surveys as part of your course work. Sometimes, you can work as a research assistant with a professor on their funded project. You'll also discover how to develop and administer a research questionnaire.

Data Analyst

An epidemiologist is knowledgeable in terms of conducting research and analyzing epidemiologic data. It adds to your skills if you take special interest in learning more about some data analyzing software programs, such as SPSS, SAS, Epi Info, Stata, and others. Take advantage of opportunities at summer programs that offer courses on SAS or SPSS to prepare for the job market! A great deal of epidemiologic research, especially research related to the environment, now requires geographic information systems (GIS) for knowledge about spatial analysis.

GIS tools are computer-based tools used to store, visualize, analyze, and interpret geographic data. Geographic data (also called *spatial*, or *geospatial data*) identifies the geographic location of variables. One of the tools used in GIS is called a *dot map*, in which each dot in a geographic map represents a case, a death, or an exposure data.

Program Manager

At a certain level of experience you may assume a position of a program manager with a degree in epidemiology. A project manager directs and manages technical support for conducting risk assessments on environmental stressors and developing state-of-the-art methods for human health risk assessments.

Some essential responsibilities include

>> Manages and tracks several concurrent active projects

>> Prepares plans for new projects

>> Manages subcontractors and performs overall program oversight to ensure projects are completed on-schedule, within budget, and of high quality

Chief Medical/Quality Officer

With the increasing demand of public health (and especially so for epidemiology), many healthcare professionals (MDs, Dos and nurses), want to get a second degree in public health. Most of them try to become a Chief Executive Officer (CEO) or a program manager of a hospital. For them, some schools offer a special master's of public health program, called Executive MPH. You may also get a regular MPH degree with a concentration in epidemiology or some other fields.

Data and Research Coordinator

The primary job of a data and research coordinator is to help in hospital-based or community-based research and grant writing.

Here are some essential responsibilities:

>> Develops data management protocols and oversight of data management systems

>> Undertakes research projects, analyze data, and summarize findings

>> Performs in SAS, SPSS, and/or basic statistical analysis

>> Assists in preparation of research reports, abstracts, and presentations

>> Assists clinical director in grant writing and submission

>> Conducts manuscript preparation and submission with research collaborators

>> Assists staff in operations of data collection, management, and database training

Chapter **21**

Ten Tips for Acing Your Epidemiology Classes

S tudents learn three aspects of epidemiology:

» **Concepts:** As an epidemiologist, you must know the basic concepts of distribution and determinants of diseases and events in humans.

» **Skills:** You discover how to develop skills on how to conduct an epidemiologic research, how to control epidemics, how to conduct a surveillance, how to know if an association of factor is causal for a disease or not, and how to analyze data and make valid conclusions from the data.

» **Applications:** You must try to apply the classroom knowledge in real-life situations.

Exams test your knowledge of these three aspects. This chapter shows you some tips for doing well in epidemiology.

Ask and Answer Questions in Class

Some professors invite questions, so ask away. When your professors ask questions you're not sure, participate and answer. Even when your answers aren't correct or are only partially correct, most of the time your professor will appreciate your thought and attempt.

REMEMBER

Don't feel shy or silly asking questions. Someone else in your class may have the same question, and by asking it, you can start a class discussion that helps not only you, but also your fellow classmates. The only dumb question is the one not asked.

Practice, Practice, and Practice

My best advice for you to ace your epidemiology course is to practice, practice, and practice some more. Nothing can replace actually doing the work and seeing what you miss. Only that way can you figure out what you need to focus on.

REMEMBER

Even if you're confident because your professor has walked you through a problem and showed you how to solve it, that doesn't mean you're ready for the exam. When you're doing the problem yourself, you may discover that you've missed a step or don't understand a part of the problem that you thought was quite easy to do. That's why practice can help you reinforce your knowledge of the material.

Take Good Class Notes

You don't learn just by reading a book. You also can learn from class lectures and discussions. You can't miss a class because in most situations, your professor explains ideas in a different way than the textbook does. In fact, a good professor tries to clarify and simplify the readings. Furthermore, a professor sometimes gives practical examples of some theoretical concepts that they experienced in their life. Students may have questions that spark classroom discussion.

TIP

To do well in your epidemiology studies, take detailed notes of not only your readings but also classroom lectures and discussions. When taking notes, use highlighted markers or develop your own system to identify important concepts. You never know what's going to be included on the exam.

Get Information Online

In this era of the Internet, you can find plenty of information and, more importantly, updated information by searching online. Medicine is constantly changing as researchers conduct more studies. What's true today may be different tomorrow. The good news is you can stay current by referring to these sources for epidemiologic information:

>> **Centers for Disease Control and Prevention:** www.cdc.gov

>> **World Health Organization:** www.who.int

>> **Mortality Morbidity Weekly Report:** www.cdc.gov/mmwr

>> **American Journal of Public Health:** http://ajph.aphapublications.org/

Apply the Knowledge

Look for opportunities to apply your classroom knowledge into practice. You'll better understand concepts and skills more when you apply the knowledge gathered through your class into your day-to-day life.

When I teach epidemiology, I ask my students to do a literature search related to some of the topics discussed in class. For example, when I cover different types of epidemiologic research, I offer one assignment to find an article on one of the following: a cohort study, a cross-sectional study, or a case-control study. I ask them to summarize the study and talk about the study design and the statistics used for the data (odds ratio, relative risk, prevalence, and so on; refer to Chapter 17 where I discuss some of these statistics).

Sometimes you read or hear about a disease outbreak in your locality. If so, discuss the event, how it happened, how many people are affected, and any information about the characteristics of the people (school children, grades, adults, occupation, and so on). Here's an example: www.cdc.gov/listeria/outbreaks/monocytogenes-06-22/index.html.

When you read about an unusual number of cases of suicides or suicidal attempts in a high school, the news may trigger your intent to discover more about the cause of the epidemic. You may discuss it further with your professor and your fellow students, which is a good way to learn about applications of your classroom knowledge.

Make a Cheat Sheet

I advise my students to write down all the formulas they've learned in class by creating a cheat sheet and keeping it handy. At the end, they're prepared and ready for the final exam. They can use the cheat sheet and practice problem solving.

Use a Scientific Calculator

A scientific calculator is invaluable in solving problems in epidemiology. Many features in a scientific calculator can make your life easy when making calculations in your epidemiology courses.

REAL LIFE EXAMPLE

Imagine how difficult calculating the following would be without the help of a scientific calculator:

>> $\sqrt{29} = 5.3852$

>> $\text{Log}\,62 = 1.7924$

>> $7! \div 3! = 840$

Furthermore, if you want to calculate some descriptive statistics such as mean and standard deviation of a set of data, a scientific calculator helps you avoid the steps of using the formula. Most scientific calculators come with a function of entering data. All you have to do is enter all the data one at a time by pressing that data entering key. It's just that easy!

Although most smartphones have functions of a calculator, they have limitations for advanced calculations. Furthermore, most professors don't allow you to have a phone during a test.

Memorize Some Definitions and Steps

Sometimes the best way to learn important definitions and terms is to memorize them in case you encounter them on an exam. For example, you may be tested to ensure you understand the words "epidemiology," "epidemiologic transition," "demographic transition," "notifiable disease," "incubation period," "epidemic," "pandemic," "pathogenicity," "virulence," and so on.

As for problems, a good starting point to learn problem solving is to follow steps. For example, if you want to investigate a disease outbreak, follow the step-by-step guide from Chapter 14. You can't conduct a field investigation without getting your team ready, training them, setting the existence of an outbreak, establishing the case definition, and so on.

Get Involved in Research

Take what you've studied and learned in class and apply it to a real-life situation. To do so, get involved in a health research project with a professor. You're fortunate if you're asked to conduct a survey or a cross-sectional study in a population as part of your classwork. You may also volunteer to take part in a research conducted by one of your professors.

Participate in Group Work

Learning sometimes is teamwork, so get engaged in group study. If you're preparing for the final exam, gather a few people together, make a study group, have coffee, and discuss. If you have difficulties in understanding any specific topic, know who you can call for help. Use your fellow students as resources to better understand concepts, skill, and applications. If you're working on a class project that allows you to complete the project in teams, group work may be a better option.

Glossary

accuracy: The lack of random and systematic error.

acquired immunity: A type of immunity that develops when a person's immune system responds to a foreign substance or microorganism or that occurs after a person receives antibodies from another source.

active immunity: When exposure to a disease organism triggers the immune system to produce antibodies to that disease. Active immunity can be acquired through natural immunity or vaccine-induced immunity.

acute disease: A disease that begins and worsens quickly and lasts for a short period of time. The disease requires urgent or short-term care.

agent: A factor that causes a disease, such as bacteria, virus, parasite, fungus, ticks, mites, and so forth.

airborne infection: Infections or infective agents that are carried or transmitted by air, such as a droplet infection.

alternative medicine: A range of medical therapies that aren't regarded as conventional by the medical profession, such as Ayurveda medicine, acupuncture, herbal medicine, homeopathy, and spiritual therapy.

analogy: A comparison of two things, typically used for the purpose of explaining "if one thing can happen, it's likely to have another condition of similar nature." For example, if there is one birth defect, it's possible to have another birth defect. Analogy is one of Hill's criteria of causal association.

analytic studies: These types of studies test a hypothesis about exposure-and-outcome relationship. They measure the association between exposure and outcome.

antigen: A foreign substance or a toxin that induces an immune response in the body, especially the production of antibodies.

area map: Also called *distribution maps*; they display one or multiple entities on a map, used in a geospatial information system (GIS).

attack rate: The number of new cases of a disease per the number of the healthy population at risk of the disease.

attributable risk among the total population: The proportion of the incidence of a disease in the total population (exposed and unexposed) that's due to exposure.

attributable risk in exposed population: The proportion of the incidence of a disease in the exposed population that is due to exposure.

bias: A systematic error in the study design or conduct of a study that causes an erroneous association between the exposure and disease.

biological gradient: Also called *strength of association.* It's one of Hill's criteria of causation, which states that if the strength of association increases, the situation is more likely to be causal.

case-control study: A type of retrospective epidemiologic study in which the exposure history is recorded for both cases and controls.

case-fatality rate: A ratio of deaths among the number of cases of a disease. It's used most commonly to describe an epidemic.

cause-specific mortality rate: A mortality rate calculated for a disease or event (such as cancer mortality rate or suicide rate) among 100,000 population.

census: A complete enumeration of the entire population. The U.S. Census, mandated by Article I, Section 2 of the Constitution. counts every resident in the United States every ten years.

chance: *See* **probability.**

cluster: An accumulation of cases of a disease or condition, such as cancer or birth defect, that are closely grouped in time and place.

coherence: One of Hill's criteria of causation. It states that the cause-and-effect relationship is consistent with generally known facts of the natural history or biology of the disease.

cohort: A segment of the population that has similar characteristics.

community intervention: In epidemiology, drug trials or interventions are conducted in a community setting called a *community intervention.*

component cause: In Rothman's pie of multiple causality, each factor of a causal pie is called a *component cause.*

confounding variable: A third variable that influences both the disease and the exposure.

consistency: When similar findings are observed in repeated studies.

crossover trial: A type of experimental study (such as clinical trial) where two or more study treatments are administered one after another to each group of individuals participating in the trial.

cross-sectional study: Also called *prevalence study,* it's one of the most commonly used epidemiologic studies. In a cross-sectional study, both the exposure(s) and disease are measured simultaneously.

crude birth rate: The number of births occurring in a specified population (usually per mid-year population or the total population) in a year; expressed as births per 100,000 population.

crude death rate: The number of deaths occurring in a specified population (usually per mid-year population or the total population) in a year; expressed as deaths per 100,000 population.

cumulative incidence: The proportion of a population at risk that develops the disease over a specified time period.

demographic transition: The change from high birth rates and high death rates to low birth rates and low death rates of a population over time.

demography: The study of population characteristics such as birth, death, migration, income, and so forth.

descriptive epidemiology: A branch of epidemiology that describes the characteristics of the people in terms of time, place, and person.

dose-response: One of Hill's criteria of causation that describes that the disease increases (or decreases) with the increase (or decrease) of the exposure dose. For example, lung cancer increases with an increasing dose of smoking.

double-blind study: A study where neither the investigator nor the participants know the treatment type.

droplet infection: Some infective particles, such as aerosols, bacteria-carrying skin cells, dust, or small microbe-carrying particles are often discharged in the air by sneezing and coughing. They're suspended in the air in the form of minute particles and can infect others. These minute particles are called *droplets,* and the infection is known as a *droplet infection.*

ecological fallacy: An issue in the interpretation of data from an ecological study, where data of exposure and the disease that arise from an entire population are inaccurately considered to deduct conclusions about an individual.

ecological study: A study that evaluates the relationship between outcome and exposure at the population level (such as a country population) instead of at the individual level data.

emerging infectious diseases: Infectious diseases that have newly appeared in a population.

endemic: A disease that's present most of the time but at a low number in a given place or a geographic area.

epidemic: An unexpected increase in the number of cases of a disease in a specific geographical area at a given time.

epidemiologic transition: Changes from acute and infectious diseases to chronic and noncommunicable diseases.

epidemiology: The study of the distribution and determinants of human diseases or events.

external validity: The extent to which you can generalize the findings of a study to other situations, people, settings, and measures.

fertility rate: Also called *total fertility rate*, the average number of children that a woman will give birth to over her lifetime.

fetal death rate: The number of fetal deaths divided by the number of live births and fetal deaths, expressed as 1,000 population.

genetic epidemiology: A field of epidemiology that focuses on how genetic factors influence human health and disease.

genotype: The genotype of an organism is its complete set of genetic material. A person's genotype refers to the two alleles (alternative forms of a gene) a person has inherited for a particular gene.

healthy worker effect: An observation that working class people tend to have lower disease mortality than the general population. This is a special type of selection bias, typically seen in observational studies with improper choice of comparison group.

herd immunity: Resistance (or immunity) acquired by the entire population in which a large proportion of the people is immune to a disease because of receiving a vaccination or being exposed to the disease.

host: A person (or animal) who can get the disease.

hypothesis: Usually a statement (or supposition) about a disease that's evaluated by conducting a study.

inapparent infection: A type of infection that doesn't show any clinical or obvious symptoms.

incidence: An occurrence of a new disease.

incubation period: A period from the point of infection to when clinical symptoms appear.

induction period: A period from the point of introduction of a risk factor to the time of initiation of a chronic disease. This term is applied to the case of chronic diseases such as cancer, heart disease, diabetes, and so forth.

infant mortality rate: The number of infant deaths divided by the total of births, expressed per 1,000.

infection: The introduction of a disease-causing agent to the human body; it may or may not cause a disease.

infectivity: The capacity of an infective agent to enter and multiply in a susceptible host.

information bias: Includes recall bias and interviewer bias. Information bias occurs due to measurement error in the assessment of exposure and the disease in study participants.

lead time bias: An erroneous perception that a screening-detected individual has a longer survival than an unscreened individual of the same disease simply because the screened case was identified earlier.

life expectancy rate: The number of years a person is expected to live.

maternal mortality rate: The number of maternal deaths during pregnancy or within one year of the end of pregnancy out of total live births.

molecular epidemiology: The field of epidemiology that studies biomarkers (such as DNA fingerprints) to establish exposure-disease associations.

multiple causality: Also called *multifactorial etiology;* for chronic diseases, the causal factors (or risk factors) are multiple. For example, heart disease and cancer.

necessary cause: In Rothman's causal pie, this one factor is always present.

neonatal mortality: The number of infant deaths younger than 28 days of age divided by the total live births.

nested case-control study: A special type of case-control study, in which both cases and controls come from a cohort of the population. This study is powerful in controlling bias.

odds ratio: A measurement of case-control studies; the odds of getting a disease among the exposed population compared to the unexposed population.

pandemic: When a disease spreads out in an unexpectedly large number and affects several countries simultaneously. Examples of pandemics are HIV/AIDS and Covid-19.

pathogenicity: The capacity of an agent to cause a disease.

perinatal mortality rate: The number of fetal deaths older than 28 weeks of gestation plus infant deaths within 7 days of birth divided by the total live births plus the number of fetal deaths.

period prevalence: The number of existing cases (old plus new) in a given time period.

point prevalence: The number of existing cases (old plus new) in a given point of time.

prevalence: The total number of existing cases (both old and new) out of the population at risk.

primary prevention: Preventive measures taken before a disease occurs.

probability: Also refers to *chance,* a number that lies between 0 and 1.

proportion: An equation in which the numerator is included in the denominator.

quasi-experimental study: In this type of experimental design, the initial assignment of subjects or groups isn't randomized, but the treatments are randomized.

randomization: An unbiased process of selection of subjects in which every member has an equal chance of being selected. The process is operated by using random numbers.

ratio: A fraction in which the numerator isn't included in the denominator.

relative risk: Also called *risk ratio*, the risk of having a disease among the exposed population compared to that in an unexposed population; a measurement used in cohort studies.

reliability: The ability of a measuring instrument to produce consistent results on repeated trials.

screening: A test to identify diseases in an apparently healthy person.

seasonality: The changes of disease events in different times of a year; for example, the flu appears in the winter season.

secondary attack rate: Applied for infectious diseases; the calculation using the number of persons infected from the contact of the primary (or index) case.

secular trend: The gradual change of diseases over a long period of time.

selection bias: The type of systematic error that occurs because of the faulty choosing of samples.

sensitivity: A measurement of the quality of a screening test; the proportion of cases detected as diseased among those who are actually disease positive.

spatial clustering: The concentration of cases of a disease in a particular geographic area.

specificity: A measurement of the quality of a screening test; the proportion of people detected as disease-free out of the total people who are actually disease-negative.

standardized mortality ratio (SMR): A ratio of the number of deaths observed in a population over a given time to the number of deaths that would be expected if the study population had the same age-specific rates as the standard population. Two methods of SMR calculations are direct method and indirect method.

surveillance: A systematic and continuous method of collection, analysis, and reporting of cases (or deaths) of a disease.

temporality: One of Hill's criteria of causation; the disease follows the exposure.

trend analysis: A technique that attempts to predict future disease incidence and deaths based on recently observed trend data.

validity: The identification of the truth in a population.

virulence: The capacity of an agent to cause serious complications including deaths.

washout period: In clinical trials (especially in a cross-over trial), the length of time that someone enrolled in one type of treatment must not receive another treatment. A gap of few days after which a second treatment is started.

Index

Numerics

2x2 contingency tables, 63–64
10-day measles, 204, 215

A

accuracy, 26, 251, 357. *See also* validity
ACIP (Advisory Committee on Immunization Practices), 219
acquired immunity, 202, 357
active immunity, 202–203, 357
active surveillance, 227–228
activity monitoring, 226–227
acute clinical cases, 80
acute disease, 29, 357. *See also* epidemiologic triangle
Adam House Suicide, 246
adult T-cell leukemia/lymphoma (ATL), 37
Advisory Committee on Immunization Practices (ACIP), 219
Aedes Aegypti mosquito, 89, 115, 116, 222
age factor
  Alzheimer's disease, 179
  as confounder, 269–270
  diseases and age groups at risk, 119
  health consequences of aging, 10
  rotavirus diarrhea, 179
agents
  bacteria, 107
  chain of infection, 79
  defined, 8–9, 357
  fungus, 107

parasite, 107
virus, 107
air quality, 110
airborne infections, 91–92, 357
Airs, Waters, and Places (Hippocrates), 19, 41–42
alimentary tract, 83
alternative medicine, 32–33, 341, 357
Alzheimer's disease, 10, 179
American Cancer Society, 253, 264, 270
American Demographics magazine, 154
American Journal of Public Health, 49
American Public Health Association (APHA), 52
American Sociological Association, 154
anal cancer, 210, 211
analogies, 284, 357
analytical epidemiologic studies
  case study, 118
  defined, 9, 18, 117, 357
  why and how questions, 9, 288
anemia, 23
animal reservoirs, 80
anonymity and confidentiality, 338
anthrax, 46, 80, 99
antibiotics, 139
antibodies, 202
antigenic drift, 132
antigenic shift, 132
antigens, 196, 248, 254, 357
APHA (American Public Health Association), 52

Are Our Winters Getting Warmer? (Webster), 44
area maps, 126–127, 357
arsenic case study, 279
arsenic poisoning (arsenicosis), 90, 101
artificial active immunity, 203
artificial passive immunity, 203
artificially acquired immunity, 11
asbestosis, 123
asthma, 121
ATL (adult T-cell leukemia/lymphoma), 37
at-risk population, identifying, 151–154
attack rates, 238–240, 244–246, 357
attributable risk among the total population, 358
attributable risk in exposed population, 357
attrition rate, 308
autonomy, 341
avian influenza A (H5N1), 132

B

B cells, 201
Bacillus Calmette-Guerin (BCG), 213
bacteria
  cancer-causing, 213
  diseases caused by, 107
bacterial vaginosis, 96
bagassosis, 123
Baker, Josephine, 50
BCG (Bacillus Calmette-Guerin), 213
Belmont Report, 336

N

nasopharyngeal cancer, 36, 212

National Center for Complementary and Alternative Medicine (NCCAM), 33

National Center for Health Statistics (NCHS), 37–38

National Commission for the Protection for Human Subjects, 335–336

National Institute of Health (NIH), 33

National Institute on Mental Health, 33

National Notifiable Disease Surveillance System (NNDSS), 11

National Vital Statistics System (NVSS), 39

Nation's Health, 49

natural active immunity, 11, 203

natural history of disease, 83–85

natural immunity, 202

natural passive immunity, 203

Nazi medical experiments, 331

NCCAM (National Center for Complementary and Alternative Medicine), 33

NCDs (noncommunicable diseases), 9, 34–35, 49. *See also* epidemiologic transition

NCHS (National Center for Health Statistics), 37–38

necessary causes, Rothman's causal pie, 285, 361

negative predictive value (NPV), 259

neonatal mortality rate (NNMR), 171–172, 361

nested case-control study, 302–304, 361

newborn screening, 255–256

niacin (vitamin B-3), 65

Nightingale, Florence, 43, 47

NIH (National Institute of Health), 33

Nipah virus, 99

nitazoxanide, 214

NNDSS (National Notifiable Disease Surveillance System), 11

NNMR (neonatal mortality rate), 171–172, 361

noncoercive disclaimer, 338

noncommunicable diseases (NCDs), 9, 34–35, 49. *See also* epidemiologic transition

Non-Hodgkin's lymphoma, 211

nonmaleficence, 341

nonsteroidal anti-inflammatory drugs (NSAIDs), 116

norovirus, 88

notifiable diseases, 87–88

NPV (negative predictive value), 259

NSAIDs (nonsteroidal anti-inflammatory drugs), 116

nuisance variables. *See* confounders

numerators, formula, 179

Nuremberg Code of Ethics, 334

nutrition, diet and nutrition

NVSS (National Vital Statistics System), 39

O

OAM (Office of Alternative Medicine), 33

Oastler, Richard, 56

obesity, 146

observational bias, 319

observational studies, 289–290

odds ratio (OR), 276, 361

Office of Alternative Medicine (OAM), 33

On Epidemics (Hippocrates), 42

On the Mode of Communication of Cholera (Snow), 62

onchocerciasis (river blindness), 94

one-to-one interviews, 224–225

online surveys, 224

open-ended questions, questionnaire, 311–312

option to withdraw, 338

OR (odds ratio), 276, 361

osteoporosis, 121

OTC (over-the-counter) medication, 30–31

outbreak investigation, 12, 29–30. *See also* epidemic investigation

    cholera case study, 242

    makeshift hospitals, 242–243

    mass suicides, 246

    pharyngitis case study, 244–246

    surveillance, 235–241

outbreaks, 12, 133. *See also* epidemics

outcome monitoring, 227

overmatching, 296, 327

over-the-counter (OTC) medication, 30–31

P

Pacini, Filippo, 65

pandemics, 131–132, 361. *See also* Covid-19; HIV/AIDS

Pap smear, 253–254

Papanikolaou, Georgios, 253

paper surveys, 224

parasites, 93–95, 107, 214

Parasitism and Disease (Smith), 105

Park, William H., 50

passive immunity, 202–203

passive surveillance, 228

Pasteur, Louis, 45–46, 65

pasteurization, 46, 52

pathogenicity, 19, 84, 361

pathophysiology, 282

pellagra, 65–68

pelvic inflammatory disease (PID), 96

People's Temple Suicide, 246

perinatal mortality rate (PMR), 173–174, 361

period prevalence, 182, 361

permethrin, 221

person factors, descriptive epidemiology, 118–125

personal habits, 123

personal protective measures, 113

personnel, epidemic investigation, 235

person-years at risk, 166

pertussis, 190, 216

Pettenkofer, Max Joseph von, 272

Pfeiffer, Richard Friedrich Johannes, 65

pharyngitis case study, 244–246

phenylketonuria (PKU), 256

physical (one-to-one) interviews, 224–225

physicians, 27–30

PID (pelvic inflammatory disease), 96

pinworm, 94

PKU (phenylketonuria), 256

place factors, descriptive epidemiology, 125–128

placebo effect, 322

plague, 10, 92, 99

Plasmodium falciparum parasite, 112, 214, 220, 283

PMR (perinatal mortality rate), 173–174, 361

pneumococcal disease, 190

pneumonia, 10, 119

PNNMR (post-neonatal mortality rate), 172–173

point prevalence, 182, 361

point source epidemic. *See* common source epidemic

polio, 10
  herd immunity, 204
  inapparent infections, 81
  target to eradicate, 22
  transmission of, 216
  vaccine, 190, 217

Poor Law Commission, 55, 56

population density, 152–154

population projections, 158–162

population pyramid, 155–157

Population Reference Bureau, 155

population surveys, 154

portals of exit, 82–83

positive predictive value (PPV), 259

post-neonatal mortality rate (PNNMR), 172–173

Pott, Percivall, 275

practical hygiene, 272

praziquantel, 214

predictive values, 259–261

pre-exposure prophylaxis (PrEP), 97–98

pregnant women
  reducing risk of malaria, 113–114
  vaccines, 207–208

prenatal care, 191–193

prescription medication, 30–31

prevalence, 182, 292, 361

prevalence studies. *See* cross-sectional studies

prevention. *See* disease prevention

primary hypertension, 142

primary case (index case), 51

primary disease prevention. *See also* vaccines
  defined, 24, 361
  health education, 191
  prenatal care, 191–193
  proper nutrition, 193–195
  vaccines, 189–191
  WASH program, 195–196

Principles of Sanitary Science and the Public Health (Sedgwick), 51

probability, 258, 317, 361

process monitoring, 226–227

progressive fibrosis of the lung, 123–124

project managers, 349–350

propagated source epidemic, 25, 35–36, 131, 232

proportion, 165, 361

proportionate mortality rate, 179–181

prospective cohort studies, 305, 306–307

prospective studies, 291

prostate cancer, 177

prostate-specific antigen (PSA) test, 196, 248, 254

prostatitis, 254

public health
  in England, 54–56
  milestones in, 59–76
  program evaluation, 26–27
  in US, 49–54

Public Health Act, 55

public health nurses, 53

Pure Food and Drug Act, 52

p-value (statistical significance), 276

Q

quality assurance, 26

quality control, 26–27

quasi-experimental study, 361

questionnaires, 26, 310–312

R

rabies, 46, 84

racial and ethnic disparities, 122–123

Ramazzini, Bernardino, 48

randomization, 326, 362

About the Author

With more than four decades of research and 25 years of teaching in public health, **Dr. Amal Mitra** has grown to become an internationally recognized scientist and leader in public health. He earned his bachelor's degree in medicine from Dhaka Medical College in Bangladesh, and his Master of Public Health (M.P.H.) and Doctor of Public Health (Dr.P.H.) degrees from the University of Alabama at Birmingham (UAB).

At his current position as Professor of Epidemiology and Biostatistics at Jackson State University (JSU) School of Public Health, College of Health Sciences, Jackson, Mississippi, he teaches master's and doctoral programs in epidemiology. With his secondary appointment as Director of Global Health Initiatives for Southeast Asia and Western Pacific Regions at JSU SPH, Dr. Mitra collaborates on research with a number of institutions around the world. He helped develop public health programs in several countries including Bangladesh, Malaysia, Hong Kong, and Kuwait. He recently volunteered offering an online certificate program in research methodology and biostatistics for medical graduates in Bangladesh. He helped develop online master's certificate programs in Epidemiology and in Biostatistics at JSU. He also has guided numerous graduate students in research and publications.

Dr. Mitra has authored and co-authored more than 120 peer-reviewed research papers. He is a member of the American Public Health Association and the Delta Omega Honorary Society in Public Health. He is the editor of the textbook, *Statistical Approaches for Epidemiology: From Concept to Application*. As a guest editor, Dr. Mitra served on five special issues of MDPI journals.

He is the recipient of many awards including the Fulbright-Nehru Academic and Professional Excellence Award in 2022–2023 (India), Tropical Medicine and Infectious Disease John M. Goldsmid Award in 2018 for the best published paper, the Lifetime Achievement Award in 2013, the Fulbright U.S. Scholar Award in 2007–2008 (Bangladesh), the Rotary Grant for University Teachers in 2009, the Innovation Award for Applied Research in 2004, and the Distinguished Teaching Award in 2000.

Dedication

Ratna Mitra, you are my inspiration while I was struggling with my time crunch in writing this book. Thank you for your sacrifice throughout my life-long journey in doing research. Amlan and Paromita, my two precious children, I learned from you going out of the way to help others. Tim McGrath, a brilliant, smart, and nice man and my son-in-law, who never said no in reviewing my research papers within hours' notice. My numerous students, who always wanted to learn more. This is another special book for you to learn more than what I could tell you in my classes.

Author's Acknowledgments

Several years ago, when an acquisition editor from John Wiley & Sons, Inc. approached me about writing *Epidemiology For Dummies*, I was so excited because that idea had been inside me for a long time. The project was later abandoned because of corporate reorganization at Wiley. Years later during the middle of 2022, Lindsay Lefevere brought life back to this project. What's great is I'm more prepared now than ever before in writing this book. The Covid-19 pandemic made a dramatic paradigm shift of public health's knowledge in epidemiology and experience in dealing with a large pandemic. My research in Covid-19 supplemented writing a section of this book as well. Thank God, we hadn't published a book like this before!

Chad Sievers, I haven't found another truly helpful person such as you. I'm blessed having you as my guide. When I wasn't understanding the Dummies style very well, your attempt after attempt of review made me learn it somewhat better. I remember your assurance by saying — "I'm going nowhere." After 25 years' of teaching, I couldn't be as good a teacher as you had been with me. Thank you a lot for making the TOC almost ready-to-go.

John Wiley & Sons, Inc. Executive Editor Lindsay Lefevere (now Lindsay Berg), thank you for your patience and support when I needed it most in accepting your book proposal. Thank you Editor Vicki Adang for your insight that improved the flow of the TOC. Elizabeth Jones, my current doctoral student at JSU, I've been impressed by your research interest and editorial skills in the past. Thank you very much for tech editing the book.

Publisher's Acknowledgments

Executive Editor: Lindsay Lefevre
Project Manager and Editor: Chad R. Sievers
Senior Managing Editor: Kristie Pyles
Technical Editor: Elizabeth Jones, MPH

Production Editor: Tamilmani Varadharaj
Cover Image: © MattLphotography/Shutterstock